Human Organ Transplantation

Societal, Medical-Legal, Regulatory, and Reimbursement Issues

Human Organ Transplantation

Societal, Medical-Legal, Regulatory, and Reimbursement Issues

Edited by
Dale H. Cowan, M.D., J.D.
Jo Ann Kantorowitz, J.D.
Jay Moskowitz, Ph.D.
Peter H. Rheinstein, M.D., J.D., M.S.

Published in cooperation with
the American Society of Law & Medicine

Health Administration Press
Ann Arbor, Michigan
1987

Library of Congress Cataloging in Publication Data
Main entry under title:

Human organ transplantation.

Based on a conference held April 18–20, 1985, in Arlington, Va.; sponsored jointly by the American Society of Law & Medicine and other organizations.
Bibliography: p.
Includes index.
1. Transplantation of organs, tissues, etc.—Law and legislation—United States—Congresses. 2. Donation of organs, tissues, etc.—Law and legislation—United States—Congresses. 3. Transplantation of organs, tissues, etc.—Social aspects—United States—Congresses. 4. Donation of organs, tissues, etc.—Social aspects—United States—Congresses. 5. Medical ethics—United States—Congresses. 6. Insurance, Hospitalization—United States—Congresses. I. Cowan, Dale H. II. American Society of Law & Medicine. [DNLM: 1. Ethics, Medical—Congresses.   2. Transplantation—Congresses.   3. Transplantation—United States—Legislation—Congresses. WO 690 H918]
KF3827.D66H86   1987   362.1'9795   86-29478
ISBN 0-910701-20-2

The American Society of Law & Medicine acknowledges with appreciation the work of Sharyn Perlman in editing the manuscripts and managing this text for publication.

Health Administration Press
1021 East Huron
Ann Arbor, Michigan 48104
(313) 764-1380

For our children

Contents

APPENDIXES

Contributors

GEORGE J. ANNAS is Edward R. Utley Professor of Health Law at the Boston University School of Medicine and Chief of the Health Law Section at the Boston University School of Public Health. He is also Editor-in-Chief Emeritus of *Law, Medicine & Health Care,* a columnist for the *Hastings Center Report* and the *American Journal of Public Health,* and Chairman of the Committee on Legal Problems in Medicine. Professor Annas was Chairman of the Massachusetts Task Force on Organ Transplantation and has written or coauthored a number of books on medical-legal subjects. He received his J.D. from Harvard Law School and his M.P.H. from the Harvard School of Public Health.

CLIVE O. CALLENDER is the Vice-Chairman of Surgery and Director of the Howard University Transplant Center in Washington, D.C. He has lectured on transplantation to professional and civic organizations and appeared before the U.S. Senate to testify on the effects and results of organ transplantation. By special appointment, Dr. Callender served on the prestigious fact-finding board for the National Task Force on Organ Transplantation. He holds membership in many medical, professional, and fraternal organizations, is the recipient of numerous awards and citations, and has written prolifically on the subject of organ transplantation. Dr. Callender received his M.D. from Meharry Medical College in Nashville.

ARTHUR L. CAPLAN is Associate Director of the Hastings Center, Institute of Society, Ethics, and the Life Sciences. He is an Adjunct Associate Professor of Philosophy at the City University of New York and has taught medical ethics at Columbia University College of Physicians and Surgeons. Dr. Caplan serves as a consultant to the New York Academy of Sciences, the Office of Technology Assessment of the U.S. Congress, the National Institutes of Health, and the National Endowment for the Humanities on ethical issues in health care. He has written for such publications as the *New York Times,* the *Philadelphia Inquirer,* and the *Los*

Angeles Times; has authored ten books; and has contributed many articles to professional journals in the fields of philosophy, medicine, and the biological sciences. Dr. Caplan received his Ph.D. in philosophy from Columbia University.

THEODORE COOPER is Vice-Chairman of the Board, The Upjohn Company. His diverse career has included positions as Professor of Surgery at St. Louis University, University of New Mexico, and Cornell University Medical College; Director of the National Heart and Lung Institute of the National Institutes of Health; Assistant Secretary for Health, Department of Health and Human Services; and Dean of Cornell University Medical College. Dr. Cooper is a member of several professional organizations including the Board of Governors of the American Red Cross. He has received awards from the American Heart Association, the American Institute of Biological Sciences, and the Department of Defense. Dr. Cooper received his M.D. from the St. Louis University School of Medicine and his Ph.D. in physiology from St. Louis University.

DALE H. COWAN is a practicing physician and attorney. In addition to a private medical practice in hematology and medical oncology and the Directorship of the Division of Hematology/Oncology at Marymount Hospital in Cleveland, he participates in activities affecting health care delivery and financing. Dr. Cowan played a major role in establishing a physician-sponsored Preferred Provider Organization at Marymount Hospital, helped create the Emerald Health Network, and authored a book on Preferred Provider Organizations. He is a Clinical Professor of Environmental Health Sciences at Case Western Reserve University School of Medicine, a Fellow of the American College of Physicians and the American College of Legal Medicine, and a member of the Ohio State and American Bar Associations. Dr. Cowan received his M.D. from Harvard Medical School and his J.D. from Case Western Reserve University School of Law.

CAROLYNE K. DAVIS currently serves as National and International Health Care Advisor to Ernst & Whinney. She also serves on the Board of Directors of Beverly Enterprises, an owner and operator of nursing homes, and SmithKline Beckman, the pharmaceutical company. Dr. Davis' previous positions include Administrator of the Health Care Financing Administration (HCFA), Department of Health and Human Services; Associate Vice-President for Academic Affairs at the University of Michigan; member of the Board of Trustees of the Johns Hopkins University; and Dean of the School of Nursing at the University of Michigan, concurrent with professorships in both nursing and education. She has published numerous articles and research documents on a wide variety of issues facing the health care system. Dr. Davis received her nursing degree from the Johns Hopkins University. Her Masters degree in nursing education and her Ph.D. in administration were granted from Syracuse University.

ROGER W. EVANS is a Senior Research Scientist with the Health and Population Study Center of the Battelle Human Affairs Research Center, Seattle. He was principal investigator for both the National Heart Transplantation Study and the National Kidney Dialysis and Kidney Transplantation Study. A nationally recognized expert on organ transplantation and kidney dialysis, Dr. Evans has served as a resource person for several foreign governments and as a special consultant to numerous organizations. He has also served on several federal government task forces, participated in National Institutes of Health consensus development conferences, and served as a member of the Task Force on Organ Transplantation of the Department of Health and Human Services. Articles by Dr. Evans have appeared in the *New England Journal of Medicine,* the *Journal of the American Medical Association,* and other medical journals. Dr. Evans received his Ph.D from Duke University.

SAMUEL GOROVITZ is Dean of the College of Arts and Sciences and Professor of Philosophy at Syracuse University. Previously he was a Professor of Philosophy and Affiliate Professor of Public Affairs at the University of Maryland. Dr. Gorovitz has been a frequent consultant to the National Institutes of Health, the National Center for Health Services Research, and various other governmental agencies. In 1985, he was visiting scholar-in-residence at Beth Israel Hospital in Boston. He is also the author of *Doctors' Dilemmas: Moral Conflict and Medical Care* (Oxford University Press, 1985) and is at work on another book, tentatively titled, *Hospital Philosopher.* Dr. Gorovitz received his Ph.D. in philosophy from Stanford University.

BERNADINE P. HEALY is Chairman of the Research Division of the Cleveland Clinic Foundation. She has also served as Director of the Coronary Care Unit of the Johns Hopkins University Hospital; Deputy Director of the Office of Science and Technology Policy at the White House; and President of the American Federation of Clinical Research. She is on the Board of Directors of the American Heart Association and has served on the Board of Governors of the American College of Cardiology; was a member of several advisory committees to the National Heart, Lung and Blood Institute; and was on the Cardiovascular Devices Committee of the Food and Drug Administration. Dr. Healy is the author or coauthor of nearly 200 medical and scientific articles and is a member of several honorary societies. She received her M.D. degree from the Johns Hopkins University School of Medicine.

NATHAN HERSHEY is Professor of Health Law, Graduate School of Public Health at the University of Pittsburgh. He is also of counsel to the law firms of Markel, Schafer & Means, Pittsburgh; and Post & Schell, Philadelphia. Mr. Hershey is a member of the New York, District of Columbia, and Pennsylvania Bar Associations; a member of the Institute of Medicine of the National Academy of Sciences; and past president of both the American Academy of Hospital Attorneys and the Society of Hospital Attorneys of Western Pennsylvania. He has coauthored *Hospital Law Manual, Human Experimentation and the Law,* and *Hospital-Physician Relationships: Case Studies and Commentaries on Medical Staff Problems.* Professor Hershey received his LL.B. from Harvard Law School.

BETTY C. IRWIN is the Clinical Nurse Specialist for Transplantation at the Johns Hopkins University Hospital in Baltimore. She works with patients undergoing renal, pancreas, heart, heart-lung, and liver transplantation. In addition to her nursing responsibilities, Ms. Irwin has been involved in nursing education, especially in the area of end-stage renal disease patient care. Author of several scholarly papers on nursing practice, she is a member of numerous clinical and professional societies. Ms. Irwin received her M.S. in nursing from the University of Maryland, Baltimore.

DAVID L. JACKSON is former Director of the Ohio Department of Health. He has also been a Professor of Medicine at Case Western Reserve University School of Medicine, a National Institutes of Health Site Visitor on the Reye's Syndrome Project, and a White House Fellow in the Environmental Protection Agency. A member of several professional societies and the recipient of numerous awards and honors, Dr. Jackson received his Ph.D. in physiology from Johns Hopkins University and his M.D. from Johns Hopkins University School of Medicine.

CHARLES R. McCARTHY is Director of the Office for Protection from Research Risks. He was also Staff Director for the Department of Health and Human Services (HHS) Ethics Advisory Board and an Adjunct Associate Professor of politics at George Washington University and Catholic University of America. Dr. McCarthy is HHS liaison to the President's Commission for the Study of Ethical Problems in Medicine and Biomedical and Behavioral Research and has authored many articles on the subject of biomedical ethics. Dr. McCarthy received his Ph.D. from the University of Toronto.

BARBARA W. MAYERS is a partner in the Health Law Department of McDermott, Will & Emery (Chicago office). She is a former Associate Counsel of the Blue Cross and Blue Shield Association and specializes in legal matters concerning health care services, alternative delivery systems, insurance, and employee health benefit plans. Ms. Mayers is admitted to practice before the Illinois Supreme Court, the U.S. District Court for the Northern District of Illinois, and the U.S. Court of Appeals for the Seventh Circuit. She is a member of the Chicago Bar Association and the National Health Lawyers Association. Ms. Mayers received her J.D. magna cum laude from DePaul University College of Law.

RICHARD E. NOLAN is a Partner in the firm of Davis Polk & Wardell in New York City. He is a Fellow of the American College of Trial Lawyers and a member of the New York Bar where he was admitted to practice in 1958. Mr. Nolan received his A.B. (cum laude) from Holy Cross University and his LL.B. from Columbia University School of Law where he was Notes Editor of the *Columbia Law Review.*

THOMAS D. OVERCAST is a consultant with a private law practice. He has been a research scientist for the Battelle Human Affairs Research Center, Science and Government Study Center; a legal analyst for the National Heart Transplantation Study; a legal affairs consultant for the American Psychological Association; and the Deputy Director of the National Center on White-Collar Crime. He is also on the Editorial Board of *Perspectives in Law and Psychology.* Dr. Overcast received both his J.D. from the College of Law and his Ph.D. in psychology from the University of Nebraska, Lincoln.

WHITNEY LAWRENCE SCHMIDT is an Associate at Davis Polk & Wardell in New York City. He is a member of the New Jersey and New York Bars where he was admitted to practice in 1980 and 1982, respectively. Mr. Schmidt received his B.A. (cum laude) from Harvard College. He was graduated from Vanderbilt University School of Law in 1980 where he was Associate Articles Editor of the *Vanderbilt Law Review* and a member of the Order of the Coif.

FRANK E. YOUNG is Commissioner of the U.S. Food and Drug Administration. He has also been Chairman of the Executive Hospital and

Medical Advisory Committees as well as pathologist at Strong Memorial Hospital; Dean of the School of Medicine and Dentistry and Director of the Medical Center of the University of Rochester; and served on the faculty of Case Western Reserve University. As FDA Commissioner, Dr. Young was a member of the U.S. Delegation to the World Health Assembly in Geneva and led the delegation to the third U.S./Israeli Symposium of Health in Jerusalem. Dr. Young received his M.D. from the Medical Center of the State University of New York and his Ph.D. from Case Western Reserve University.

Introduction

This volume is a compilation of papers and background materials presented at a conference on the Legal and Ethical Issues Surrounding Organ Transplantation. The conference was held April 18–20, 1985, in Arlington, Virginia. It was sponsored jointly by the American Society of Law and Medicine, the American College of Legal Medicine, and the National Heart, Lung, and Blood Institute of the National Institutes of Health (NIH) in cooperation with seventeen associations and organizations representing interested medical professionals and institutions, government, business, insurance, and private interest groups.

The goal of the conference was to promote an informed and scholarly discussion on the societal, medical-legal, regulatory, and reimbursement issues affecting human organ transplantation. To focus the debate, leading experts were invited to present papers that addressed these issues. Each speaker was also asked to provide a perspective that could serve as the basis for future decision making. Thus, it was hoped that the conference would provide a forum in which individuals concerned with different aspects of human organ transplantation could exchange ideas and begin the process of developing a consensus for resolving the difficult ethical, societal, legal, and financial problems related to this complex and promising technology.

The chapters in this volume represent most of the conference presentations. Each author provided a manuscript that was subsequently edited for publication by the American Society of Law & Medicine staff. Major credit for organization of the conference papers belongs to A. Edward Doudera, Esq., former executive director of the American Society of Law & Medicine, who was instrumental in obtaining the support of the cooperating sponsors and in enlisting the participation of many of the speakers, and to Sharyn Perlman who did the lion's share of the manuscript editing.

Part I of this volume is divided into five sections, the first of which consists of papers addressing societal issues. The section begins with a thoughtful and probing overview by Arthur Caplan, of the Hastings

Center, of the issues that pertain to obtaining and allocating organs for transplantation. In particular, Dr. Caplan addresses the problem of the relative scarcity of donor organs, schemes for alleviating this shortage, and the ethical issues related to the allocation of scarce resources. The second chapter is by Theodore Cooper, Vice-Chairman of the Upjohn Company and formerly Assistant Secretary of Health in the Department of Health and Human Services. Dr. Cooper discusses the broad social and political considerations attending the development of a national policy for organ transplantation in light of present and anticipated medical knowledge and technological advances.

Roger Evans, of the Battelle Human Affairs Research Center, presents the findings of the study on transplantation commissioned by the Federal Task Force on Organ Transplantation and discusses societal and medical considerations that affect the selection of both donors and recipients. The section ends with a chapter by Clive O. Callender, chairman of the heart transplant program at Howard University Medical School. Dr. Callender reviews many of the issues related to transplantation from the perspective of the transplant team, and discusses the availability of transplantation as a treatment modality for members of minority groups and economically disadvantaged individuals.

The second section focuses on medical-legal issues. Thomas Overcast, an attorney with the Battelle Human Affairs Research Center who helped draft the report on transplantation for the Federal Task Force, discusses the legal issues related to the definition and determination of death of potential donors of nonpaired organs, such as heart, liver, and pancreas, and the problems associated with obtaining informed consent from the relatives or guardians of dying or deceased patients. His discussion forms a basis for the development of appropriate policies that may protect the integrity of the potential donor yet allow for the expeditious harvesting of viable organs. Nathan Hershey of the University of Pittsburgh School of Public Health analyzes in detail the sources of liability for both practitioners and institutions that conduct and manage transplantation programs. His analysis provides additional considerations for the development of institutional policies that can minimize the liability potential for providers of transplant services by safeguarding the interests of both donors and recipients.

Whereas transplantation of organs such as the kidney and the heart has attained the status of accepted medical practice, the transplantation of other organs, such as the liver and pancreas, remains experimental. Charles McCarthy, Director of the Office of Protection from Research Risks of the National Institutes of Health, reviews the federal regulations pertaining to research with human subjects and the role of local institutional review boards in reviewing and approving research protocols for studying transplantation. The section concludes with a discussion by Betty Irwin of the role of the nursing professional in organ transplantation. Ms. Irwin emphasizes the pivotal role that nursing personnel have in managing the care of dying patients who are potential organ donors, counseling relatives of these patients, and participating in the selection and care of prospective recipients.

Section three addresses the regulatory issues affecting human organ transplantation. An overview of the regulation of medical practice is offered by Dale Cowan, a physician-attorney specializing in health law and a former member of the National Advisory Council of the National Heart, Lung, and Blood Institute (NIH). Dr. Cowan distinguishes standard medical practice from innovative practice and reviews the legal and regulatory restraints affecting each. He proposes a scheme for regulating innovative practices and their passage into standard practice.

Although natural human organs are not (at least yet) subject to regulation by the Food and Drug Administration (FDA), artificial organs and the drugs used to suppress rejection are subject to FDA regulation. Frank Young, Commissioner of the FDA, discusses the role of the FDA in regulating organ transplantation. He raises an intriguing question— whether natural organs might be considered "devices" for purposes of regulation and, if so, the policy considerations that might arise.

Richard Nolan and Whitney Schmidt, attorneys whose practices encompass products liability, present a probing and provocative review of the application of product liability law to transplantation of both natural and artificial organs. They raise the interesting question of whether natural organs are "products" for purposes of product liability law and whether the transplant team or the donor can be held liable for an allegedly defective organ.

Governmental regulation of the procurement of organs and the selection of prospective recipients is discussed by David Jackson, former Director of the Ohio Department of Health, and George Annas, Professor of Health Law at the Boston University School of Public Health. Dr. Jackson describes the role of government in addressing the question of fairness in allocating scarce resources to ensure equal access to expensive life-saving technologies. He reviews the highly innovative procedure adopted and implemented by institutions in Ohio under the auspices of the Ohio Department of Health. Dr. Annas, who chaired the Massachusetts Task Force on Organ Transplantation, discusses the findings and recommendations of that group and considers how government can promote policies that sustain the delicate balance between complex legal and ethical issues.

The fourth section focuses on the costs for transplantation and how these costs can be fairly apportioned. The section begins with an analysis by Samuel Gorovitz, Dean of Arts and Sciences at Syracuse University, of the ethical considerations and implications of policies affecting payment for transplantation and other expensive medical procedures. This is followed by a review by Carolyne Davis, former Administrator of the Health Care Financing Administration, of considerations taken by the federal government in determining whether or not to pay for transplantation under Medicare. Since her chapter was written, the Department of Health and Human Services has authorized payment under Medicare for a limited number of heart transplants performed in designated transplantation centers.

The role of private insurers in paying for organ transplantation is discussed by Barbara Mayers, formerly of the general counsel's office of the Blue Cross/Blue Shield Association. Ms. Mayers considers the need for private insurers to be responsive to the concerns of their policyholders, the consequences of reimbursement decisions on policy design, and the use of transplantation as a treatment modality. The section concludes with an overview by Bernadine Healy, former Associate Director of the White House Office of Technology Policy, on federal policy pertaining to transplantation and the role a coherent federal policy plays in influencing policy determinations by both government and the private sector.

Part II of this volume contains a compilation of reports and articles prepared and published during the past several years that address many of the issues presented in Part I. A reader interested in probing any of the issues in greater depth will find that these articles provide data and a spectrum of opinions that can serve as a valuable resource. Additionally, the appendixes include executive summaries of the National Task Force Report and the Report on Immunosuppressive Drugs, as well as the summary and conclusions from the Presidential Commission Defining Death; guidelines for the determination of death; state organ transplantation and required consent statutes; and a statement by Senator Albert Gore, Jr. A selected bibliography for further research ends the volume.

It is hoped that the extensive and varied materials provided in this volume will serve as a comprehensive source of information to all individuals interested in and concerned with the social, ethical, legal, regulatory, and political issues that surround human organ transplantation.

The Editors

Part I

Conference Presentations

Section 1

Societal
Issues

1

Obtaining and Allocating Organs for Transplantation

Arthur L. Caplan

This chapter presents an overview of four areas of organ transplantation that raise interesting ethical and policy questions. Three of the topics—cost, assessment, and allocation—are closely related. The other is the procurement of organs, which has a direct bearing on matters of cost and rationing.

When one sees the kind of success rates that are being attained today with the transplantation of solid organs and tissues such as bone marrow and corneas, one must be impressed with the progress that medicine has made in a relatively short period. Transplant surgeons have made remarkable advances in the ability to transplant tissues and organs successfully from both live and cadaver sources.

However, transplantation is expensive. Depending on whom you ask, prices are said to range from $100,000 to $250,000 for a liver transplant. One sees figures between $100,000 and $150,000 for a heart transplant and costs in the neighborhood of $50,000 for a pancreas transplantation.

With such large sums of money involved, the public, insurance officials, and policymakers are concerned that, while we are now able to transplant many organs and tissues successfully, we may not be able to afford to do so. The issue of cost dominates much of the contemporary discussion of public policy regarding transplantation.

COST AND RATIONING

It is sometimes said by people in the transplant field that the question of payment should not be the concern of the transplant surgeon, the person procuring the organ, or the patient or the patient's family. Money, or more accurately, profit, should not be an objective for transplantation, either for those undertaking the procedure or for those charged with determining access to this kind of surgery.

However, despite these claims, when one looks at the situation in the United States today, it is obvious that the way our society has decided to cope with the large costs of transplantation—at least for the time being—is to ration access by means of the ability to pay. The burden of costs has resulted in the development of a number of criteria, both formal and informal, for rationing access to transplantation.

The major way in which this is done is by using what might be called a "green screen." The green screen basically involves restricting access to transplants to those who can pay or can guarantee payment. There are a number of medical centers in the United States which simply will not admit someone to their waiting list for a transplant unless he or she has the financial resources to pay for the procedure. If someone does not have the money, that person is simply not eligible to be considered for a transplant at many centers. Moreover, it is alleged that at some centers preference is given to those who can pay in cash. So certainly one way that has evolved for coping with the enormous costs of many forms of transplantation is not only by requiring that people have the ability to pay, but by making them pay prior to being considered eligible for transplantation.

If one looks at the available estimates of need for transplants, it becomes clear that these figures vary a great deal. Published estimates are that anywhere between three and four hundred livers per year are needed to meet the demand for livers in this country. Other sources give estimates in the thousands. Some estimates in the literature of the demand for kidney transplants are in the neighborhood of seven thousand per year; others range as high as twenty-five thousand. It quickly becomes evident that these "objective" empirical estimates are very much a function of both cost and organ availability.

Based on this information, a second way of containing costs is to ration access to expensive forms of transplantation by age. People over age fifty-five or sixty are deemed ineligible for many types of transplantation. Their ineligibility is not based on a determination that none of those in older groups can benefit from transplants. Rather, the current scarcity of organs and the prohibitive costs of the procedures are seen as barriers to including older persons in most estimates of need.

Infants and children are also often excluded from consideration for transplants for similar reasons. For example, children under the age of one are rarely considered in estimates of need for heart transplants, not solely because of limits of medical or technical ability, but also because age exclusion is a policy that helps providers cope with the allocation problems raised by high costs and the scarcity of organs. A direct relationship exists between currently established age limits used to determine the need for transplants and both the availability of organs for transplant and the cost of these procedures. If changes were to occur in the cost or in the availability of organs, corresponding changes would occur with respect to age limits and, thus, estimates of need for these procedures.

How else is rationing accomplished? There is what might be called the "mediagenicity" criterion. People who are willing to go public, who are squeaky wheels—especially those who, in the eyes of the media, are particularly attractive and cogent squeaky wheels—oftentimes get the necessary attention. If someone does not have funds to meet the requirements of access which prevail at many centers, he or she may be able to generate money through car washes, bake sales, and other forms of personal fund-raising. And it may be possible to get TV time or newspaper space to plead a person's case to obtain the resources needed to enable a transplant to take place.

People who do not relish publicity or who are not particularly attractive in the eyes of the media do not fare so well in the race to attract private money for expensive transplant procedures. The ability of those in need to manipulate the media, to make their cases heard, and to command public attention in obtaining resources, and their willingness to do so, are critical factors in determining who is able to gain access to transplantation.

Geography and social status also play roles in rationing. Many centers give priority of access to those in need who live nearby. Some may give priority of access to those who are wealthy or have prominence within the local community. Numerous reports have appeared in the popular press concerning favoritism shown to those persons who can make significant contributions, either monetary or in terms of favorable publicity, that will benefit the medical centers where transplants are performed.

Some rationing is also known to be done by means of the etiology of organ failure. Alcoholics have a more difficult time getting access to liver transplants than persons who have suffered liver failure as a result of congenital diseases. In attempting to provide reimbursement coverage for expensive forms of medical care such as transplantation, it is simply easier to focus public attention and elicit legislative concern for those who are perceived to be the victims of nature and chance than it is for those who are seen as the victims of their own behavior.

One final way in which cost is used to allocate access to transplantation (often quietly and somewhat surreptitiously) is by imposing other limits on settings and practitioners defined as reimbursible. Certain medical procedures are reimbursed only if they are done in a hospital. Other procedures are not reimbursed if they are done in the home or on an outpatient basis. This means that the reimbursement for necessary drugs such as cyclosporin will occur only if the drug is given in a hospital setting. It is clear that such reimbursement policies are entirely a function, not of the benefit to the patient nor of the quality of care that can be delivered, but of the source liable for incurring the cost of delivering the care.

While it is often popular to claim that no one in our society is denied necessary care because of a lack of money, or that rationing does not exist in our health care system, this is plainly false. A great deal of rationing has occurred and continues to occur with respect to organ transplants. Our society has chosen, or at least tolerates, rationing according to ability to pay, age, mediagenicity, geography, disease etiology, and the setting in which care is delivered.

The Morality of Rationing Access to Organ Transplants

This author believes that the present mechanisms for rationing access to needed transplants—subtle, surreptitious, not publicly discussed forms of rationing—are ethically wrong. There are five conditions that, if fulfilled, would seem to require that society remove cost barriers from those seeking access to organ transplants. These are: (1) if a procedure is known to be efficacious, if it is known to be life saving or life extending; (2) if a procedure has a reasonable chance of success, if there is at least a reasonable chance that providing a particular form of care will restore function or extend life; (3) if a reasonable quality of life is afforded the patient who receives the procedure; (4) if the procedure is desired by the patient; and (5) if there is no severe decrease in the availability of existing services in a community or an institution by making a new service available.

If all of these conditions can be met, a very powerful case can be made for positing a moral obligation to ensure that cost not be a barrier to access. If these conditions are met, either government (at the federal or state level) or third-party payers have an obligation to make sure that cost is not an obstacle to access.

If those in medical need do not have the means to get coverage through insurance or government programs, then an insurance pool or other system should be available to make sure that these indigent and uninsured are covered. If various forms of organ transplantation can satisfy the five conditions cited, a strong moral obligation exists to make them available to help people, to extend their lives, and to provide them with a good quality of life—one that they view as acceptable and desirable. Medicine as a profession has such an obligation. Society, if it cares about the weak and the vulnerable and the needy, has such an obligation.

TECHNOLOGY ASSESSMENT

How do we know if any particular medical intervention meets the five conditions outlined above? This question can be answered only through a systematic and thorough system of technology assessment. Unfortunately, current public policy and planning are especially weak with respect to technology assessment in general, and organ transplantation in particular.

How do we know whether a particular type of transplant is life saving, provides a reasonable quality of life, is desired by a patient, or does not severely distort access to the existing services that a hospital or institution is already giving? It is true that some medical centers that perform transplants of different types do report information in the professional literature which bears upon these questions. It is also true that government agencies such as the Health Care Financing Administration occasionally release data on programs such as the End-Stage Renal Disease (ESRD) program that provide information about the efficacy and outcomes associated with various forms of organ transplantation. There are also registries in the United States and certain foreign countries that contain relevant information about the costs, outcomes, and efficacy associated with some forms of organ transplantation.

However, the fact remains that it is very difficult to provide reasonable answers to any of the conditions suggested herein as preconditions for obligating society to reimburse the costs of transplantation without some system of standardized, centralized data collection. Unfortunately, no mandatory data collection exists for either established or evolving transplant procedures. In fact, no system exists for conducting assessments of most medical procedures and technologies of any sort.

No government agency says, "If you are going to try a pancreas transplant, you have to report the results to a central place in a standardized fashion so that the data can be analyzed. Moreover, you must follow a specific research protocol to facilitate the analysis of data from different centers." No laws or regulations exist that require those in the field of organ transplantation to produce standardized data. Our society has no means of collecting and storing such data in ways that would be useful for medical professionals or policymakers. And our nation lacks any sort of mandatory reporting requirement to ensure that someone or some agency is responsible for tracking the developments in the organ transplantation field. Incredibly, a nation that spends over $400 billion on health care spends far less than 1 percent of that amount to monitor the spending of that money and its effect on the health of U.S. citizens.

Moreover, we also lack independent, regular monitoring or assessment at the state and federal level of new technologies such as liver or pancreas transplants. While it is true that many in health care do report progress in their particular area of transplantation in the professional literature or at professional conferences, this is not "independent" assessment, particularly when many of the studies that are reported are done by the very people who are conducting the transplants and who have a personal stake in the outcome of their work.

In order to have the information necessary to formulate rational standards of efficacy, outcome, quality, and impact on the overall health care system, an agency should be created either at the federal or the state level to collect, analyze, and disseminate information. If no one is collecting information in a standardized fashion, in a centralized way independent from those promoting or performing new procedures, we will never be able to answer the questions of what is a "reasonable" chance of success; what is life saving; what is a "reasonable" quality of life; and whether resource availability for other beneficial medical services is being unduly distorted by making a particular transplant procedure available.

Assessment is the basis on which to decide whether to pay, when to pay, and how much to pay. Unless a system of assessment is created, the question of cost will be answered with rationing by means of the individual's ability to pay, geography, age, etiology of disease, and so on. If we want to continue with these forms of rationing access to contain cost, we can. It would make much more sense for our society to move toward a prudent and efficient approach to the question of cost by having the information available that would allow us to make reasonable and intelligent choices about providing reimbursement for those in need.

ALLOCATION OF SCARCE RESOURCES

What if—in an ideal future world—all of the requisite information were available: we knew the survival rates under different drug regimens of different forms of organ transplantation; we understood exactly what was going on when different centers reported different rates of success for the same procedures; we even had basic information on what happens to people who have had transplants from live and cadaver sources in terms of their ability to return to work, to avoid complicating infections, to live at home, and the various other factors that might be considered part of a reasonable quality of life? If we had all of these answers and we found out that transplantation was still too expensive to cover the costs for everyone or, more likely, that there still were not enough organs and tissues available for all of those in need, what might we do then? How would we make our choices?

There are questions that would have to be considered even if an adequate system of technology assessment were to exist and a policy were established that did not allow money to be used as the primary means to ration services. Allocation questions would likely remain. Who should resolve them, and what criteria should be used? The question of who shall decide really divides into two proposals: should providers decide or should patients?

A number of proposals have been made, especially by medical organizations, suggesting that the best way to handle rationing decisions is by committee. These so-called "ethics committees" are appearing all over the United States. Such committees are usually composed of public representatives, health care professionals, administrators, and sometimes hospital risk managers. This combination of persons is brought together to deliberate about the procedure to establish for situations where rationing seems, or is de facto, unavoidable.

Unfortunately, history shows that committees have had a very poor track record with respect to bias. An old joke about the Seattle Dialysis Committee of the late 1960s put it this way—the Pacific Northwest was no place for a Ralph Waldo Emerson to get renal failure. Given his reluctance to conform to societal norms, Emerson would not have received high priority among those seeking access to dialysis from a committee dominated by members of the middle and upper classes.

Committees often represent a narrow and unrepresentative cross section of the communities they serve. They are often made up of health care professionals—people from the upper strata of society—and are usually white males.

These biases have historically been very evident in the outcomes associated with all sorts of committees, both patient-selection committees for dialysis and others. Selection committees for cardiac transplantation at Stanford in the 1960s tended to favor employed white men. The Institutional Review Board (IRB) committee system governing human experimentation also reflects this bias. Given the extremely small number of persons who have come a cropper of the IRB in the past twenty years, it is not a system that can be characterized as being overly aggressive in monitoring and penalizing the wayward and the lax.

Peer review by committee often results in bias, but there are other problems facing committees. Committees cannot act quickly; they simply are not always easy to convene, thus creating an obstacle to the fast action that rationing often demands. Committees are not readily held accountable. Part of the reason people like committees is not because they will make better ethical decisions, but because committees distribute the responsibility for tough decisions in ways that diffuse personal responsibility.

One of the few ways to ensure thoughtfulness in any decision-making context is to make sure that those who make the decision are held responsible and liable for their actions. Decision makers should be held accountable. If rationing decisions are to be given to committees and if committees are willing to take on such decisions only by being secretive, indemnified, and protected against either public scrutiny or lawsuits, then sound ethical decisions are not likely to be made.

There is another reason for skepticism about committees. No committee can function for very long in allocating access to scarce resources unless it has explicit criteria for making such decisions. Committees cope with objections concerning bias by formulating uniform rules, principles, and criteria, and following them. Such rules permit allocation decisions that are publicly available, subject to scrutiny, and accountable.

If rules and criteria for rationing are agreed upon, however, then there is no need for committees. The rules and criteria can be given directly to the doctors and patients and allowed to function. There may be some argument for a committee to supervise, monitor, and perhaps play an educational role for those who have to make decisions. But if the criteria exist, and if agreement is possible on how best to ration, decisions can be handled just as well by individuals as by groups.

If negotiations about rationing should take place between doctor and patient, is it the doctor who should make the tough calls in deciding who should get access when rationing must occur—when some can receive a transplant and others cannot?

This author does not think physicians should make these decisions; my argument is that doctors should act as advocates for their patients, not as the rationing agents of society.

In today's cost-containment climate it has become popular to arm doctors with price lists and to hold seminars for them so they know exactly what everything costs. It has also become fashionable among physicians to volunteer to assume the burden of fiscal responsibility, of trying to prevent uncontrolled escalation of costs.

Fiscal constraint at the bedside is a very poor ethical basis for medical practice. If it is true that the relationship between doctor and patient is a fiduciary one, patients must believe that physicians give their interests the highest value. Who wants his or her physician thinking, "Well, Art Caplan would cost a fortune to treat and, after all, the State of New York is in poor financial shape, and the national deficit continues to grow, so maybe I will not treat Art Caplan; I've got moral responsibilities to my society and my community." Any such thinking undermines the ethics of the doctor-patient relationship. Physicians cannot be asked to make these kinds of rationing choices. Those physicians who put themselves forward as accepting the role of rationer will eventually undermine the relationship of trust that now prevails. They will destroy the possibility of honesty and candor that are the foundation of fiduciary relationships.

Moreover, doctors cannot maintain a public system of rationing for too long. They will have to disguise rationing by means of talk of "medical suitability" and "medical indications." The clearest evidence that this kind of obfuscation inevitably occurs when physicians ration lies in the allocation decisions made by physicians who are forced to ration dialysis in the British National Health Service.

Basically, physicians in England have deluded themselves into believing that they can handle questions of access to expensive forms of medical technology under limited resources by resolving matters simply on the basis of empirical facts. British physicians state that they will not dialyze people who are over age fifty-five. They will not dialyze people who have other forms of serious and debilitating illnesses, such as diabetes or cardiovascular problems, or who have psychiatric ailments. They give lower priority to those who are orphans or those who are not able to speak English, since these people have a more difficult time learning to dialyze themselves. All of this is done by describing these individuals as "medically unsuitable" for dialysis.

These examples of medical contraindications for dialysis have been published in the medical literature. The list cited above comes from a 1982 *British Medical Journal* BMA report on nephrology, in which the inability to speak English, psychiatric conditions, diabetes, and age over fifty-five were all mentioned as contraindications for dialysis.

What is going on? British nephrologists know that some hard choices must be made; and since they are unwilling to come forward and state that certain people must die, or because they cannot face making quality-of-life judgments about their patients, they have convinced themselves, despite the fact that there is plenty of American literature and literature from other Western European countries to the contrary, that people over age fifty-five cannot tolerate dialysis. Even with ample evidence to the contrary, British physicians are telling us that the old, the mentally ill, and the diabetic are inappropriate, unsuitable, and medically contraindicated for dialysis.

We can have this system of rationing here, if we like, leading inevitably to the imposition of value judgments under the guise of medical objectivity—a situation difficult to detect and even more difficult to reverse.

What is the alternative? If we must ration because of limits on the availability of organs or limits on money or social resources; if we are not willing to pursue technology assessment aggressively in order to ensure that people have access to desired, life-saving procedures that provide a reasonable quality of life and are proved not to overburden the rest of the health care system—if we are unwilling to take these steps, and if we therefore have to ration, then a two-step process of allocation should be employed.

First and foremost, the patient must always want what is being offered. The person who needs to be consulted first regarding whether he or she wants what medical science can avail is the patient (or in the case of an incompetent patient, the patient's family or surrogate). The patient should make an informed choice, wherein he or she understands the risks and benefits, the quality of life, the consequences of receiving a transplant, how it will influence personal lifestyle, what it will mean to the family, and what it will mean in terms of health. The first place to start and try to decide how to ration is with patient desires and patient wants—not with whims, but with informed choices.

Then, if scarcity still exists, a rationing decision is necessary. Doctor and patient must work together to try to make sure that the procedure being offered can readily provide the kind of extension of life, quality of life, and benefits that the patient seeks. This can happen only by providing adequate, realistic information. Intuition, hunch, or tradition should play no role in trying to make such an assessment. What is needed is hard evidence that in a given medical center with a particular level of expertise and with the resources that the center can commit to the procedure the desired goals can be achieved. The less information available, the more other criteria will necessarily be used to ration.

Finally, if no decision is reached, if the patient wants the transplant and understands what is reasonable to predict as the outcome of surgery, then the optimal moral choice is a system of randomization. This country ought not to have public policies that say one person is more worthy or deserving of care than another. If we limit eligibility to those who want transplants, and try to determine what they can reasonably expect, that is the best we can do. From that point on we should follow a chance or random means of allocation.

There is also a fourth obligation, and this leads to the last subject. What can be done to avoid rationing?

ORGAN PROCUREMENT

Unfortunately, the current public policy in this country simply does an unacceptable job of generating an adequate supply of organs and tissue. Following the generally accepted figures in the field, there are somewhere between 20,000 and 25,000 people who are declared brain dead each year. Our present system obtains organs from only between 10 percent and 15 percent of that pool; this is simply too low, particularly for those kinds of transplants, such as cornea and kidney, which have already passed every reasonable standard of efficacy.

Our present system is built upon voluntary choice, encouraged by advertising and education or what could be termed "encouraged voluntarism." This system is not working. Most people do not carry donor cards. Most donor cards do not reach the hospital. When they do, they are often not found or are not acted upon. Most disturbingly, health care professionals do not always ask next of kin about organ donation.

Encouraged voluntarism may have been adequate when it was instituted in 1968 in each state as exemplified in the Uniform Anatomical Gift Act. It is no longer adequate. What ought to be done?

One suggestion is that we take a very simple step that is consistent with the values reflected in encouraged voluntarism, a policy of the right to choose to give and the right to choose not to give. The policy we should institute is what often is called "required request" or "routine inquiry."

Since most people, according to public opinion surveys, either want to give or would give permission to have organs taken from their next of kin, since families play a pivotal role in controlling what happens in organ donation, and since health care professionals do not like to ask about organ donation, every state should institute a policy wherein, as part of the pronouncement of death and the making out of the death certificate, someone will be required to certify that an inquiry about the willingness of the family to consent to organ donation was made.

This is a very simple policy that has several merits. One merit is to ensure that donor cards will likely be found, because the persons most likely to know about the written directives and wishes of a deceased or dying person are family members. The chance of discovering written directives is increased if every family is routinely asked about organ donation.

Routine request will also help remedy a serious problem under the present system, that of suspect consent. Organ procurement specialists now approach bereaved and grieving persons under terrible circumstances, asking difficult questions about donation of families that often have not thought about the subject, have not discussed it, and are not prepared for the request. Occasionally, pressure is exerted to secure a donation, which may lead to a less than perfect consent on the part of the family.

If each state had a system whereby each hospital was responsible for routinely and customarily inquiring about organ donation, then the public would soon come to understand that this is part of what it means to die in a hospital. Requests would be expected, just as people understand that when someone dies under suspicious circumstances, there is an autopsy and that when a person dies, under any circumstances, someone fills out a report on that death.

In other words, if we routinize what is now haphazard and contingent, we can encourage families to discuss this issue before a tragedy occurs, so that they will be prepared to cope with the decision if the need arises. Routine or required request encourages health professionals to implement guidelines so that people who seek consent will understand how to do it and will not approach families at terrible moments as awkward strangers.

There is every reason to believe that routine request would increase the supply of tissue and organs available for transplantation. This policy respects the rights of people to say no if they do not want to be involved in donation. It does not jeopardize the right of every individual to leave a written directive or to make an oral statement about his or her wishes, and, in fact, it provides protection for those wishes by trying to involve family members, surrogates, and others who might speak for the deceased, to ensure that these wishes are known, found, and honored.

Most important, routine or required request respects the right of people to be altruistic. We depend upon people's altruism in making the so-called gift of life to procure organs. We are not going to be very successful in capturing that altruism unless we ask for it. Very few people are altruistic enough to motivate themselves to make a gift. That is particularly true of the dying and the dead. However, if we adopt a policy of asking at the time of tragedy, if we educate the public to expect this kind of question, if we try to integrate into our system a routine and customary way for dealing with the terrible tragedy of sudden, unexpected death, then we will improve the supply of organs and tissue available to all while respecting individual choice.

What are the prospects for this policy's adoption? There are now three states that have adopted required request legislation—California, New York, and Oregon—and twenty more that are considering such legislation. And if those who have the power to do so can agree that we ought to try to think of ways to reform or revamp our organ procurement policy, and if we can see to it that in those states that do not have this kind of legislation pending it is at least being considered, then we will be on the right track.

Will this help us answer the difficult questions already raised concerning payment, assessment, and allocation? The answer is yes. We can reduce some of our current anxiety about allocation by increasing the supply of organs and tissues. We can reduce some of our anxiety about payment, at least in the area of dialysis and kidney transplantation, if we can do something to increase the number of transplants that are done and decrease the amount spent on dialysis. We can certainly help ourselves cope with the issue of rationing if we have more tissue and organs to allocate.

Is more efficient organ procurement the long-run solution? The answer, sadly, is no. Inevitably, we will still face the problem that there are not going to be enough organs. We are then faced with having to address, in a careful and systematic way, not in the haphazard fashion that has characterized public policy to date in this area, the issues of cost, assessment, and allocation. Morally, an obligation exists to provide reimbursement. Cost should not be a barrier to transplantation when the transplant procedures or, for that matter, any other procedures, meet certain standards. The only way we will have a chance to answer the question, "Do they meet the standards?," is to create a system of technology assessment. This system must be capable of collecting standardized data, of analyzing it, and of making it available for analysis by independent parties. Ultimately the answer to issues of allocation, cost, and reimbursement ought not rest with either committees or physicians. The hard choices about these matters must involve the joint efforts of legislators, patients, providers, and the public to make the moral choices that are required.

2

Survey of Development, Current Status, and Future Prospects for Organ Transplantation

Theodore Cooper

Any one of the numerous issues pertaining to organ transplantation could be the subject of lengthy debate. The diverse issues include scientific, legal, medical, educational, and regulatory aspects of transplantation. The difficulties must be clearly defined because, as H. L. Mencken observed, "For every problem there's a solution that's neat, simple, and wrong."

This chapter presents a review of what has happened in the area of organ transplantation, speculates about the future, and ventures into the question of what to do with a medical technology whose time has come.

A caveat is in order. The data concerning transplantation are fluid and are subject to a number of variables. Therefore, the material presented here should not be viewed as a final assessment, but rather as an indication of both the scope of the problem and the extent to which medical needs must still be met.

Organ transplantation as a therapeutic modality is a fairly recent phenomenon. In fact, if one accepts the American Council on Transplantation's definition of a "successful" transplant to be one that results in normal organ function one year after the transplantation, then the first successful organ transplant was done in 1954, at Peter Bent Brigham Hospital in Boston. That operation involved the transfer of a kidney from one twin to another, and the kidney functioned for nine years. The first successful transplant of a postmortem kidney took place in 1962, also at Peter Bent Brigham Hospital. The first successful liver transplant was performed at the University of Colorado in 1967. That was also the year that Dr. Christiaan Barnard successfully transplanted a heart in South Africa; that operation has become one of the most famous. In 1969, a postmortem pancreas was transplanted at the University of Minnesota, and in 1981, a successful heart-lung transplant took place at Stanford University in California. In 1984, a heart-liver transplant was successfully performed by Dr. Thomas Starzl and his colleagues in Pittsburgh.

One can see that in the past thirty years organ transplantation has greatly progressed. Kidneys can be called the "flagship" of organ transplants. More than 70,000 such operations have been done worldwide, of which 30 percent involved kidneys from living donors and 70 percent involved postmortem kidneys. The success rate in kidney transplants rose dramatically after the introduction of cyclosporin, an immunosuppressive agent that has mitigated the problem of graft rejection. Dr. Starzl reported that his patients' survival rates had increased to 80 percent with the introduction of cyclosporin and to 90 percent when its use became more widespread. Other centers using the drug found their success rates with postmortem kidneys approaching that previously achieved only with kidneys from living donors.

The American Council on Transplantation also reports normal kidney function for more than twenty years in patients who received kidneys from relatives and normal kidney function for over sixteen years in patients who received postmortem kidneys. During 1983, however, approximately 4,000 postmortem transplants were performed, which is only a slight increase from the 3,400 performed in 1980. This slight increase is more perplexing when one considers that at least 10,000 Americans are awaiting kidney transplants, the bulk of whom would use postmortem organs. This disparity between supply and demand is worthy of attention and will be discussed later in this chapter.

Organ transplantation is no longer an arcane procedure restricted to one or two medical centers. At the same time, however, organ transplantation is not and should not be within the reach of every sizable medical center or hospital. These conclusions are reached by examining the state of the art in five major types of organ transplantation—kidney, heart, liver, heart-lung, and pancreas.

Kidney transplantation has clearly made the transition from experimental to therapeutic. There are 173 renal centers in the United States today, and those using cyclosporin are experiencing success rates of over 90 percent. In addition, tissue compatibility has been improved by transfusing recipients with blood from donors. This transfusion technique could widen the donor pool because it enables unrelated individuals—spouses, for example—to donate kidneys to each other at potentially the same success rate found in donations by living blood relatives. Recent improvements in organ preservation provide a better opportunity to match recipients to donors. To prove that kidney transplantation is now considered therapeutic, one need only ask the question, "Is it reimbursible?" The answer is a definite and justifiable "Yes." The passage of the National Organ Transplant Act and the success of the End-Stage Renal Disease Program buttress the argument that kidney transplantation is therapeutically valid.

With regard to heart transplants, more than 800 such operations have been performed since the historic transplant in South Africa. An estimated 225 transplants were performed in the United States in 1984 at the thirty designated heart transplant centers. As in the case of kidney transplantation, cyclosporin has contributed to the accelerating success rates in heart transplantation. Some estimates put the one-year postoperative success rate at 80 percent and the five-year rate at 60 percent.

The reimbursement policies for heart transplants, which can show whether insurers view the procedure as experimental or therapeutic, are less clear than those for kidneys. Heart transplants were once performed regularly, but then some medical centers suspended these operations. The Health Care Financing Administration (HCFA) was reimbursing the Stanford University Medical Center for heart transplants performed on Medicare beneficiaries. In 1980, HCFA's parent organization, the federal Department of Health and Human Services, sponsored the National Heart Transplantation Study on the issues surrounding heart transplants, and suspended reimbursement for Medicare heart transplants until the study was completed. HCFA has received this report, compiled by Dr. Roger Evans and his colleagues at the Battelle Human Affairs Research Centers, but has not yet acted on it. And action is indeed needed; one of the findings in the study was that as many as 50,000 people could benefit from a heart transplant.

Numerous other data and indicators show that heart transplants have progressed beyond the purely experimental stage. Fifteen years ago, Stanford University reported that 22 percent of its patients had normal organ function at one year. That figure has now climbed to 80 percent. In 1983, Stanford's Dr. Norman Shumway, testifying in a congressional hearing, said that transplantation of the heart was equally as therapeutic as transplantation of the kidney. He pointed out that medical centers throughout the world are beginning to perform heart transplants again and that many of these clinics are approaching or matching Stanford's 80 percent success rate.

More than 500 liver transplants have been performed since the first successful effort in the late 1960s. In 1984 alone, 308 such procedures were done at the twenty liver transplant centers in the United

States. Survival rates, using the one-year criterion, have improved considerably and are now estimated to be 65 percent. One young woman has survived fifteen years with a liver transplanted when she was four years old.

While liver transplants have not achieved the same success rate as kidney and heart transplants, they are improving rapidly. The number of liver transplants increased 500 percent between 1981 and 1983. Between 1979 and 1984, there was a 100 percent increase in the success rate. Given the difficulty and the complexity of liver transplantation, the progress made in this area is impressive.

Because of this progress, liver transplantation was endorsed during a consensus development conference sponsored by the National Institutes of Health (NIH). At the end of two and one-half days, the consensus panel concluded that liver transplantation is a therapeutic modality for end-stage liver disease deserving of broader application.

Lung transplantation has not been as successful. Actually, it is now thought that a heart-lung transplant is the preferred procedure because the heart acts as the monitor of the immunological events surrounding the cardiopulmonary axis. After previous failures with transplanting the lung alone, the heart-lung procedure is beginning to meet with some success. There have been fifty such operations to date, including seventeen in the United States last year. A 50 percent survival rate has been reached, and one patient has even lived for four years following a heart-lung transplant. There are currently an estimated 500 to 1,000 potential candidates for a heart-lung transplant.

Approximately 400 pancreases have been transplanted worldwide, 218 of which occurred in the United States in 1983. The success rate is currently 35 percent to 40 percent in the United States, and the longest-surviving patient has reportedly been insulin independent for six years. The Battelle study estimated that some 5,000 persons could benefit from a pancreas transplant.

A complicating factor in transplantation reimbursement is the very high cost of organ transplants. Public health policy is consumed with cost containment. Legislation to encourage the spread of expensive operations cannot coexist with legislation to reduce overall costs. Table 2.1, which shows current transplant costs, presents them as a range because a variety of factors differ from hospital to hospital and from patient to patient. The expense of these procedures figures into all discussions of organ transplantation, whether the discussion is regulatory, medical, or legal.

There are, however, encouraging signs in the regulatory and reimbursement sectors that organ transplantation can be further developed.

Table 2.1: The High Costs of
Organ Transplantation

Organ	Average Cost
Heart	$57,000–$110,000
Kidney	$25,000–$30,000
Liver	$135,000–$238,000
Pancreas	$30,000–$40,000

For instance, the Food and Drug Administration (FDA) has already approved the three areas in which cyclosporin has had the most dramatic effect—the kidney, the heart, and the liver. It is encouraging that the FDA is acting on such recent medical progress in transplantation. Furthermore, even though the federal government has been reluctant to approve reimbursement for anything other than kidney transplants, other insurance carriers have gone much further. In March 1985, Blue Cross-Blue Shield of Michigan announced that it would start to cover a number of organ transplants on a trial basis. The Metropolitan Insurance Companies cover kidney, heart, heart-lung, and liver transplants.

The progress of the near future will probably be as exciting as that of the recent past. Transplant teams will continue to grow in number, although this growth will be cautious. New pharmacological agents even more effective than cyclosporin will be developed. We can anticipate further advances in drug combinations to reduce or eliminate the graft rejection problem. There are also many reasons to be optimistic about future developments in tissue preservation and matching methods. In short, most, if not all, of the technology issues surrounding organ transplantation are progressing satisfactorily.

Despite all of these encouraging signs, many problems remain, and their progress is less certain. Of these, one stands out—the supply and demand problem. In April 1985, the waiting list for transplants was: kidney—7,000; heart—40; liver—175; pancreas—30.

In 1983, the *Bulletin* of the American College of Surgeons stated that the number of kidney transplants performed yearly should increase from approximately 5,000 to between 15,000 and 18,000. Today it is thought that as many as 25,000 patients could benefit from kidney transplants. Given the current shortage of organs, this goal far exceeds our reach.

A number of factors explain the shortage of donor organs, but the problem certainly does not lie with *potential* donors. Nearly 60,000 people die from automobile accidents each year. The Centers for Disease

Control estimate that 12,000 to 27,000 of these deaths take place in hospitals, which greatly enhances the chance of organ retrieval. Furthermore, most people know that organ transplantation is possible and that there is a need for donor organs. The key here is educating both the public and the health professionals.

Meeting the challenges of improving and extending organ transplantation will take considerable effort and resources, more than any one organization can muster. The formation of the American Council on Transplantation (ACT) should encourage further growth in the field. Another encouraging development is the Task Force on Organ Transplantation. One of its major purposes is to strengthen the loosely knit link between organ procurement agencies and organ transplant centers to improve coordination of the organ procurement system. The Office of Organ Transplantation in the Department of Health and Human Services will work with the Task Force and ACT to improve procurement networks and to forge powerful alliances.

ACT was formed in the belief that the complex challenge of improving and extending organ transplantation could be addressed more effectively by a consolidation of interests than by many competing or overlapping ones. Nearly every major organization with an interest in organ transplantation is represented on ACT's board of directors. The Task Force on Organ Transplantation issued two reports to Congress and the secretary of Health and Human Services. The first report, which came out in August 1985, helped to resolve general issues regarding safety and efficacy as well as to provide a basis for improving the availability and reimbursement of long-term immunosuppressive drug therapy. The second report, published in January 1986, addressed the numerous problems surrounding the procurement and allocation of organs. These reports will probably form a solid foundation for organ transplantation through the rest of the 1980s. [The executive summaries of these reports appear in Appendixes A and B of this volume.]

The capacity of our present system will be strengthened by the Office of Organ Transplantation within HHS. Among its other functions, the office will work with the regional organ procurement organizations and conduct a much-needed public information program. Also important will be the coordination of procurement efforts under the auspices of the End-Stage Renal Disease Program, which has already made significant improvements in the field of kidney transplantation. One significant aspect of the program is that it pays all hospitalization costs for donors. Since its inception in 1974, the program has boosted the number of transplants from 1,500, which was 17 percent of the total that year, to 6,100, which, due to increased numbers of kidney transplants, was 8 percent of the total.

Finally, there exists a good model for a coordinated approach to improving and extending organ transplantation in this country. The National High Blood Pressure Education Program, which began as an effort within what was then the Department of Health, Education, and Welfare, has now grown to include nearly every organization and group with an interest in detecting and treating hypertension. The key to the success of the National High Blood Pressure Education Program has been the coordination of efforts and the marshaling of resources. The same will hold true for efforts in the field of organ transplantation.

Although we have more to learn about organ transplantation, today's technology exceeds our ability to apply it. Our most important immediate challenge is to catch up with technology; thus, we must tackle the legal, ethical, and regulatory issues that can either help or hinder our efforts.

BIBLIOGRAPHY

Editor's Note: Because this chapter is a transcription of a keynote address, the following bibliography is provided for reference.

Abram, H. S., Vander Zwaag, R., Johnson, H. K., *Physicians' Attitudes Toward Organ Donation,* SOUTHERN MEDICAL JOURNAL 68(4) (April 1975).

Banta, H. D., Assistant Director for Health and Life Sciences, Office of Technology Assessment, Statement before the Subcommittee on Investigations and Oversight, House Committee on Science and Technology, Congress of the United States (April 27, 1983).

Bart, K. J., Macon, E. J., Humphries, A. L., *A Response to the Shortage of Cadaveric Kidneys for Transplantation,* TRANSPLANTATION PROCEEDINGS 11(1) (March 1979).

Brandt, E. N., Jr., Statement before the Subcommittee on Investigations and Oversight, House Committee on Science and Technology, Congress of the United States (April 27, 1983).

Council on Scientific Affairs, *Organ Donor Recruitment,* JOURNAL OF THE AMERICAN MEDICAL ASSOCIATION 246(19) (November 1981).

Davis, C., Former Administrator, Health Care Financing Administration, Statement before the Subcommittee on Investigations and Oversight, House Committee on Science and Technology, Congress of the United States (April 27, 1983).

Denny, D. W., Director of Organ Procurement Transplant Foundation, University of Pittsburgh, Testimony on Organ Procurement and Distribution for Transplantation before the Subcommittee on Investigations and Oversight, House Committee on Science and Technology, Congress of the United States (April 13, 1983).

Evans, R., *Health Care Technology and the Inevitability of Resource Allocation and Rationing Decisions, Part I,* JOURNAL OF THE AMERICAN MEDICAL ASSOCIATION 249(15) (April 1983).

Evans, R., *The Present and Future Need for and Supply of Organs for Transplantation.* Prepared for the Surgeon General's Workshop on Solid Organ Procurement for Transplantation: Educating the Physician and Public (June 7, 1983).

Evans, R., Anderson, A., Perry, B., *The National Heart Transplantation Study: An Overview,* HEART TRANSPLANTATION 2(1) (November 1982).

Evans, R. W., Garrison, L. P., Manninen, D. L., *The National Kidney Dialysis and Kidney Transplantation Study: Description, Statement of Objectives, and Project Significance,* CONTEMPORARY DIALYSIS (June 1982).

The Gallup Organization, *Attitudes and Opinions of the American Public Toward Kidney Donation, Executive Summary.* Prepared for the National Kidney Foundation, Washington, D.C. (February 1983).

Iglehart, J. K., *Transplantation: The Problem of Limited Resources,* HEALTH POLICY REPORT 309(2) (July 14, 1983).

Koop, C. E., *A Time and Place for Wisdom,* Keynote Address to the Surgeon General's Workshop on Solid Organ Procurement for Transplantation: Educating the Physician and Public (June 7, 1983).

Koop, C. E., *Remarks of the Surgeon General,* before the Surgeon General's Workshop on Solid Organ Procurement for Transplantation: Educating the Physician and Public (June 9, 1983).

Koop, C. E., Surgeon General, Testimony on the Surgeon General's Workshop on Solid Organ Procurement for Transplantation: Educating the Physician and Public, before the Subcommittee on Investigations and Oversight, House Committee on Science and Technology, Congress of the United States (April 13, 1983).

Lasagna, L., *Editorial: Rationing Human Life,* JOURNAL OF THE AMERICAN MEDICAL ASSOCIATION 249(16) (April 22, 1983).

Liver Transplantation, NATIONAL INSTITUTES OF HEALTH CONSENSUS DEVELOPMENT CONFERENCE SUMMARY 4(7) (June 20–23, 1983).

Mack, W., President, North American Transplant Coordinator's Organization, Testimony before the Subcommittee on Investigations and Oversight, House Committee on Science and Technology, Congress of the United States (April 27, 1983).

Michigan Blues to Cover Organ Transplants, American Medical News (March 8, 1985).

Najarian, J. S., *Immunologic Aspects of Organ Transplantation,* HOSPITAL PRACTICE (October 1982).

ORGAN TRANSPLANTATION FACTS (American Council on Transplantation, Washington, D.C.) (1983).

Overcast, T., *Problems in the Identification of Potential Organ Donors: Misconceptions and Fallacies Associated with Donor Cards.* Prepared for the Surgeon General's Workshop on Solid Organ Procurement for Transplantation: Educating the Physician and Public (June 7, 1983).

Pfaff, W., Director of the Kidney Transplantation Program of the University of Florida, Testimony Concerning Organ Sharing in Transplantation, before the Subcommittee on Investigations and Oversight, House Committee on Science and Technology, Congress of the United States (April 13, 1983).

Prottas, J., *Encouraging Altruism: Public Attitudes and the Marketing of Organ Donation*, MILBANK MEMORIAL FUND QUARTERLY 61(2):278–306 (1983). (September 1982).

Shumway, N. E., Heart and Heart-Lung Transplantation (Speech), Stanford University (1983).

Starzl, T. E., University of Pittsburgh, Testimony before the Subcommittee on Investigations and Oversight, House Committee on Science and Technology, Congress of the United States (April 13, 1983).

Starzl, T. E., Iwatsuki, D. H., *et al.*, *Evolution of Liver Transplantation*, HEPATOLOGY 2(5) (1982).

Surgeon Calne Tells Transplanters Cyclosporin A Saves Grafts, Medical World News (August 4, 1980).

Tennessee, University of, Testimony on Organ Procurement Program at the University of Tennessee, before the Subcommittee on Investigations and Oversight, House Committee on Science and Technology, Congress of the United States (April 27, 1983).

Waltzer, W. C., *Procurement of Cadaveric Kidneys for Transplantation*, ANNALS OF INTERNAL MEDICINE 98 (1983).

3

Social and Medical Considerations Affecting Selection of Transplant Recipients: The Case of Heart Transplantation

Roger W. Evans
Junichi Yagi

The selection of transplant recipients is one of the more significant problems faced by cardiac transplant teams. Although a relatively uniform set of patient selection criteria has evolved over the past few years, it is still uncertain to what extent these criteria have been followed. For example, one criterion stipulates that patients over the age of fifty not be considered for transplantation; in practice, however, patients who are age fifty-five or older are occasionally accepted as transplant candidates. Inconsistencies between stated criteria and actual practice underscore the fact that patient selection criteria are still evolving. As transplantation technology improves, relaxation of the criteria by which patients are selected will continue. It is also reasonable to argue that so-called "selection criteria" are merely guidelines for the selection of transplant recipients, and rigid adherence to such guidelines by transplant teams should not be expected. However, due to pressures from public and private insurers, if reimbursement is to follow, it is quite possible that teams will be expected to comply with specifically stated criteria for the selection of transplant recipients.

The shortage of donor hearts for transplantation presents us with a moral and ethical dilemma in selecting transplant recipients similar to that which existed when kidney dialysis became a reality.[1] In the late 1960s, selection criteria were created for dialysis patients for two reasons: (1) funds were unavailable to pay for treatment, and (2) the number of available kidney dialysis machines was inadequate to treat all needy patients. Both of these problems were eventually resolved through federal government intervention.[2] Patients with end-stage renal disease (ESRD) are no longer precluded from dialysis on the basis of any criteria. Patients may, however, choose to forgo treatment.

Today, no artificial device is available to treat patients with end-stage cardiac disease (ESCD) and, as a result, it is inappropriate to argue that an analogy exists between the treatment of ESRD and that of ESCD. The only connection between the treatment of these two conditions is the historical significance of patient selection. Medicare coverage of kidney dialysis and kidney transplantation has removed the moral and ethical dilemma of selecting ESRD patients for treatment. It is noteworthy that a similar decision concerning coverage of heart transplants, however, will not alleviate the ethical dilemma of selecting heart transplant recipients. In the absence of a viable long-term artificial device, many patients with treatable ESCD will die because of an inadequate supply of donor hearts. We currently estimate that as many as 15,000 people who might have benefited from some form of cardiac replacement die each year.[3] We further estimate that under the existing organ procurement system, only 400 to 1,000 donor hearts become available each year.

Other constraints may also preclude patients from transplantation benefits. These include the inequitable availability of reimbursement (not all public and private insurers pay for heart transplants) and a possibly inadequate number of centers with transplantation capabilities for all of the donor organs that may become available.[4]

One must conclude that patient selection will be a constant problem associated with heart transplantation.[5] Bluntly stated, the problem is one of deciding who will benefit when not all can; this is one of the most fundamental issues facing medicine today and in the foreseeable future. Medical triage is not a new problem, it is a growing problem.

Most people find patient selection unpalatable. Ethicists have offered numerous proposals to resolve the patient selection issue, but most of these have negative consequences and vary only in the degree to which they are distasteful.[6] Most neutral, perhaps, is the usual lottery proposal, which is problematic because of its inability to ensure that scarce resources are put to the best available use.

It seems that it would be useful to provide an empirical basis for the selection of patients according to preestablished selection criteria. The object would be to demonstrate that the criteria used are clearly associated with positive patient outcomes, such as survival.[7] In this regard, it could be argued that, although patient selection criteria are unpalatable, they are justifiable. Their use would accomplish two basic objectives: (1) making the best use of scarce resources and (2) ensuring that patients have the highest probability of successful operations. The objective of this chapter is to provide a preliminary empirical basis for the selection of heart transplant recipients. Using this approach, it is possible to develop a patient selection protocol that would meet the two forementioned objectives.

CURRENT PATIENT SELECTION CRITERIA

The patient selection criteria currently followed by cardiac transplant teams are provided in Table 3.1. These criteria are a mix of medical and social considerations.[8] From both a legal and an ethical perspective, some of these criteria, as demonstrated by Merriken and Overcast,[9] have questionable validity. Both the Age Discrimination Act and Section 504 of the Rehabilitation Act call into question the use of these criteria.[10] In the past, these criteria went unchallenged because heart transplantation was offered to patients as an experimental procedure. As the procedure has gained acceptance, however, the legal status of these criteria has become unclear.

There is some confusion concerning the use of criteria listed in Table 3.1. Broadly stated, the criteria used to select heart transplant recipients are intended to ensure the success of the transplant in terms of patient survival and to maximize the probability that the recipient will be able to adapt successfully to the transplant. The medical criteria are related to survival, while the social criteria clearly have implications for adaptation and adjustment. Accumulated evidence shows that transplant recipients frequently encounter both a medically and a socially complicated posttransplantation course. Some patients, and their families, have a greater ability to adapt to the transplant experience than others.[11]

The current use of an age criterion is questionable from both legal and ethical perspectives. Patients over age fifty-five are not considered good candidates for many organ transplant procedures, particularly heart transplantation.[12] In practice, however, physiological rather than chronological age is the primary indicator of suitability. Age serves as a reasonable, although indirect, indicator of the patient's health status as well as the patient's ability to tolerate the transplant procedure and postoperative treatment. Older patients are likely to have significant co-morbidity that will preclude transplantation. In addition, it is commonly asserted that older patients are less able than younger patients to tolerate long-term immunosuppressive therapy.[13] All transplant recipients remain on immunosuppressive therapy for the remainder of their lives to

Table 3.1: National Heart Transplantation Study Criteria Against Patient Selection

1. Advancing age, for example, beyond the age (normally about 50) at which the individual begins to have a diminished capacity to withstand postoperative complications

2. Severe pulmonary hypertension as reflected, for example, by a pulmonary artery systolic pressure over 65–70 mm Hg and exceeding pulmonary artery wedge pressure by about 40 or more mm Hg, or a calculated pulmonary vascular resistance above approximately 6 Wood units (applicable to orthotopic cardiac transplantation because of the limited work capacity of a normal donor right-ventricle)

3. Irreversible and severe hepatic or renal dysfunction (because of the likelihood of early postoperative exacerbation and because of interference with immunosuppressive regimens)

4. Active systemic infection (because of the likelihood of exacerbation with initiation of immunosuppression)

5. Any other systemic disease considered likely to limit or preclude survival and rehabilitation after transplantation

6. A history of behavior pattern or psychiatric illness likely to interfere significantly with compliance with a disciplined medical regimen (because a lifelong medical regimen is necessary, requiring multiple drugs several times a day with serious consequences in the event of their interruption or excessive consumption)

7. Recent and unresolved pulmonary infarction or pulmonary roentgenographic evidence of abnormalities of unclear etiology (because of the likelihood of pulmonary infection or its exacerbation with initiation of immunosuppression under such circumstances)

8. Insulin-requiring diabetes mellitus (because of exacerbation by chronic corticosteroid therapy)

9. Symptomatic or documented severe asymptomatic peripheral or cerebrovascular disease (because of observed accelerated progression in some patients after cardiac transplantation and on chronic corticosteroid treatment)

10. Acute peptic ulcer disease (because of the likelihood of early postoperative exacerbation)

11. The absence of adequate external psychosocial supports for either short- or long-term bases (because such support is generally necessary during the inevitable waxing and waning of the clinical status of the patient and for adherence to the lifelong medical regimen).

Source: *Federal Register* 46(14):7072–7074, Thursday, January 22, 1981.

combat rejection of the transplanted graft. The major drawback of immunosuppressive therapy is that it increases the patient's susceptibility to a variety of infections. In short, the two primary evils associated with transplantation are infection and rejection.

Despite these concerns, it is apparent that patient selection criteria for heart transplantation are becoming increasingly liberal. The age factor, although important, has been relaxed somewhat from age fifty to age fifty-five. In addition, some transplant teams now accept patients who have significant comorbidities, such as diabetes. Perhaps a more alarming trend in recipient selection is the tendency of some programs to accept healthier patients. Generally, patients accepted for heart transplantation have a prognosis for survival of less than six months.[14]

The timing of the transplant procedure has always been a debated topic. On the one hand, the transplant team does not want to impose an undue risk upon the patient by performing the transplant on him or her too early, when the risk of the procedure itself may shorten the patient's life. On the other hand, if the team waits too long to perform the procedure, the patient may not benefit because he or she is too weak. The current trend suggests that transplants may be performed earlier rather than later.

There is no evidence to suggest that cardiac transplant teams inherently discriminate when selecting transplant candidates. Although the majority of heart transplant recipients are white males, it is evident that the conditions for which heart transplantation is appropriate are more prevalent among white males. Data from the National Heart Transplantation Study suggest that women and minorities are slightly underrepresented in the recipient pool.[15] We do not consider this misrepresentation to be based on intentional discrimination.

MATERIALS AND METHODS

In an effort to justify empirically the use of transplant recipient criteria, data from the National Heart Transplantation Study have been used to examine one significant outcome of transplant recipients—survival. The analyses pursued here are necessarily preliminary, but they are also highly instructive and suggest that it is possible to subject allegedly value-laden criteria to empirical analyses to ascertain their utility as predictors of patient outcome. The primary goal of transplantation, unlike that of some surgical procedures, is to prolong life, not simply to relieve symptoms. Thus, survival is the most suitable outcome indicator for the proposed analyses.

DATA

The National Heart Transplantation Study provided a unique opportunity to collect extensive data on the survival experiences of heart transplant recipients.[16] Although data were obtained on a total of 441 heart transplant recipients, only 414 patients have been included in these analyses. Of these 414, 242 received their heart transplant at Stanford, while the other 172 received their transplant at the remaining five transplant centers that participated in the study.

METHOD OF ANALYSIS

The current consensus is that the Cox proportional hazards model, with transplant status as a time-dependent covariate, is the most powerful method available for the analysis of heart transplant survival data.[17] A proportional hazards model is partially nonparametric in that no assumptions are made regarding the functional form of the baseline hazard functions, whereas the multiplier is parameterized linearly in a logarithmic scale. Its semiparametric nature makes it possible to control for known or potentially confounding effects of concomitant factors simultaneously, while producing bias-free estimates of the coefficients of interest.

VARIABLES

A number of potential risk factors were incorporated into the Cox proportional hazards regression model to determine how they affected patient survival and to ascertain whether they increased the risk of mortality. In addition to age at transplant, possible covariates for survival included: transplant period, gender, race, age, and functional impairment prior to transplantation (Karnofsky Index). These variables are fully described in the final report for the National Heart Transplantation Study.[18]

The foregoing variables have been coded and recoded in various ways to facilitate data analysis. For example, the year of transplant is grouped into three categories; hereafter this variable is referred to as the transplant period and includes three time periods: 1968 through 1973, 1974 through 1979, and 1980 through 1983. The reason for this is twofold. First, the immunosuppressive drug cyclosporin was introduced in 1980, and second, considerable technological advances in heart transplantation have occurred since 1973. The Karnofsky Index is used to measure a patient's functional impairment prior to transplantation. A score of 1 on this index stands for the normal ability to function physically, while higher scores represent increasingly impaired functional ability. Race is considered to be binary because of the small numbers of patients in the nonwhite subcategories.

As with most multivariate statistical techniques, estimation of the proportional hazards model is hampered by missing data for one or more covariates included in the model. The larger the number of explanatory variables included, the greater the chance that missing data may hinder the analysis. Possible covariates missing for some patients include race, diagnosis, functional impairment prior to transplantation, cyclosporin, and HLA-matches (i.e., tissue-typing data). When these five covariates are included in the full statistical models, 62 of the total 420 observations are excluded from the analysis. If the HLA-matches variable is deleted, then only eleven observations are excluded. The loss of these cases for analysis has not affected the results.

RESULTS

The first step in the analysis involved an extensive examination of the effect of gender on cardiac transplant recipient survival. Numerous other variables were included in the model, although they were treated as nuisance factors. These variables were included in the Cox proportional hazards model only to ensure that the estimate of the regression coefficient was rendered free of other confounding effects. Ultimately, no specific meaning is attached to the coefficients of these nuisance factors.

Determining which other variables should be controlled in the regression analysis is not as straightforward. Generally, one would like to include all of those variables that a priori are considered appropriate. According to Breslow,[19] even statistically nonsignificant variables should be included in the model, if inclusion of such variables changes the estimated coefficient of the variables of interest—in this case, patient gender—to any appreciable degree. If the model is saturated with the effects of all possible confounding factors, the estimated coefficient of the variable (gender) is said to reach equilibrium. As shown in Table 3.2, the estimated coefficients associated with gender changed dramatically from Model 1 to Model 3, although none of these coefficients is statistically significant. After the third model, the estimates reached a state of equilibrium. Based on this, it is reasonable to conclude that an unbiased estimate of the effect of gender is approximately 0.265 with a ζ score of 1.35 or 1.38.

Precision in the estimation process is lost when a model includes

Table 3.2: Results of Fitting Cox Regression Models—All Heart Transplant Patients ($N = 414$)

Model	1	2	3	4	5†	6†	7†	8†
Number of Parameter	2	3	6	7	2	5	5	6
Log Likelihood	−1263.55	−1262.86	−1246.18	−1246.10	−1167.97	−1151.55	−1151.64	−1151.39
Gender	0.038 (0.202)*	0.037 (0.195)	0.261 (1.35)	0.266 (1.38)				
Race		0.291 (1.123)	0.181 (0.696)	0.191 (0.735)	0.289 (1.112)	0.173 (0.663)		0.182 (0.697)
Year of transplant			−0.044 (−2.63)			−0.044 (−2.64)		
Transplant period: 1968–1973								
Transplant period: 1974–1979				−0.382 (−2.15)			−0.391 (−2.18)	−0.388 (−2.17)
Transplant period: 1980–1983				−0.486 (−2.66)			−0.491 (−2.68)	−0.489 (−2.67)
Age at transplant			0.021 (3.08)	0.022 (3.24)		0.021 (3.06)	0.022 (3.21)	0.022 (3.14)
Functional impairment just before transplant			0.148 (3.21)	0.151 (3.27)		0.147 (3.16)	0.151 (3.25)	0.150 (3.23)

*b/s.e. (b).

†Stratified Cox model by gender:

$\lambda_1(t; Z) = \lambda_{01}(t) \cdot \exp (\beta \cdot Z)$; male

$\lambda_2(t; Z) = \lambda_{02}(t) \cdot \exp (\beta \cdot Z)$; female

extraneous variables. Such variables have either nonsignificant coefficients or coefficients whose magnitude is smaller than the standard deviation of the estimate. At this point in the analysis, however, the primary concern was not to achieve precision in the estimation process, but rather to control the potential confounding effects of the nuisance factors.

Similarly, the effects of other variables, such as race, transplant period, and so forth, can be taken into consideration. As shown in Table 3.2, a comparison of the maximized log-likelihood between the second and third models reveals that an improved fit of the data with the model corresponds to the inclusion of three additional variables, namely, transplant period, age at transplant, and functional impairment just before transplant.

$$[X^2_3 = 2(1262.86 - 1246.18) = 33.36, p < 0.0001]$$

The third and fourth models fit equally well, as their log-likelihoods are -1246.18 and -1246.10, respectively. In the fourth model, an additional variable—transplant period—has been included. Three specific time periods have been identified in an attempt to ascertain the extent to which improvements in cardiac transplant technology might contribute to a better fit of the Cox model.

The subsequent models in Table 3.2 are stratified by gender, the immediate effect of which is to make the incidence ratio of mortality of individuals characterized by explanatory variables ζ and $\zeta 0$ at posttransplant time t proportional with gender. In other words, the regression coefficient β is invariant for both sexes and, therefore, so is the relative risk for a given pair of covariates.

As revealed in Table 3.2, stratification improved the overall fit of the models when they are compared with their corresponding nonstratified models; yet the regression coefficients themselves changed very little. This can be seen, for example, by comparing Model 3 with Model 6 and Model 4 with Model 8.

Cox regression coefficients for Model 4 contained in Table 3.2 are presented in Table 3.3, together with the 95 percent confidence limits for each variable. Variables are significant at the .05 level if the confidence interval does not contain zero. As can be seen from Table 3.3, year of transplant, age at transplant, and functional ability prior to transplant are all statistically significant. Race and gender, however, are not statistically significant.

Based on the regression coefficients reported in Table 3.3, it is possible to compute the risk of death, as a function of time after transplantation, and to determine the influence of covariates (such as age and gender) on this risk. Table 3.4 summarizes the relative risk of mortality

Table 3.3: Estimates of the Cox Regression Coefficients Based
on the Fourth Model

Beta	Estimates	Standard Deviation	Lower†	Upper
Gender	.2659	.1931	−.1126	6444
Race	.1910	.2603	−.3191	.7011
Transplant period*				
Year 2	−.3816	.1783	−.7312	−.0321
Year 3	−.4861	.1832	−.8452	−.1271
Age at transplant	.0218	.0069	.0082	.0333
Functional impairment	.1513	.0462	.0607	.2419

*Year of heart transplant = 1968–1973, if Year 2 = 0, Year 3 = 0,
1974–1979, if Year 2 = 1, Year 3 = 0, and 1980–1983, if Year 2 = 0, Year
3 = 1.
†95 percent confidence limits.

after heart transplantation in relation to various risk factors included in
the proportional hazards analyses, controlling for all other risk factors
included in the regression equation. Thus, since all of the relative risks
are adjusted for each other, they can be interpreted independently.

For example, it is possible to compute the relative risk of death for
males compared with females. Based on the Cox regression coefficient
estimates reported in Table 3.3, the estimated coefficient of the gender
variable is .2659. Thus, the relative risk of death for females is given by
$\exp[.2659(1 - 0)] = 1.30$, compared with a relative risk of 1.0 for males.
Similarly, 95 percent confidence limits of the relative risks are obtained
by using the lower and upper estimates of the regression coefficients
(as reported in Table 3.3).

The relative risks, as shown in Table 3.4, indicate that the risk of
death for females is 1.3 times greater than for males; the risk for whites
is 1.2 times greater than for nonwhites. However, with Chi-square statistics of 1.90 and 0.54, respectively, neither difference is statistically
significant.

With respect to the other risk factors (transplant period, age at
transplant, and functional impairment), some interesting differences can
be observed. The relative risks of mortality associated with the transplant period clearly show a decreasing risk associated with more recent
transplants. Compared with a risk of 1.0 for the baseline period (1968
through 1973), the relative risk is only .68 for the period 1974 through
1979 and .62 for the period 1980 through 1983. The Chi-square statis-

tics (4.62 and 7.08, respectively) show that these differences are highly significant, confirming the fact that transplantation technology has improved and, therefore, that survival rates have indeed increased in more recent years.

Finally, a comparison of relative risks shows that patients with less functional impairment prior to transplantation have a lower risk of death following transplantation. Table 3.4 shows that those patients who were reported to have a Karnofsky Index of 10 (moribund, fatal processes progressing rapidly) have a relative risk of death that is almost four times as great as those who were in better health prior to the transplant. Indeed, it is clear that the relative risk of death increases steadily as the condition of the patient deteriorates. These statistically significant differences in the relative risks of mortality after transplantation (with respect to both functional impairment and age at transplant) provide strong support for the use of patient selection criteria in allocating the limited supply of donor organs.

DISCUSSION

In the absence of an adequate supply of donor organs, the selection of transplant recipients will remain a complex legal and ethical problem. Only in the case of renal transplantation has the patient selection dilemma been largely eliminated, given the availability of a mechanical substitute—maintenance dialysis. Unfortunately, a patient with end-stage cardiac disease or end-stage hepatic disease does not have a viable mechanical option. As a result, if referred to a transplant program, and accepted as a transplant candidate, such a patient will either receive a scarce organ or die waiting for one.

Transplant recipient selection is often decided on by a mix of clinical and social criteria. While the clinical criteria often go unchallenged in the legal and ethical literature, considerable debate surrounds the use of social criteria, particularly those that reflect social worth. In the early days of kidney dialysis, the use of social criteria was often questioned.[20] Now, the extension of Medicare benefits to patients with end-stage renal disease largely eliminates the access problem. Nonetheless, over the years it has become apparent that social criteria for patient selection have some merit. Patients with unstable home environments often adapt poorly to the strict treatment regimens. Certain behavioral problems in patients are exacerbated with the onset of dialysis or following transplantation. It is most unfortunate that no empirical basis has been provided to evaluate the validity of social criteria in patient selection.

Table 3.4: Relative Risks of Mortality After Heart Transplant in Relation to Various Potential Risk Factors—Results of Proportional Hazard Analyses Controlling for the Other Risk Factors

| Risk Factors | Number of Recipients | | Relative Risk | 95 percent CL | $\chi^2(1)$ | p-Value |
	Dead	Alive				
Gender						
Male	208	152	1.00		1.90	1.25
Female	34	26	1.30	0.896–1.904		
Race						
Nonwhite	15	20	1.00		0.54	0.25
White	224	158	1.21	0.727–2.016		
Transplant period						
1968–1973	58	5	1.00 (1.61)		4.62	0.05
1974–1979	89	41	0.68 (1.47)	0.484–0.969	7.08	0.01
1980–1983	95	132	0.62 (1.00)	0.730–0.881	10.50†	0.001
Age at transplant*						
–20	17	20	1.00			
20–30	23	33	1.25			
30–40	48	47	1.55			
40–50	103	65	1.93			
50+	51	13	2.41			
Functional impairment					10.69†	0.001
1	0	1	1.00			
4	5	8	1.57			
5	14	12	1.82			
6	29	26	2.13			
7	69	62	2.88			
8	38	15	3.35			
9	64	35	3.35			
10	22	17	3.89			

*Based on a restrictive proportional hazards model.
†Score test for linear trend.

While most people find medical and clinical criteria less distasteful, they, too, have not been subjected to systematic empirical analyses. Most people have simply accepted the use of clinical criteria. These criteria, however, are worthy of further empirical analyses to determine their validity as predictors of successful patient outcomes, such as survival.

In the National Heart Transplantation Study, Overcast and Merriken have considered thoroughly the legal implications of using certain social criteria—namely, age and potential for rehabilitation.[21] Their conclusion: in the absence of an empirical basis, the value of social criteria for purposes of patient selection is debatable. While legislative action may ease the problems associated with the use of such criteria, an empirical basis must still be provided for their use.

In this chapter we have described a method by which the merits of patient selection can be evaluated using empirical data. Although considerable data must be accumulated to ensure the feasibility of this approach, it is apparent that there is no better basis available for validating the various patient selection criteria. Until such data are accumulated on all variables of interest, it is inappropriate to criticize transplant teams as being discriminatory in their patient selection deliberations. If teams have a reasonable basis for the use of any criterion, they should not be chastised for such use. However, transplant teams must be willing to exercise some flexibility in the patient selection process to assure that the merits of various selection criteria can be assessed.

In conclusion, the process by which patient selection criteria can be validated will be both controversial and lengthy. To assure an expeditious validation process, however, emotional controversy should be set aside in favor of objective scientific inquiry.

NOTES

1. Evans, *et al.*, *Implications for Health Care Policy: A Social and Demographic Profile of Hemodialysis Patients in the United States*, JOURNAL OF THE AMERICAN MEDICAL ASSOCIATION 245(5):487 (February 6, 1981) [hereinafter cited as *Implications*].
2. U.S.C. Title 42, §1395rr(b)(2)(a) (1976).
3. R. W. EVANS, *et al.*, THE NATIONAL HEART TRANSPLANTATION STUDY: FINAL REPORT, Volumes 1–5 (Battelle Human Affairs Research Centers, Seattle, Wash.) (1985) [hereinafter cited as NATIONAL TRANSPLANTATION STUDY].
4. *See generally,* Iglehart, *Transplantation: The Problem of Limited Resources*, NEW ENGLAND JOURNAL OF MEDICINE 309(2):123–28 (July 14, 1983).
5. Christopherson, *Heart Transplants*, HASTINGS CENTER REPORT 12(1):18, 19–20 (February 1982).

6. Examples include systems run on a first-come, first-served basis, by lottery, or in which the sickest are treated first.

7. Aitkin, *et al., A Reanalysis of the Stanford Heart Transplant Data,* JOURNAL OF THE AMERICAN STATISTICAL ASSOCIATION 78(382):264, 270–73 (June 1983); J. D. KALBFLEISH, R. L. PRENTICE, THE STATISTICAL ANALYSIS OF FAILURE TIME DATA (John Wiley, New York, N.Y.) (1980) at 135–40; Crowley, Hu, *Covariance Analysis of Heart Transplant Survival Data,* JOURNAL OF THE AMERICAN STATISTICAL ASSOCIATION 72(357):27 (March 1977); Griepp, *et al., Increasing Patient Survival Following Heart Transplantation,* TRANSPLANTATION PROCEEDINGS 9(1):197, 198–99 (March 1977); Schroeder, *et al., Cardiac Transplantation: Review of Seven Years of Experience,* TRANSPLANTATION PROCEEDINGS 8(1):5 (March 1976); Mantel, Byar, *Evaluation of Response-time Data Involving Transplant Status: An Illustration Using Heart Transplant Data,* JOURNAL OF THE AMERICAN STATISTICAL ASSOCIATION 69(345):81 (March 1974); Gail, *Does Cardiac Transplantation Prolong Life? A Reassessment,* ANNALS OF INTERNAL MEDICINE 76(5):815–17 (November 1972); Clark, *et al., Cardiac Transplantation in Man: VI. Prognosis of Patients Selected for Cardiac Transplantation,* ANNALS OF INTERNAL MEDICINE 75(1):15 (July 1971).

8. *See generally,* Thompson, *Selection of Candidates for Cardiac Transplantation,* HEART TRANSPLANTATION 3(1):65–69 (November 1983).

9. Merriken, Overcast, *Age Discrimination in Patient Selection for Heart Transplantation,* UPDATE REPORT NUMBER 9: NATIONAL HEART TRANSPLANTATION STUDY (Battelle Human Affairs Research Centers, Seattle, Wash.) (1982).

10. Age Discrimination Act 42 U.S.C. §§6101–07 (1976); Rehabilitation Act 29 U.S.C. §§701–94 (1976).

11. Watts, *et al. Psychiatric Aspects of Cardiac Transplantation,* HEART TRANSPLANTATION 3(3):243–47 (May 1984); Christopherson, *et al., Rehabilitation After Cardiac Transplant,* JOURNAL OF THE AMERICAN MEDICAL ASSOCIATION 236(18):2082, 2083 (November 1, 1976): Kraft, *Psychiatric Complications of Cardiac Transplantation,* SEMINARS IN PSYCHIATRY 3(1):58, 61–9 (February 1971); Lunde, *Psychiatric Complications of Heart Transplants,* AMERICAN JOURNAL OF PSYCHIATRY 126(3):369, 371–73 (September 1969).

12. *See generally,* Thompson, *supra* note 8.

13. HEART TRANSPLANTATION (D. W. Cooper, R. P. Lanza, eds.) (MTP Press Ltd., The Hague, Netherlands) (1984) at 18.

14. Baumgartner, *et al., Cardiac Homotransplantation,* CURRENT PROBLEMS IN SURGERY 16(8):2, 50 (August 1979); *see generally,* Copeland, Stinson, *Human Heart Transplantation,* CURRENT PROBLEMS IN CARDIOLOGY 4(8):1–51 (November 1979).

15. NATIONAL TRANSPLANTATION STUDY. *supra,* note 3, at 9-4.

16. *Id.* at 21-1; Evans, *et al., The Need for and Supply of Donor Hearts for Transplantation,* HEART TRANSPLANTATION 4(1):57–62 (November 1984); Evans, *Heart Transplants and Priorities,* LANCET 1(8381):852–53 (April 14, 1984); Evans, *Organ Transplantation,* SCIENCE 222(4621):234 (October 21, 1983); Evans, *et al., The National Heart Transplantation Study: An Overview,* HEART TRANSPLANTATION 2(1):85, 86 (November 1982).

17. Anderson, *et al.*, *Linear Nonparametric Tests for Comparison of Counting Processes with Applications to Censored Survival Data*, INTERNATIONAL STATISTICAL REVIEW 50(2):219, 220 (1982); Anderson, Gill, *Cox's Regression Model for Counting Processes: A Large Sample Study*, ANNALS OF STATISTICS 10(4):1100–01 (November 1982); KALBFLEISH, *supra* note 7, at 142; Breslow, *Covariance Analysis of Censored Survival Data*, BIOMETRICS 30(1):89, 97–98 (March 1974); Cox, *Regression Models and Life Tables*, JOURNAL OF THE ROYAL STATISTICAL SOCIETY, SERIES B 34(2):187, 202–03 (1972). *See generally*, D. R. COX, D. OAKES, ANALYSIS OF SURVIVAL DATA (Chapman and Hall, New York) (1984).

18. NATIONAL TRANSPLANTATION STUDY, *supra* note 3, at 21-10.

19. Breslow, *Discussion III: Design to Optimize Combined-Modality Therapy and Selection and Verification of Prognostic Factors*, CANCER TREATMENT REPORTS 64:497– 98, 1980.

20. *See generally, Implications, supra* note 1.

21. NATIONAL TRANSPLANTATION STUDY, *supra* note 3, at 32-1.

4

Legal and Ethical Issues Surrounding Transplantation: The Transplant Team Perspective

Clive O. Callender

MEDICAL QUESTIONS

When organ transplantation is mentioned within the context of law and ethics, the following medical questions emerge:

1. Who can and who cannot donate?
2. Who can and who cannot have a transplant?
3. Will the organ come from a cadaver or from a living (whether related or unrelated) donor?

THE TRANSPLANT DONOR

In this decade, the most important question about organ transplantation revolves around whether the donation will be from a living (related or unrelated) donor or from a cadaver donor. Living related donors must be between the ages of fifteen and eighty. It is essential that these donors are willing and healthy, have two normal kidneys, and are medically compatible with the recipient. Cadaver donors are preferably brain dead with the heart beating. They need to have normally functioning kidneys without infection or metastatic cancer and, in most instances, they need to be younger than age fifty-five.[1]

If the brain-dead potential donor's condition deteriorates and the heart stops beating, the vascularized organs must be removed from the body and cooled within sixty minutes of cessation of the heartbeat. Most other tissues for transplantation need to be obtained within three to twelve hours of cessation of the heartbeat.[2]

THE TRANSPLANT RECIPIENT

In 1954, the first successful American kidney transplants were performed in Boston by Dr. David Hume and others. However, only when Dr. Thomas Starzl (the father of clinical kidney and hepatic transplantation) reported the first one-year graft survival results of 70 percent in 1963, did the era of successful kidney transplantation begin.[3] Today, the criteria for transplant recipient candidacy are liberal. Any sufferer of end-stage organ failure (heart, heart-lung, kidneys, or liver) who can tolerate surgery and who does not have infection or cancer is an acceptable organ transplant recipient. Restrictions on recipients of tissue transplants are even less stringent. Each recipient of a whole organ transplant is evaluated by the transplant team who then makes a determination of transplantability. Of utmost importance in this decision process is the patient's willingness and motivation to undergo the transplant operation.

CADAVERS AND LIVING DONORS

Kidney donation can be of two types—cadaver or living (related or unrelated). Prior to the advent of cyclosporin, the difference between the success of transplants from living donors related to recipients and of transplants from cadavers was over 20 percent. In most transplant centers this made transplantation from living related donors the preferred choice.

Since the introduction of cyclosporin in 1982 and the subsequent early improvement in cadaver (CAD) graft survival—the survival rate after one year is now 70 percent—the gap between cadaver and living related one-year graft survival has narrowed.[4] This may culminate in an even further decrease in the reliance on living related donor (LRD) transplantation. Living related donors are very attractive to the transplant team because of the superior short- and long-term graft survival rates: LRD transplantation has a survival rate at one year of greater than 90 percent, and CAD has a survival rate at one year of 50 to 70 percent; LRD five-year survival rates are greater than 80 percent, compared with CAD five-year survival rates of 45 to 50 percent.[5,5a] This represents a difference in survival of greater than 20 percent in favor of the LRD transplant. It must be remembered that because cyclosporin therapy is a relatively new therapy, five-year and ten-year results are not yet available. The early results, however, suggest that the cyclosporin era is just the beginning of a major immunosuppressive drug breakthrough that may revolutionize transplantation.[6]

Immunosuppressive drugs may obviate some of the reliance upon organs from living related donors. Although no data have been published, there have been rumors that living related donors who were otherwise healthy have died after surgery. Some centers are, therefore, greatly reluctant to use living related donors even though the benefit-risk ratio and the favorable survival rate from living related donors do not currently warrant this reluctance.

Living unrelated donors may be used in circumstances where cadaver organs are not readily available, when the transplant recipient's condition cannot tolerate the long wait for a cadaver organ, and when no living related donor is available. The fact that the living unrelated donor is healthy and the fact that the success rate is likely to be no better than that of a cadaver organ transplant are among the reasons why this voluntary donor is not used more often. In addition, when the motives for donation are other than altruism, the use of these donors is questioned.

NONMEDICAL QUESTIONS

Nonmedical (i.e., legal and ethical) issues exert an ever-increasing influence on whether organ and tissue transplants will be performed. The following nonmedical questions are commonly asked:

1. How much does the transplant cost?
2. Can the patient afford it?
3. Can the hospital afford it?
4. Can society afford it?
5. Is saving the patient worth the effort?
6. Is it justifiable to spend so much money for transplantation instead of treating other medical illnesses?

While some of these questions seem to require the wisdom of Solomon, a simple response is available for others.

THE PROBLEM OF COST

The costs of transplanting human organs are as follows:[7]

Organ	Approximate Hospital Cost
Kidney	$30,000.00†
Heart	$80,000.00*
Liver	$150,000.00†

*These hospital costs are identified by Dr. Roger Evans in unpublished data from the Battelle Research Institute[8] and refer to all in-hospital costs of keeping these patients alive (nursing, drugs, ICU, etc.); they do not include the surgical fee.
†The costs of these operations at Howard University Hospital.

Who can afford a transplant? The answer depends upon whether the patient is destitute, in which case medical assistance programs are likely to pay the cost. If one has health insurance and if the organ transplantation procedure is not considered experimental, the health insurance provider is likely to pay. In such instances, 80 percent of the expense is usually provided. If the transplant is not covered by a third-party carrier, then the cost will have to be borne by the potential organ recipient. Most liver and cardiac transplants are in this category, thereby restricting access to transplants by minority and impoverished groups; the typical hospital will not admit a patient with a disease that will cost $80,000 to $150,000 if there is no hope of remuneration.

Recently, questions that are more policy oriented (see questions 4, 5, and 6 in the list of nonmedical questions on page 44) have been raised: How can American society afford not to help sick and dying patients? Which of these people will we let die? Who will make these decisions?

How can spending so much money for transplantation be justified? The same rationale that is used for spending so much money for the Acquired Immune Deficiency Syndrome (AIDS), a disease which received funding when it seemed to affect a very narrow group of people but which now can potentially affect a large number of Americans, should be used in justifying moneys spent for transplantation. Similarly, organ transplantation, which began with kidney transplants, may result in many other successful organ transplantations such as the pancreas which, if successful, could be the major breakthrough in one of the most common diseases of all—diabetes mellitus.[8] Society cannot afford to let money stand in the way of these major breakthroughs. A reimbursement method compatible with the national economy must be developed.

For many reasons, nonmedical (legal and ethical) issues surrounding organ and tissue transplantation have surfaced. For instance:

1. The cost of House Resolution No. 1 (HR-1) funding, which became the ESRD Medicare Bill that paid for dialysis and transplantation effective July 1, 1973, has far exceeded expectations. The payments for subsequent dialysis and kidney transplantation as treatment for end-stage renal disease (ESRD) since July 1973 has cost over $2 billion and has nearly bankrupt the Medicare system.
2. The cost of health care has risen dramatically during the past decade.
3. Physicians' and surgeons' incomes have risen during the past decade.
4. The media have brought attention to Medicare's finances and to the cost of health care.
5. The media have heightened public awareness of the miracle of transplantation and of its cost.
6. Today's society is more cost conscious.
7. The Reagan administration has emphasized the cost-reduction effort, especially in the area of health.

THE TRANSPLANT TEAM'S SPECIAL CONCERNS

It is virtually impossible to respond to all of the questions asked of the transplant community, but this chapter will address some of the most common ones from the perspective of a member of the transplant team.

Independent publications by Childress, Evans, and Bart have made it clear that there are more than enough deaths of potential donors in the United States[8a,b]—20,000 of two million deaths per year are of potential donors.[8c,9] What is lacking is a satisfactory method of bringing these cadavers into the donor pool. There were approximately 2,150 cadaver kidney donations in 1981,[8c] which is far short of the need; 6,000 to 8,000 dialysis patients are waiting for renal transplants. This is irrespective of the numbers of potential recipients of other organs, such as heart, heart-lung, liver, and pancreas.[5b]

Since there are so many potential donors, why have so few people donated? A recent Gallup Poll, authorized by the National Kidney Foundation in 1983, indicated that while 93 percent of those questioned were aware of organ transplants, only 40 percent were either very or somewhat likely to want their own kidneys donated after their death.[10] Even worse, Childress has pointed out that only 15 to 19 percent of people have actually signed donor cards.[8a] Perhaps this figure is so low because it is inconvenient for individuals to sign organ donor cards. If so, this problem can be solved by including the option to donate on driver's license applications.

Another factor affecting the low rate of organ donation is the mistake, after an individual signs a donor card, of not discussing this with family members.[11] Indeed, the most appropriate use of the organ donor card is for family discussion before the donor's death. Families find it very difficult to discuss organ donation after the death of a loved one, especially if they have not discussed the topic previously with the deceased. When the transplant team asks for organs under such circumstances, the request is often met with hostility, anger, frustration, and despair. The explanation that this benevolent act may weaken the "sting of death" and that in the midst of death there can be life often is unappreciated when the "gift of life" talk is first heard upon the death of a loved one. Physicians and other health care professionals, when they are members of such families, are no more inclined to donate than others. And in their professional roles, health care professionals are reluctant to discuss organ donation with bereaved families. These facts emphasize the desperate need for public and professional education to overcome some of the obstacles to organ and tissue donation.

Two special minority groups have recently received much attention related to organ transplantation. The first is the foreign national who comes to the United States for a kidney and competes with United States citizens. In some states, these individuals form a significant minority. This problem can be alleviated by availing organs and tissues to foreigners only when there are no suitable matched resident recipients on the waiting list. The presence of foreign nationals on waiting lists and the possibility of their receiving transplants ahead of Americans are potential major deterrents to organ donation programs.

The second group is the black minority which makes up 10 percent to 12 percent of the American population. According to the National Kidney Foundation's Gallup Poll of 1983,[12] blacks are 10 percent less knowledgeable about transplantation than are whites. Blacks are also two-thirds less likely to donate organs after death, according to the same poll. At the Howard University Transplant Center, which is 97 percent black, only seven of sixty-three donated cadaver kidneys were from blacks. In a study conducted at the center, the most common reasons for blacks not donating were ignorance, superstition, distrust of the medical community, and racism (i.e., the reluctance of blacks to donate without assurance that their organs would be used for other blacks).[13] The D.C. Organ Donor Project was initiated to combat this problem in 1982; by 1986, the results of this project should be evident.

Efforts to improve the supply of organs and tissues to keep pace with the demand for them will probably result in hospitals requesting consent of the next of kin at the time of each death, as suggested by Caplan, Childress, and Evans.[14]

Many questions are raised by laypersons about using living related donors. Living related donors are the source of organs in 30 percent of all kidney transplants in the United States. As discussed earlier in this chapter, the success rate among the recipients of these organs is at least 20 percent better than the success rate among recipients of cadaver organs.[15] The risk these donors are exposed to is slight. Nevertheless, it is certainly possible for the kidney donor to be traumatized by the operation or to become ill and lose his or her remaining kidney due to an unrelated cause. Since this is very unlikely and because the risk-benefit ratio is so greatly in favor of the benefit, most kidney transplant centers consider the use of living related donors to be a sound medical decision.

A similar conclusion is reached by those who perform experimental pancreatic transplants. The risk-benefit ratio of using cadaver organs versus organs from living related donors, according to Sutherland and Najarian at the University of Minnesota, greatly favors the use of living related donors.[16]

The advent of cyclosporin promises to improve the success rate of cadaver organ transplants. Should cyclosporin be as effective in the five- to ten-year follow-up period as it is in some centers now, the use of living related donors could become obsolete.

Some individuals wonder why transplantation, which is such an expensive treatment modality, is used. The transplant teams view kidney, heart, and liver transplants as the preferred therapeutic modality for many patients with end-stage organ failure. Not only are the one-year and five-year graft survival rates of these organ transplants highly competitive with alternative therapies, but the cost of alternative therapy is occasionally higher than transplantation when diseases of these organs are in their terminal stages. For example, costs for hospital care and renal transplantation are approximately $30,000 the first year and $1,000 to $2,000 per year thereafter, in contrast to hemodialysis which costs $20,000 to $25,000 per year.[17] Liver transplantation (including hospital care) costs $150,000 to $200,000 the first year; the comparative cost of keeping the patient with end-stage hepatic disease alive is difficult to determine.[18] Hospital and cardiac transplantation costs are $80,000 the first year and $2,000 to $3,000 per year thereafter, in contrast to the cost of care for cardiac cripples, including in-hospital intensive care and frequent hospital readmissions, estimated to be $16,000 per month, or $192,000 per year.[19]

Where all the moneys to pay for the treatment of so few will come from is another question, one this chapter must sidestep. But the money must come from somewhere. And it will, even if our social consciences must first be pricked by emotional appeals and affected by the positive support of national leaders and the media.

THE MEDIA—FRIEND OR FOE?

Transplantation and implantation have become the darlings of the media and as such have received extremely positive exposure. The media can be a vehicle for the elimination of myths and superstition—the major obstacles to organ tissue donation. The media's role in public and professional education cannot be overemphasized. However, if the transplant field should be viewed as exploitive in its use of this very powerful force, the media can become an unrelenting and unfriendly adversary.

The media have been used to publicize individuals' needs for transplantation and organs; without such publicity many recipients would have died. Prior to the intervention of the White House and the press, patients without the funds for extrarenal transplantation were denied hospital admission and died. Many people feel, however, that there has been unequal access to the media and can point to few media reports in which minorities plea for organs. They allege that black, Hispanic, and borderline middle-class patients are often denied equal access to extrarenal and renal transplantation and to new advances in immunosuppression, such as cyclosporin, because their ability to raise funds and attract media attention is not as effective as other groups. Unfortunately, needy patients who try to use the media for their own purposes have as unequal an access to the media as they have to transplantation. Despite this, the media have been helpful allies; much of the success and popularity of transplantation today is owed to their positive support.

The problem of unequal access—which has recently been addressed by the creation of the United Network for Organ Sharing (UNOS)—can be alleviated with such a national organ-sharing network. This network, with the cooperation of the North American Transplant Coordinators Organization (NATCO) and its umbrella organization, the American Council on Transplantation (ACT), may soon make individuals' access to renal and extrarenal organs more equitable. The problems of unequal access to transplantation and immunosuppressive drug therapy (cyclosporin) are also the prime target of the recently selected National Task Force on Organ Procurement and Transplantation. The Task Force responded to the Congress of the United States in August

1985, with its first report and in January 1986, with its final report. The executive summaries of these reports appear in Appendixes A and B of this volume.

Organ and Tissue Transplantation: Where Do We Go from Here?

As of 1984, 173 hospitals were approved by the End-Stage Renal Disease Program and certified by the secretary of Health and Human Services as transplant centers (according to Health Care Financing Administration data).[20] In addition, approximately 22,000 patients (of 65,000 patients on dialysis) are potential kidney transplant candidates, although only 10 percent of the patients on dialysis (6,000 to 7,000 per year) receive transplants.[21] If the success of transplantation continues to improve, and if new immunosuppressive drugs such as cyclosporin and monoclonal antibodies further prolong graft and patient survival, the need for organs is likely to increase. It was estimated by Evans and others that there would be a potential yearly need for 50,000 hearts, 5,000 livers, 22,500 kidneys, and 5,000 pancreases if the immunity problems of transplantation could be overcome (and many of them have been since those 1979 estimates were made).[22] Needed, then, to achieve maximum utilization of transplantation would be:

—Financial resourcefulness
—More efficient methods of organ procurement to lessen the gap between need and supply
—Public and professional education
—A more efficient national organ procurement system with well-integrated regional systems
—Training of more extrarenal transplant surgeons to meet the increased demand for extrarenal transplantations
—The creation of more regionally based extrarenal transplant centers
—Strategies for dealing with the long-term solution to the problem of organ scarcity, including the reassessment of xenografts and the financing of research on the expansion and the use of artificial organs.

In conclusion, a myriad of ways are possible to examine the legal and ethical issues surrounding transplantation. This transplant surgeon has presented the transplant team's views and responses to many of the questions being raised as the price of this new technology threatens to bankrupt the nation's health care system.

NOTES

1. *See* Simmons, *et al.*, *Section II: Technique, Complications and Results,* in TRANS-
PLANTATION (J. S. Najarian, R. L. Simmons, eds.) (Lea and Febiger, Philadelphia, Pa.) (1972) at 448 [hereinafter referred to as TRANSPLANTATION].
2. *See, e.g.*, Harris, Rathbun, *Ocular Tissues*, in TRANSPLANTATION, *supra* note 1,
at 615.
3. T. E. STARZL, EXPERIENCE IN RENAL TRANSPLANTATION (W. B. Saunders Co.,
Philadelphia, Pa.) (1964).
4. Krakauer, Eggers, Grauman, Unpublished data from the National Institute
of Allergy and Infectious Disease and the Health Care Financing Administration (Baltimore, Md.) (1985); (4a) Stiller, *et al.*, *A Randomized Clinical Trial
of Cyclosporin in Cadaveric Renal Transplantation,* THE NEW ENGLAND JOURNAL
OF MEDICINE 309(14):809–15 (October 6, 1983).
5. Ferguson, *et al.*, *Cyclosporin A in Renal Transplantation: A Prospective Randomized
Trial,* SURGERY 92(2):175, 177 (August 1982); (5a) Hakala, *et al. Cadaveric
Renal Transplantation with Cyclosporin A and Steroids,* TRANSPLANTATION PRO-
CEEDINGS 15(1):465, 466 (March 1983); (5b) Evans, The Present and Future
Need for Supply of Organs for Transplantation (Prepublished Data) (1983);
(5c) R. W. EVANS, *et al.*, THE NATIONAL HEART TRANSPLANTATION STUDY:
FINAL REPORT (Battelle Human Affairs Research Centers, Seattle, Wash.)
(1984) at ch. 4.
6. *See* Krakauer, Eggers, Grauman, *supra* note 4; Ferguson, *et al.*, *supra* note 5,
at 180; Hakala, *et al.*, *supra* note 5, at 468.
7. EVANS, *supra* note 5.
8. EVANS, *supra* note 5; Childress, The Gift of Life: Ethical Problems and Policies in Obtaining and Distributing Organs for Transplantation (Unpublished Data) (1983): T. L. BEAUCHAMP, J. F. CHILDRESS, PRINCIPLES OF
BIOMEDICAL ETHICS (Oxford University Press, New York) (2d ed. 1983) at
202; Bart, *et al.*, *Increasing the Supply of Cadaveric Kidneys for Transplantation,*
TRANSPLANTATION 31(5):383 (May 1981).
9. Childress, *supra* note 8; EVANS, *supra* note 5.
10. The Gallup Organization, *Attitudes and Opinions of the American Public Towards
Kidney Donation* (Prepared for the National Kidney Foundation, Washington,
D.C.) (February 1983) (GO 8305).
11. Overcast, *Problems in the Identification of Potential Organ Donors: Misconceptions
and Fallacies Associated with Donor Cards,* JOURNAL OF THE AMERICAN MEDICAL
ASSOCIATION 251(12):1559, 1561 (1984).
12. Gallup Poll, *supra* note 10.
13. Callender, *et al.*, *Attitudes among Blacks Toward Donating Kidneys for Transplantation: A Pilot Project,* JOURNAL OF THE NATIONAL MEDICAL ASSOCIATION
74(8):807–09 (August 1982).
14. Caplan, *Ethical and Policy Issues in the Procurement of Cadaver Organs for Transplantation,* THE NEW ENGLAND JOURNAL OF MEDICINE 311(15):981, 983 (October 11, 1984); EVANS, *supra* note 5; *Childress, supra* note 8.
15. Krakauer, *et al.*, *supra* note 4; Ferguson, *et al.*, *supra* note 5, at 177.

16. Sutherland, *et al.*, *Effect of Donor Source Technique, Immunosuppression and Presence or Absence of End State Diabetic Nephropathy on Outcome in Pancreas Transplant Recipients*, TRANSPLANT PROCEEDINGS 17(1):325–30 (February 1985).
17. *Supra*, note 11 *re* renal care costs.
18. EVANS, *supra* note 5; Bart, *supra* note 8.
19. *Id.*
20. Krakauer, Eggers, Grauman, *supra* note 4.
21. EVANS, *supra* note 5; Childress, *supra* note 8.
22. Childress, *supra* note 8.

Section 2

Medical-Legal Issues

5

Legal Aspects of Death and Informed Consent in Organ Transplantation

Thomas D. Overcast

While the frequency of organ transplantation has increased dramatically in recent years,[1] transplant professionals have not experienced a corresponding increase in professional liability claims—a situation in stark contrast to that of health care professionals working in other areas of specialty practice. However, the evolution of transplantation procedures into standard medical practice may portend more uncertain times. As more centers and professionals engage in transplant practice and as patients' expectations about transplant outcomes rise, an increasing number of liability claims can be expected. Although these claims will result from relatively unique situations, existing legal principles will provide some—but probably not all—of the answers for many of the issues involved. For example, the organ donation and retrieval process presents a number of interesting, and only partially resolved, questions that involve the responsibilities and potential liability of transplant centers and professionals. These include:

1. How far does the Uniform Anatomical Gift Act's (UAGA) grant of "good faith" immunity for transplant professionals extend?
2. May a physician be held criminally or civilly liable for his or her determination that death has occurred and that organ retrieval may proceed?
3. What effect do autopsy statutes have on organ retrieval efforts, and what is required of the transplant professional under these laws?

Similarly, the referral and care of transplant recipients may also raise unique and highly complex legal dilemmas. For example:

1. May health care providers be held liable if they fail to refer persons with heart conditions amenable to treatment by transplantation to transplant programs?
2. What role does—or should—informed consent play in transplant practice?
3. What types of malpractice actions involving transplant providers can be anticipated?
4. What exposure to liability does the provider have for transplantation of a defective or diseased organ?

This chapter outlines some of the current legal developments and issues that confront medical centers and professionals involved in retrieving and transplanting hearts.

LIABILITY FOR ACTIONS TAKEN WITH RESPECT TO THE DONOR

Cases involving organ donation from living donors have generated a great deal of legal and ethical discussion. The courts have addressed the problem of defining under what conditions relatives may give legally valid consent for organ removal from children or mentally incompetent individuals in order to save the life of another family member.[2] In some cases, plaintiffs have unsuccessfully asked the courts to determine whether a living donor may recover damages for organ removal by claiming that the donation was necessitated by negligent treatment of the donee.[3] Although issues involving live donors are not relevant in cardiac transplantation, cadaveric organ retrieval raises some unique legal questions of its own; these questions have garnered much less attention in both the courts and the legal literature. Three important issues affecting providers involved in cadaveric organ retrieval are the validity of the donor's consent for the use of the organ and compliance with the terms of the UAGA, the timeliness of the determination of the donor's death, and the removal of organs when death is by violent means and the medical examiner or coroner has jurisdiction over the body.

CONSENT UNDER THE UNIFORM ANATOMICAL GIFT ACT

One of the most pressing issues in the early years of heart transplantation was whether the removal of tissues from cadaveric donors could result in civil or criminal liability for those involved.[4] The National Conference of Commissioners on Uniform State Laws developed the Uniform Anatomical Gift Act in 1968, in part to remove concern over potential legal liability for organ retrieval.[5] Section 7(c) of the Act states:

> A person who acts in good faith in accord with the terms of this Act or with the anatomical gift laws of another state (or foreign country) is not liable for damages in any civil action or subject to prosecution in any criminal proceeding for his act.

Although this good faith exemption is intended to protect the physician from legal action associated with the removal of organs from a dead person, there is disagreement over whether the exemption protects the physician against torts such as "wrongful death" or "premature declaration of death," or whether the exemption refers to cases where organ donation may itself cause "death" as it is traditionally defined.[6]

In only one reported case has a court considered the tort liability of a physician or hospital in connection with the organ or tissue transplant procedures performed upon a donor who had been declared dead prior to removal of his or her organs or tissues. In *Williams* v. *Hofman*,[7] a treating physician informed the husband of a patient that his wife had died and obtained the husband's consent to remove her kidneys for transplantation. Two days later, after a mortician reported that he could not locate the body, the husband learned that his wife's body was functioning through life support techniques, and officially had not yet been pronounced dead. He attempted to contact the physician to stop removal of the kidneys only to discover that, as he acted, his wife was declared dead, and her kidneys were removed.

The husband attempted to recover damages—against the physicians involved in the transplant operation and the county in whose hospital the operation had occurred—for the charge of mutilation of the corpse and for negligence in communicating an erroneous and premature death message. The Wisconsin Supreme Court held that the good faith exemption constituted an affirmative defense against the actions brought by the husband in his individual capacity. However, the court also held that the good faith defense did *not* apply to actions brought by the husband in his capacity as administrator to recover damages for assault and battery and negligence. The court pointed out that the UAGA concerned only the mechanics of giving and receiving anatomical gifts, the determination of the time of death, and the procedures following death, but did not extend to treatment of the donor prior to death, nor to the treatment of the live transplant donee.

No plaintiff has alleged that physicians have acted in bad faith and, thus, are not immune under section 7(c) of the UAGA. Generally, the good faith standard of care connotes a state of mind involving honesty of purpose, freedom of intent to defraud, and a faithfulness to one's duty.[8] In a medical setting, this translates into good intention and the honest exercise of the physician's best judgment regarding the patient's needs.

The question of whether a transplant provider has acted in good faith is always one of fact and is determined on a case-by-case basis. However, the individuals involved in obtaining the consent of the family, and the physician who removes the organs, should carefully observe the procedures for valid donation as delineated in the UAGA. If they do not, providers are open to charges of bad faith and may not be entitled to the immunity from liability detailed in the UAGA.

Priority

One way a physician might lose immunity would be to accept a donation from a relative of the deceased with the knowledge that a closer relative to the donor or the donor him- or herself objected to the donation. The UAGA establishes a prioritized list of persons who may consent to the donation of a deceased person's organs. The list provides that a person in one class may donate only in "the absence of actual notice of contrary indications by the decedent or actual notice of opposition by a member of the same class or a prior class," and that "[i]f the donee has actual notice of contrary indications by the decedent or [if] a gift is opposed by a member of the same or prior class, the donee shall not accept the gift."[9] Thus, if a provider involved in retrieving the organ has actual notice of a valid objection to the gift, then notice exists of a procedural defect in the gift, and the provider may not be immune from suit.

"Stale" Consent

Another way the health care provider could lose immunity would be to act knowingly on a "stale" consent, that is, a consent that is obtained from an appropriate family member a considerable length of time before the actual death of the donor and which may, therefore, be invalid. The UAGA stipulates that relatives or individuals other than the deceased may make the gift "after or immediately before death."[10]

Because there are no easy rules to guide the practitioner, the determination of the amount of time that must pass before a consent may be considered stale will depend on the individual circumstances. In general, the physician should be alert to any change in circumstances that might result in a change of mind on the part of a relative who had previously consented to donation. Common sense suggests, for example, that a new consent be obtained if a patient is readmitted to the hospital after some extended period of time at home or in a nursing facility. Similarly, if a patient lingers near death for several weeks, it would be advisable to confirm the next-of-kin's intentions by obtaining a new consent. The lack of specific guidelines means that the practitioner should take every precaution to have a clear picture of the validity of the consent under which he or she intends to proceed.

Revoked Consent

The most obvious example of bad faith is to proceed with organ removal knowing that the gift of the organ has been validly revoked.[11] Failure to act in accordance with the terms of the UAGA does not, in and of itself, establish criminal or civil liability. Rather, it simply results in the loss of immunity from civil or criminal action.[12]

DETERMINATION OF DEATH

One of the most difficult medical-legal problems in transplant practice involves determining the moment of the donor's death. The UAGA leaves that determination to the attending physician and makes no attempt to define the uncertain point when life terminates,[13] even though the issue of exact time of death, thus allowing the removal of the organ, is critical to the transplant process. One commentator has noted: "To delay too long, so that metabolism ceases and tissue is damaged, can be fatal to the recipient. To act precipit[ously], when there is still a possibility of restoration of the donor, is unthinkable."[14] If the donor is not legally dead at the time the declaration of death is made, the physician pronouncing death may be open to charges of wrongful death or homicide.

The potential for liability has been exacerbated by the fact that "legal" and "clinical" definitions of death are not always the same. In *Tucker* v. *Lower*,[15] the brother of an organ donor brought suit against a transplant surgeon for $100,000, alleging, in part, that the donor's heart and kidneys had been removed before the donor was legally dead. As evidence that the donor was not legally dead, he pointed to the fact that his brother's heart was still beating when death was declared. At the time, Virginia had not yet adopted a standard of death based on the discontinuance of brain function. The trial judge initially refused to dismiss the case against the transplant surgeon, stating that death was to be determined under the "cessation of bodily functions" standard developed by the common law. At the end of the trial, however, the judge instructed the jury:

> In determining the time of death ... under the facts and circumstances of this case, you may consider the following elements, none of which should necessarily be considered controlling, although you may feel, under the evidence, that one or more of these conditions are controlling: the time of the total stoppage of the circulation of the blood; the time of the total cessation of the other vital functions consequent there to, such as respiration and pulsation; the time of complete and irreversible loss of all function of the brain; and whether or not the aforesaid functions were spontaneous or were being maintained artificially or mechanically.[16]

Although the jury found for the surgeon, the case nevertheless prompted the Virginia Medical Society to support a statute (later adopted) recognizing cessation of brain function as one ground for declaring death.[17]

Uncertainty over the appropriate definition of death continues to create problems for health care providers. Another incident arose in 1980, but apparently did not result in legal action.[18] After a neurologist pronounced a seventeen-year-old woman who had suffered severe head injuries as dead, the parents consented to organ donation. While the daughter was being maintained on a respirator pending organ removal, a second neurologist examined her and decided that she was not legally dead. In the resulting confusion, the parents withdrew their consent for donation. The patient was declared legally dead some time later.

In 1975, a New York hospital sought a declaratory judgment to clarify uncertainties over the application of neurological brain death criteria. In *New York City Health and Hospital Corporation v. Sulsona,*[19] the hospital asked a court to construe the meaning of the provisions concerning the time of death in the New York Anatomical Gift Act in light of the fact that New York had no statutory standard for determination of death.[20] The pertinent section provided only that "[t]he time of death shall be determined by a physician who attends the donor at his death, or, if none, the physician who certifies death." Although the comments to the Uniform Anatomical Gift Act state that it is not intended to define when death occurs, the trial judge held that "[t]he context in which the term 'death' is used in [the UAGA] ... implies a definition consistent with the generally accepted medical practice of doctors primarily concerned with effectuating the purposes of this statute."[21]

The uncertainties produced by the gap between the varied legal definitions of death and the advances in modern medicine have resulted in legal movement toward the adoption of "brain death" as the legal standard of death. Legislators in half the states have enacted laws that permit reliance on brain-related criteria for determining death.[22] In addition, courts in several states have judicially recognized brain-death standards in the absence of statutory recognition.[23] However, the standards adopted in the various states are not uniform. At least six varying standards exist, many of which have been criticized as unworkable or outmoded.[24]

Legal recognition of brain-death criteria does not end liability concerns for physicians who determine that death has occurred. For example, physicians may be challenged if they use brain-death criteria that are more liberal than those contained in the relevant statute, or if they make an error in assessing whether, in fact, legal death has occurred. While the UAGA clearly protects the surgeon who in good faith relies upon another's declaration of death and removes an organ, it is not at all clear that immunity extends to the physician who makes the actual determination of death.

Arguably, the good faith immunity provision in section 7(c) of the UAGA would not bar legal claims against a physician determining death. First, a court or a jury may be unlikely to find that a physician who acted negligently by making a premature declaration of death could meet the good faith standard required for immunity under section 7(c). Second, a premature declaration of death would not be in accord with the UAGA, since it specifies that it is not intended to override the statutorily or judicially enacted standards for determining death. Finally, it can be argued that the statute was intended to immunize physicians from civil and criminal liability only for actions taken *after* the donor is dead.[25]

On the other hand, Jeddeloh and Chatterjee[26] argue that the good faith defense would apply to physicians who make the determination of death. They state:

> To suggest . . . that the treating physician's decision as to time of death, critical in the transplant procedure, is not covered is to ignore important protection of the Act. While it is true that gifts under the Act do not take effect until after death, the Act discusses considerably more than just the mechanics of a gift. Section 7(b) directs that the time of death is to be determined by the treating physician, and, therefore, when he determines the time of death, he is acting pursuant to the Act. Since section 7(c) protects anyone who acts pursuant to the Act from both civil and criminal liability, the treating physician is so protected when he determines the time of death.[27]

Although to date, no cases have dealt directly with this issue, one court has implied that the section 7(c) exemption for physicians acting in good faith in accordance with the terms of the UAGA applies to physicians making a determination of death.[28] Whether the good faith defense applies to determinations of death, and to what extent it may shield physicians from suit for premature declaration of death, are as yet unclear and will remain so until case law develops.

MEDICAL EXAMINER AND CORONER CASES

A large number of heart (and other organ) donors are victims of traumatic injuries, usually to the head. These injuries often occur under violent or suspicious circumstances in which a police investigation and/or autopsy may be considered. Because of rapid tissue deterioration, the time delay normally inherent in these processes rules out use of the victim's organs for transplantation. In addition, organ removal prior to investigation by the medical examiner or coroner's office may lead to questions about whether evidence relating to the causes or circumstances of the death has been destroyed.[29]

Under the UAGA, organ retrieval has a lower priority than the requirements of autopsy and investigation by the medical examiner; section 7(d) specifies that the UAGA is subject to all laws regarding autopsies. In many cases, however, the medical examiner and the transplant team can work together to coordinate organ removal and investigation and/or autopsy.[30] For example, the medical examiner in Dade County, Florida, has established a formal program of cooperation with transplant programs.[31] The transplant team, the attending physician, or the hospital immediately notifies the medical examiner of potential deaths that fall under the jurisdiction of the medical examiner and provides that office with the medical history, the circumstances of death, and other pertinent information. The medical examiner then decides whether he or she will permit organ retrieval (with, of course, legal consent by the donor or next of kin and after a determination of death has been made).[32]

In Texas, a statute requires transplant centers to notify the medical examiner's office of a death occurring within its jurisdiction.[33] The medical examiner's office then sends a representative to the transplant facility to perform an inquest and, if necessary, an autopsy. If an autopsy is required, the organ needed for transplantation is first examined for clinical evidence and then released for transplantation.

Cooperation with the medical examiner and the local prosecutor (in suspected criminal cases) may also forestall legal difficulties in organ retrieval. In cases of potential criminal prosecution, it is particularly important to obtain the permission of both the prosecuting attorney with jurisdiction over the case and the medical examiner. While permission of the prosecutor is not legally required in most states,[34] it prevents potential charges of interference with criminal law enforcement through the destruction of evidence. Prosecuting attorneys generally will grant permission when they are assured that organ donation will not compromise the testimony regarding the cause of death.

LIABILITY ISSUES AFFECTING POTENTIAL AND ACTUAL TRANSPLANT RECIPIENTS

Transplantation practice has legal ramifications not only because it involves interventions upon a donor, but because it may affect potential and actual transplant recipients as well. As discussed below, medical malpractice and informed consent issues involving organ recipients will undoubtedly be raised as transplantation becomes more commonplace. However, this section begins with a discussion of another, rather unique question. Can a health care provider be held liable for negligently failing to advise a patient who may be a good transplant candidate of the existence of transplantation as a viable form of therapy, and for failing to refer the patient for such an evaluation?

LIABILITY FOR REFERRAL PRACTICES

As a general rule, physicians have a duty to advise their patients of alternative methods of treatment.[35] Courts have held that this duty exists even though the physician may not be competent actually to provide all of those forms of treatment. Failure to explain a standard treatment alternative, if one exists, is generally regarded as negligence.[36] The physician thus retains a duty to acquaint the patient with general information about treatment alternatives and to refer the patient to another health professional who may perform the treatment.[37]

In typical cases involving failure to inform, liability is based on the physician's failure to stay current with the advances in the medical profession.[38] One likely reason physicians may fail to recommend transplantation to patients who are nearing the final stages of organ disease is that the physicians are simply unaware of advances in transplant practice. However, transplant cases differ from the usual situation in two important respects. First, despite improving survival rates,[39] many physicians still consider transplantation to be outside the realm of standard practice. Second, unlike many forms of treatment, organ transplants may be restricted by resource scarcity. Because of the limited availability of donor organs, there is simply no guarantee that a person who is medically suitable for transplantation will be able to undergo the procedure. These two factors may influence courts regarding the question of whether or not a duty to inform exists in transplantation cases. Failure to prove that a treatment could have been obtained, even if the physician had advised the patient of it, may be a factor in determining whether the physician's failure to refer "caused" the injury to the patient. Because the likelihood of acceptance is small, even the physician who accepts the therapeutic value of transplantation may not wish to advise a potential transplant candidate of the possibility of transplantation.[40]

An initial question in any "failure to inform" case is whether heart transplantation is an option that must be disclosed to an individual who may be a good transplant candidate.[41] An important question concerns, complicating factors aside, the point at which a medical procedure becomes standard to the extent that the physician has a legal duty to advise his or her patient of its existence. This question again raises the thorny issue of how to pinpoint any meaningful dividing line between experimental and therapeutic medical care.

While a physician may not be convinced of the efficacy of the treatment, he or she probably should inform the patient of the alternative as long as reasonable medical opinion would consider it acceptable. One writer has stated:

> [W]hich risks the patient chooses to run are, in most cases, value judgments which fall entirely outside of the scope of medical decision making and involve social, economic, religious, and personal considerations that the physician cannot possibly know.[42]

Depending on their location and type of practice, the level of knowledge expected of physicians about transplantation may differ. Most health care providers today are aware of heart transplantation, but some may not be acquainted with the advances in, and increasing usage of, the procedure.

In many jurisdictions, the law may recognize that it is not realistic or fair to expect all physicians to exhibit the same level of awareness of advances in cardiology. Some courts have held that a general practitioner's duty to inform is limited to that which a reasonable general practitioner should know.[43] Likewise, the specialist's duty to inform is limited to matters that a reasonably knowledgeable specialist in that field would know.[44] For this reason, it is far more likely that a claim of failure to inform could be made against a cardiologist or cardiac surgeon than against a small-town general practitioner. However, as transplantation becomes more widely practiced and successful, perhaps even nonspecialists may incur a duty to inform cardiac disease victims of the transplant option.

Breach of a duty to inform cannot, however, be equated with legal liability. Even if the physician's failure to inform a patient of the possibility of transplantation is a breach of a duty to the patient, the patient still has to prove that the failure caused him or her some injury and damages. At this point, facts concerning the probability that the patient would have been accepted into a transplant program in time to avoid death as well as the likelihood of a successful outcome would become extremely important.[45]

INFORMED CONSENT OF THE TRANSPLANT RECIPIENT

Since the beginning of the century, courts have recognized that a physician must obtain a patient's consent to treatment. Justice Cardozo, in the famous 1914 case of *Schloendorff* v. *Society of New York Hospital*,[46] stated:

> Every human being of adult years and sound mind has a right to determine what shall be done with his own body and a surgeon who performs an operation without his patient's consent commits an assault for which he is liable in damages.[47]

During the first half of this century, the physician's potential liability was based exclusively on the tort of battery to avoid liability, and the physician merely had to obtain the patient's consent to be treated; courts were not seriously concerned with whether the patient truly understood the nature and effects of the proposed treatment.[48] However, the last twenty-five years have seen a dramatic increase in public consciousness concerning the patient's right to be actively involved in treatment decisions. Starting with a 1957 decision,[49] courts began to combine the physician's duty to secure consent with a new affirmative duty to obtain an "informed consent," that is, to disclose information prior to obtaining consent about the proposed treatment and its effects. Under this new theory, the focus of the physician's liability began to shift from battery to negligence. Currently, in most states, failure to obtain an informed consent is a type of professional malpractice subject to the standards of negligence law.[50] The courts generally hold that the physician has a duty to disclose to the patient:

—The patient's condition or problem
—The nature and purpose of the proposed treatment
—The risks and consequences of the proposed treatment
—Any feasible alternatives to the treatment
—The patient's prognosis if the proposed treatment is not given.

While health care providers have undoubtedly become more sensitive to the need to make the patient an active participant in the medical decision-making process, physicians have sometimes tended to "cut corners" in obtaining consent to treatment in an effort to bolster the often critically ill patient's confidence, especially when the treatment is a serious intervention and retains an element of unknown risk. In addition, physicians and researchers may fail to inform their patients fully of material facts, because the providers' faith in the potential benefits of a new medical procedure subtly erodes their willingness to regard the patients as full partners in the undertaking. One commentator has noted:

> This is especially true as medical procedures become increasingly complicated and a corps of specialists, rather than a lone physician, treats a patient for a catastrophic disease. The physician, often a surgeon, who is in charge of this veritable army, undeniably has the upper hand in the doctor-patient relationship. Indeed, he may be the originator of a new technique which offers a desperate patient a "chance for a cure" which he cannot get from any other practitioner. . . . Having the patient place himself entirely within the physician's hands has been an accepted part of medical ideology, justified by the physician's concern for the patient's well-being and his alleged need for complete freedom to undertake whatever steps are believed necessary to promote it. But the risk is great, especially in experimental medicine, that the patient's abdication of his decisional authority will convert him from an end in himself to a means that can be employed along with others at the physician's command to serve the goal of the procedure, as defined by the physician and his peers.[51]

When Christiaan Barnard performed the first human heart transplant on Louis Washkansky, he considerably overstated the probability of success, leading Mr. Washkansky to believe that the procedure had an 80 percent chance of success, even though that figure applied only to the chance of living through the operation itself. Dr. Barnard's justification was:

> He had not asked for odds or any details . . . he was at the end of the line. . . . For a dying man it was not a difficult decision. . . . [I]f a lion chases you to a bank of a river filled with crocodiles, you will leap into the water convinced you have a chance to swim to the other side, but you never would accept such odds if there were no lion.[52]

This account of the first "consent" to heart transplantation dramatically illustrates the temptations and rationalizations that underlie the tendency to avoid fully informing the patient.

From a purely clinical standpoint, the physician may feel strongly that the proposed intervention is the "best decision." However, it is the patient's legal and moral right to be afforded an opportunity to make a decision based upon his or her own personal values, knowledge, and beliefs. The legal principle of informed consent is designed to prevent the physician from misrepresenting or failing to present important information. The physician is in no position to weigh all of the intensely personal factors that may be of extreme importance to the patient: will the pain be worth the procedure when the chance of survival is uncertain? Will a slower, probably more peaceful death be preferable to undergoing the trauma of major surgery and a large risk of later death by organ rejection or infection? Will financial and emotional burdens on the patient and the patient's family be justifiable in light of the risks?

Against this background, the question is what information the transplant provider should disclose to the recipient in order to obtain an informed consent. The two most critical elements of informed consent to transplantation are ensuring that the patient fully understands the material risks and possible complications associated with transplantation, and the likelihood that the transplant will succeed. Beyond current legal requirements, a truly informed consent to heart transplantation may also involve acquainting the patient with the often serious fiscal and psychological ramifications of transplantation.

The Diagnosis

The duty to obtain an informed consent from the patient includes the duty to tell the patient about his or her condition or problem. Failure to disclose the diagnosis is rarely the basis for liability, however, since diagnosis is commonly discussed in the physician-patient dialogue. In the normal situation, the patient should be informed of any significant reservations about the diagnosis. Problems in this area do not generally occur in heart transplant cases, since the diagnosis of cardiac disease occurs long before the transplant is considered, and virtually all potential recipients would be aware of their diagnosis and its accuracy.

Nature and Purpose of Treatment

The physician must explain the nature and purpose of the proposed treatment to the patient in nontechnical terms. In the case of transplantation, the explanation should include not only the nature of the transplant itself, but also of pre- and postoperative treatments, including the necessary drug regimens, physical therapy, and continued care.

While this part of the informed consent process is important to the patient's truly informed and voluntary consent, it has seldom been a topic of litigation.[53] This is probably because the patient is generally curious about the diagnosis and the provider is likely to volunteer information.[54]

Feasible Treatment Alternatives

Knowledge of the available alternatives is essential to the patient's informed consent. Several courts have held that a consent is not informed unless the health care provider discloses to the patient at least those alternatives that would be generally acknowledged within the medical community as feasible in the patient's case.[55] As discussed earlier, the physician may have a duty to inform potential transplant candidates that transplantation is a viable treatment for them. However, the physician also has a duty to inform these patients of other treatment regimens, even though there are few, if any, alternative treatments for persons with end-stage cardiac disease.

Prognosis if Proposed Treatment is not Given

The final, traditional element of informed consent is a projection of what will happen without the proposed treatment. Because physicians typically utilize this information to guide patients toward a recommended treatment, cases litigating this element are rare. A dispute involving this issue is also unlikely in transplant practice since every potential recipient should be aware that his or her prognosis for long-term survival is poor in the absence of a transplant.[56]

Material Hazards and Complications of Treatment

Most of the litigation surrounding informed consent has centered on allegations of failure to inform the patient of the material hazards and possible complications associated with treatment. The most well known discussion of this element of informed consent occurred in a landmark case, *Canterbury* v. *Spence*.[57] In *Canterbury*, a surgeon failed to tell his nineteen-year-old patient that the proposed treatment, a lumbar laminectomy, carried with it about a 1 percent risk of paralysis. The patient agreed to the operation, but later suffered paralysis. He sued, claiming in part that he would not have agreed to the operation had he known of the risk of paralysis. His physician defended the decision not to inform the patient of the risk by stating:

> I think that I would not tell patients that they might be paralyzed because of the small percentage, one percent, that exists. There would be a tremendous percentage of people that would not have surgery and would not therefore be benefited by it, the tremendous percentage that get along very well, 99 percent.[58]

The court in *Canterbury*, however, set forth the principle that important information cannot be kept from a patient solely out of the belief that a physician can best weigh the risks of treatment against its beneficial effects.[59]

Not all risks, no matter now slight or remote, need to be revealed to the patient. The doctrine of informed consent holds that only material risks need be revealed. In states that use an "average patient standard," the definition of material risk is often the one first articulated in *Canterbury:*

> A risk is ... material when a reasonable person, in what the physician knows or should know to be the patient's position, would be likely to attach significance to the risk or cluster of risks in deciding whether or not to forego the proposed therapy.[60]

The courts have not attempted to define a specific probability that triggers the disclosure requirement. Generally, the necessity of disclosure is determined by weighing both the probability that the risk will occur and its potential severity. Thus, a physician may not be required to disclose that a 5 percent to 10 percent risk of greater complications could lengthen the patient's recuperation. However, one court has held that any known risk of death, however slight, must be disclosed.[61] The standard creates uncertainty for the health care provider, since he or she must often "guess" what the average person would want to know.[62]

Because heart transplantation involves both known and unknown hazards and consequences, there are many risks to the procedure that would be considered "material." Some of the several known risks of heart transplantation that would probably be considered material are discussed below.

Graft Rejection. Successful organ transplantation is limited by immunologic rejection of the transplanted organ by the recipient.[63] Successful transplantation always involves the use of immunosuppressive drugs that chemically suppress the normal bodily defense responses against pathogenic microorganisms and foreign tissues.[64] Immunosuppressive agents can prevent or delay rejection episodes in many, but not all, individuals. The incidence of mortality in cases of rejection is quite high, and there is a greater incidence of increased side effects from augmented dosages of immunosuppressive drugs. The possibility of graft rejection and of known side effects that may result from augmented doses of immunosuppressive drugs are also risks that should be made known to the patient.

Infection. One of the effects of immunosuppressive drugs is that they handicap the transplant recipient's ability to ward off infection. Infection is, therefore, one of the most frequent and serious complications of transplantation and, as a result, is a risk that should be disclosed to the patient.[65]

The Risk of Transplant-related Cancer. Immunosuppressive agents can also cause a wide variety of malignant diseases in transplant recipients.

The reported incidence of cancer in all types of transplant patients surviving more than four years after transplant approaches 25 percent.[66] Cancer can also be transplanted from the donor to the recipient. Although many transplanted cancer cells would be rapidly destroyed if planted in a healthy individual, cancer cells implanted into an individual via allograft may thrive due to the immunosuppressed state of the recipient. Cancer transfer carries some risk of malpractice claims as well, since it may be alleged that proper precautions were not taken in examining the donor and the available medical history for signs of malignancy.[67] However, due to the short ischemic time that the donor heart remains viable, failure to ascertain the presence of cancer that is not externally apparent on the organ or apparent from the donor's treatment or available records would probably not be considered malpractice.

Miscellaneous Complications of Transplantation. In general, the recipient should be made aware of possible material risks and consequences involved with transplantation, as well as any exacerbation of the usual surgical risks of transplantation. Many other risks are involved in transplantation, and most are either caused or exacerbated by the use of immunosuppressive agents. A transplanted organ may carry undetected diseases or infections into the immunosuppressed patient.[68] Other, rarer but still serious, complications include hypersplenism[69] and excessive destruction of one or more types of blood cells in the spleen, death of bone tissue in the adult,[70] death of vascular tissue and failure to grow in children,[71] and interstitial pneumonia.[72]

Heart transplant practice and treatment regimens are advancing and will continue to evolve, and transplant specialists are continually learning more about the long- and short-term risks and complications of transplantation. One of the more difficult questions concerning what should be disclosed to the recipient is how one can explain to the patient the risks of new and evolving techniques when not all is known about new aspects of treatment and their potential side effects. The informed consent literature indicates that the transplant provider should, at a minimum, candidly relate to the potential recipient that an organ transplant involves as yet unknown or little understood risks and complications beyond those already divulged. The physician has the added duty of discovering as much as possible about new techniques and regimens that have been described in the literature.[73].

Probability of Success. Another crucial element of a fully informed consent is an accurate assessment of the likelihood that the heart transplantation will be successful, in terms of both survival and degree of rehabilitation.[74] An unresolved issue that the transplant provider must determine is which survival data are used—those of all transplant centers or those of the transplant center at which the recipient will undergo treatment.[75] Whatever data are used, the tenets of informed consent dictate that the provider not skew the odds.[76]

Nonmedical Aspects of Transplantation. Courts generally have focused on medical factors when forming the requisites of informed consent. However, transplantation and other types of catastrophic disease treatment decisions may be more profoundly affected by social and psychological factors than by strictly physiological considerations. Courts may conceivably expand the list of legally "material" items that may be disclosed to the patient to include:

1. The impact of the proposed procedure on the patient's family or job situation
2. The likely cost of the proposed treatment and any necessary drug regimens and follow-up visits
3. The necessity and cost of assuming residence close to a treatment center for an extended period of time, or
4. The probability that the procedure and follow-up treatment would be covered by the patient's insurance.[77]

There may be sound arguments for not expanding the health care provider's advisory duty to include matters that are not strictly medical. However, especially in catastrophic disease treatment, many of these nonmedical considerations are of utmost concern to the patient and any one may be the deciding factor in whether he or she accepts treatment. This is particularly true with such procedures as organ transplantation, because a successful outcome cannot be assured and the potential risks are high. Courts may feel that it is the provider's duty to disclose, or at least disclaim consideration of, the social and economic effects of treatment and nontreatment of which the provider is aware.

The Requirement of Materiality and Proximate Cause

In cases asserting a lack of informed consent, liability exists upon proof that a duty was breached, and that the breach caused injury to the patient. When the breach of duty lies in not disclosing, or in misrepresenting, pertinent information to a patient, there is no liability unless the patient, had the information in question been disclosed, would have chosen a different course and would thereby have avoided the injury. This causal "link" between nondisclosure or misrepresentation and the resulting damage or injury is what is meant by the term "causation" or "proximate" cause. Providing this element can be a substantial obstacle in many types of cases. One writer has noted:

> The patient's ability to convince a court of the existence of proximate cause turns on several factors. Key among these are the severity of the patient's condition, which bears on how likely it is that the patient, as a reasonable person, would have challenged the physician's judgment, and the availability of treatment alternatives. Generally speaking, a patient who had no sensible choice but to accept the proposed treatment will not be able to prove causation.[78]

For virtually all transplant candidates, the alternative to transplantation is acceptance of palliative care and of death within a short period. In order to prevail in a case alleging lack of informed consent to transplantation, the patient (or next of kin) must show that, had all material information been disclosed, a reasonable person would have chosen palliative care over heart transplantation. Courts and juries may be unwilling to say that the reasonable patient, under any circumstances, would choose death over life after a transplant, however short and painful that life may turn out to be.[79] However, in the current era, when "death with dignity" has become an increasingly acceptable alternative, successful suits are not totally unrealistic. For instance, where the patient was not informed of the possibility of serious posttransplant malignancy, a court or jury may be willing to find that a reasonable person would choose death from end-stage cardiac disease over a prolonged, cancer-related death complicated by other transplantation effects.

In addition, if courts become more sensitive to the nonmedical implications of transplantation, they may also be willing to consider nonmedical harms as well. For example, a jury may accept the notion that a patient might not have accepted the financial and emotional hardships of transplantation had he or she been fully aware that in his or her particular case, the probability of prolonged, healthy survival was only 40 percent.

While the potential for civil liability is small, the legal (and, most would maintain, ethical) duty to disclose remains unchanged. Moreover, as Katz and Capron note, informed consent to catastrophic disease therapy serves many purposes beyond protecting the provider from liability. Its purposes include:

1. Promoting individual autonomy
2. Protecting the patient-subject's status as a human being
3. Avoiding fraud or duress
4. Encouraging self-scrutiny by the physician-investigator
5. Encouraging rational decision making
6. Involving the public.[80]

Despite the low probability of civil liability, these other values and purposes suggest that obtaining informed consent from heart transplant recipients must be emphasized.[81], [82]

NOTES

1. In 1980, 36 heart transplants, 15 liver transplants, and 4,697 kidney transplants were performed in the United States. In 1983, 172 heart transplants, 164 liver transplants, and 6,112 kidney transplants were performed. Evans, *The Need for and Cost of Liver Transplantation in the U.S., Update No. 38*, NATIONAL KIDNEY DIALYSIS AND KIDNEY TRANSPLANT STUDY (Battelle Human Affairs Research Centers, Seattle, Wash.) (1984); R. W. EVANS, *et al.*, THE NATIONAL HEART TRANSPLANTATION STUDY: FINAL REPORT (Battelle Human Affairs Research Centers, Seattle, Wash.) (1984); END-STAGE RENAL DISEASE PROGRAM HIGHLIGHTS, 1983 (Health Care Financing Administration, Baltimore, Md.) (1984).

2. *See, e.g.,* Strunk v. Strunk, 445 S.W.2d 145, 146 (Ky. 1969) (mentally incompetent adult allowed by court order to donate a kidney to his brother due in part to strong relationship between brothers and perceived harm to incompetent individual if brother died); Little v. Little, 576 S.W.2d 493, 499–500 (Tex. Civ. Ct. App. 1979) (authorizing removal of kidney from fourteen year old with Down syndrome for transplantation into brother); *Cf.* Lausier v. Pescinski, 226 N.W.2d 180, 183 (Wisc. 1975) (no kidney removal allowed from mentally incompetent adult where he would gain no benefit from donation). *In re* children without mental disability, *see, e.g.,* Hart v. Brown, 289 A2d 386 (Conn. 1972) (kidney donation allowed). *See generally,* annot., *Transplantation: Power of Parent, Guardian, or Committee to Consent to Surgical Invasion of Ward's Person for the Benefit of Another,* 35 A.L.R. 3d 692.

3. Sirianni v. Anna, 285 N.Y.S.2d 709, 712 (N.Y. Sup. Ct. 1967), Moore v. Shah, 458 N.Y.S.2d 33, 34 (N.Y. App. Div. 1982) (both courts refused to apply the tort theory of "a wrong to the victim is a wrong to the rescuer," because of the voluntary nature of the organ donations).

4. At common law, a number of actions could be maintained for taking flesh from a deceased person. A cause of action could be based on allegations such as "mayhem," "mutilation of a corpse," or "unauthorized autopsy." 25A C.J.S. Dead Bodies §80(3).

5. However, the Act does not limit liability for treatment of the live transplant recipient. Williams v. Hofman, 223 N.W.2d 844, 847 (Wisc. 1974).

6. *See* Rose, *Medicolegal Problems Associated with Organ and Tissue Transplantations,* in LEGAL MEDICINE 1982 (C. Wecht, ed.) (W. B. Saunders Co., Philadelphia, Pa.) (1982); Jeddeloh, Chatterjee, *Legal Problems in Organ Donation,* SURGICAL CLINICS OF NORTH AMERICA 58(2):245, 248 (April 1978).

7. *Williams, supra* note 5, at 845.

8. *See, e.g.,* Raab v. Casper, 124 Cal. Rptr. 590 (1975) (case dealing with good faith improvement of land). Bad faith, by contrast, is evidenced by actual

or constructive fraud, intent to mislead or deceive another, or a neglect or refusal to fulfill some duty or contractual obligation not prompted by an honest mistake as to one's rights or duties, but instead prompted by some interest or similar motive. *See also, Williams, supra* note 5, at 847.

9. The UAGA provides that a number of persons can be specified as the donee of the organ, including the intended recipient. *See* §3. If no donor is specified, the gift may be accepted by the deceased person's attending physician. However, the physician who becomes a donee in this manner cannot participate in the procedures for removing and transplanting an organ. *See* §4(c).

10. UAGA §2(c).

11. UAGA §6 outlines the means by which an anatomical gift may be revoked.

12. Such a suit would probably be grounded on a charge of interference with a corpse and would likely involve a substantial claim for damages for emotional distress. *See, e.g.,* W. PROSSER, W. KEETON, THE LAW OF TORTS (West Publishing Co., St. Paul, Minn.) (5th ed. 1984) at 63; 4 RESTATEMENT OF TORTS, 868. *See also,* Koerber v. Patek, 102 N.W. 40 (1905) (plaintiff entitled to recover where defendant was given permission to examine the decedent mother's stomach but instead removed it).

13. UAGA §7(b). The comments to §7(b) adopt the view that no clear-cut definition of death can be formulated and that "no reasonable statutory definition is possible. The answer depends upon many variables, differing from case to case. Reliance must be placed upon the judgment of the physician in attendance."

14. Stason, *The Uniform Anatomical Gift Act,* BUSINESS LAWYER 23(9):919, 928 (July 1968).

15. Tucker v. Lower, No. 231 (Richmond, Va. L. & Equity Ct., May 23, 1972).

16. *Id.*

17. *See* Va. Code §54-325.7 (Cum. Supp. 1981).

18. *See Dispute over "Death" Stirs Medical Debate,* American Medical News (October 3, 1980).

19. New York City Health and Hospital Corp. v. Sulsona, 367 N.Y.S.2d (Sup. Ct. 1975) at 691.

20. N.Y. Pub. Health Law Article 43 §§4301 *et seq.* (1977).

21. *Sulsona, supra* note 19, at 691.

22. Ala. Code 2-31-1 *et seq.* (1979); Alaska Stat. §09.65.120 (1980); Ark. Stat. Ann. §82-537-538 (1981); Cal. Health and Safety Code §§7180–7182 (1980); Colo. Rev. Stat. §12-36-136 (1981); Fla. Stat. §382.085 (1980); Ga. Code Ann. §88-1715.1 (1980); Hawaii Rev. Stat. §37C-1 (1980); Kan. Stat. Ann. §77-205 (1979); La. Rev. Stat. Ann. §9.111 (1981); Md. Ann. Code HG 5-203 (1982); Mich. Stat. Ann. §14.15 (1021–24) (1978); Mont. Code Ann. §451.007 (1979); N.M. Stat. Ann. §12-2-4 (1978); N.C. Gen. Stat. §90-323 (1979); Oka. Stat. Ann. tit. 63, §1-301(g) (1981); Or. Rev. Stat. §146.001 (1977); Tenn. Code Ann. §63-501 (1980); Tex. Rev. Civ. Stat. Ann. Art. 4447t (1980); Va. Code §54-325.7 (1981); W. Va. Code §16-19-1(c) (1980); Wyo. Stat. §35-19-101 (1979).

23. Several courts have recognized brain death standards in criminal homicide cases. *See, e.g.*, State v. Fierro, 603 P.2d 74, 77 (1979) (removal of respiratory life support system was not the proximate cause of gunshot victim's death); Commonwealth v. Golston, 366 N.E.2d 744, 749 (1977) *cert. denied*, 434 U.S. 1039 (1978) (adopting a brain death standard in criminal cases). Brain death standards have also been judicially adopted in several civil cases. *See, e.g.*, *Tucker, supra* note 15 (wrongful death action involving claim of premature declaration of death of organ donor); *Sulsona, supra* note 19, at 686 (Sup. Ct. 1975) (declaratory judgment on brain death standard under New York's Anatomical Gift Act; *In re Bowman*, 617 P.2d 731 (Wash. Sup. Ct. 1980) (judicial adoption of the Uniform Determination of Death Act).

24. *See* PRESIDENT'S COMMISSION FOR THE STUDY OF ETHICAL PROBLEMS IN MEDICINE AND BIOMEDICAL AND BEHAVIORAL RESEARCH, DEFINING DEATH (U.S. Government Printing Office, Washington, D.C.) (1981) at 62–67.

25. *See, e.g.*, Kusanovich, *Medical Malpractice Liability and the Organ Transplant*, UNIVERSITY OF SOUTH FLORIDA LAW REVIEW 5:223, 250–53 (1971).

26. *See, e.g.*, Jeddeloh, Chatterjee, *supra* note 6, at 248.

27. *Id.*

28. *Williams, supra* note 5, at 846 (good faith exemption applies to (a) the mechanics of giving and receiving anatomical gifts, (b) the determination of time of death, and (c) procedures following death).

29. In the National Heart Transplantation Study, a review of the records of 1,955 organ donors in the United States over an eight-month period revealed that among 1,291 potential heart donors, permission of the coroner was obtained for the removal of organs in 60.2 percent of the cases. Permission of the next of kin was obtained in 95.7 percent of the cases. R. W. EVANS, *et al.*, THE NATIONAL HEART TRANSPLANTATION STUDY: FINAL REPORT (Battelle Human Affairs Research Centers, Seattle, Wash.) (1984).

30. An early attempt to suggest guidelines for cooperation was made by the Committee on Forensic Pathology of the College of American Pathologists in 1969. The Committee suggested that organ retrieval not be permitted prior to autopsy in cases of:

(1) Known or suspected homicide
(2) Body trunk injuries when major organs are desired
(3) Industrial accident
(4) Suspected poisoning
(5) Possible medical malpractice cases
(6) Two or more party vehicle accidents in which there are serious questions of liability
(7) Apparent suicide in which there is serious suspicion of possible accident or involvement of another person.

Committee on Forensic Pathology of the American College of Pathologists, *Coroners Cases as Transplant Donors*, PATHOLOGIST 23(1):45–47 (1969).

31. *See* Davis, Wright, *Influence of the Medical Examiner on Cadaver Organ Procurement*, JOURNAL OF FORENSIC SCIENCES 22(4):824 (October 1977).

32. The medical examiner is generally present at the time the organs are removed. If the medical examiner is not present, then the removing surgeon must detail in writing the surgical procedures used and the absence of injury to the affected area of the body. In order to show that the declaration of death and subsequent organ removal were not independent, intervening causes of death, the following facts are documented in writing:

> (1) The circumstances surrounding the injury
> (2) The status of the victim when first viewed at the scene or examined at the hospital
> (3) The status of the victim at the hospital
> (4) Documentation of the evidence leading to the declaration of death
> (5) Documentation of absence of injury or other potential causes of death related to the donated organs
> (6) Documentation of the medical examiner's or coroner's autopsy findings.

33. Texas Code Art. 49.25(6) (1977).
34. Health Law Center, *Dying, Death, and Dead Bodies,* in HOSPITAL LAW MANUAL II (Aspen Systems Corp., Rockville, Md.) (1983) at §6–7.
35. A. R. HOLDER, MEDICAL MALPRACTICE LAW (John Wiley & Sons, New York, N.Y.) (1975).
36. *See, e.g.,* Dunham v. Wright, 4233 F.2d 940, 944 (1970); Young v. Group Health Cooperative, 534 P.2d 1349, 1352 (1975).
37. Bang v. Charles T. Miller Hospital, 88 N.W.2d 186, 190 (1958).
38. *See* Campbell v. Olivia, 424 F.2d 1244, 1251 (1970). *See generally, Failure to Keep Up as Negligence,* JOURNAL OF THE AMERICAN MEDICAL ASSOCIATION 224(10):1461–62 (June 4, 1973).
39. At the present time, approximately 80 percent of all heart transplant recipients will survive one year, and 50 percent will survive for five years. It is now projected that nearly 25 percent will survive ten years. These survival figures compare well with those for kidney transplant graft survival. See Evans, *Heart Transplants and Priorities,* LANCET 8381(1):852 (April 14, 1984).
40. Moreover, the physician may be reluctant to refer a patient to a distant center. Cardiac transplant centers tend to be clustered in metropolitan areas on the two coasts. As a result, residents of large geographical areas currently do not have ready access to a transplant center. However, the large centers typically draw patients from all over the country (and the world). If the physician reasonably should know of the possibility of recommending the patient to a transplant center, then presumably lack of proximity to such a center should not be a decisive factor in determining whether the duty to inform exists. Whether the patient chooses to travel in order to seek treatment would likely be assessed as a personal issue that falls within the patient's sphere of decision making.
41. If the physician has a reasonable belief, indicated by the appropriate medical standard of practice, that an existing treatment would not work in a particular patient's case, the physician need not suggest it. *E.g.,* Harrigan v.

United States, 408 F. Supp. 177, 189 (1976); Downer v. Vielleux, 332 A.2d 82, 92 (Me. 1974). Therefore, whether or not the physician's duty to inform is excused depends upon the reasonableness of the assessment that treatment is not feasible in light of the legally accepted level of medical practice. It is likely that the level of sophistication required in making this determination will increase as transplantation becomes more widely acknowledged as a viable treatment alternative.

42. Holder, *Physician's Failure to Obtain Informed Consent to Innovative Practice of Medical Research,* 15 P.O.F.2d 711, 725.

43. *Id.*

44. Morrison v. McKillop, 563, P.2d 220, 223 (Wash. App. 1977).

45. The shortage of donor organs has led to a situation in which demand for the procedure outstrips the supply of transplantable organs. Waiting lists for many transplant programs have developed and may continue to grow as transplantation becomes more accepted within the medical community. A physician would undoubtedly argue either that no duty existed because there was no reasonable chance of acceptance into a transplant program or that there is no causal relationship between the failure to refer and the harm to the patient, since there is no proof that the patient would have been accepted and would have survived surgery.

46. Schloendorff v. Society of New York Hospital, 105 N.E. 92 (1914).

47. *Id.* at 93.

48. *See Note: Evolution of the Doctrine of Informed Consent,* Georgia Law Review 12(3):581, 582 (Spring 1978).

49. Salgo v. Leland Stanford, Jr. University Board of Trustees, 317 P.2d 170, 181 (Cal. App. 1957).

50. Some jurisdictions, however, still treat the cases as arising out of the law of assault and battery. There are two basic standards for determining a breach of duty in informed consent cases. The first standard is commonly known as the "professional standard." It is based on the notion that the duty of a physician is limited to those disclosures that a reasonable medical practitioner would make under the same or similar circumstances. *See, e.g.,* Natanson v. Kline, 350 P.2d 1093, 1106 (Kan. 1960), *reh'g denied,* 354 P.2d 670 (Kan. 1960). The second standard, the "reasonable patient standard," bases the standard for disclosure on what the average, reasonable patient would want to know, rather than on what the average physician would disclose. *See* Canterbury v. Spence, 464 F.2d 772, 780–83 (D.C. Cir. 1972). For a discussion of the two standards, see T. Rosoff, Informed Consent: A Guide for Health Care Providers (Aspen Systems Corporation, Rockville, Md.) (1981), 34–41.

51. Capron, *Informed Consent in Catastrophic Disease Research and Treatment,* University of Pennsylvania Law Review 123(2):340, 367–68 (December 1974).

52. Annas, *Consent to the Artificial Heart: The Lion and the Crocodiles,* Hastings Center Report 12(2):20 (1983).

53. Gates v. Jensen, 595 P.2d 919, 922–23 (Wash. 1979).

54. Rosoff, *supra* note 50, at 43.

55. *See, e.g.,* Holt v. Nelson, 523 P.2d 211, 215 (Wash. Ct. App. 1974).
56. In general, persons selected as candidates for heart transplantation have a prognosis of survival that is less than six months. At Stanford University, the average duration of survival of patients selected for heart transplantation who fail to receive one due to the unavailability of a donor is forty-five days. *See* Baumgartner *et al., Infra.* A similar figure is reported in the National Heart Transplantation Study, based on data derived from six heart transplant programs. *See* J. W. Evans, *et al.,* The National Heart Transplant Study: Final Report (Battelle Human Affairs Research Centers, Seattle, Wash.) (1984).
57. *Canterbury, supra* note 50, at 783–84.
58. *Id.* at 794.
59. *Id.* at 787.
60. *Id.*
61. Cobbs v. Grant, 502 P.2d 1, 11 (Cal. 1972).
62. However, if a particular patient is proved to have been aware of certain risks, they cannot form the basis of a claim of nondisclosure.
63. Transplant recipients may experience several varieties of rejection. These are generally discribed at (1) hyperacute, (2) acute, and (3) chronic. *See* Wood, Renal Transplantation: A Clinical Handbook (1983); Kidney Transplantation: Principles and Practice (P. J. Morris, ed.) (1979). Ignoring these distinctions, it was determined in the National Heart Transplantation Study that the majority of patients experience an average of 2.46 episodes prior to their deaths. Evans, *supra* note 56.
64. Immunosuppression is accomplished by infusing the donor's tissue with concurrent or properly timed immunosuppressive drugs. There are three general groups of immunosuppressive drug regimens:

    (1)   Antiproliferative, antimetabolic, and antimotic agents that act on cells in their reproductive cycle; examples include methotrexate, cyclophosphamide, and vincristine
    (2)   Agents that affect lymphoid tissues: cyclosporin A is the most promising agent recently introduced
    (3)   Agents with specific immunosuppressive properties.

    See Floersheim, *Pharmacologic Immunosuppressive Agents,* Transplantation Proceedings 12(2):315, 316–19 (June 1980); Penn, *Lymphomas Complicating Organ Transplantation,* Transplantation Proceedings 15(4, Supp. 1):2790, 2791 (December 1983); Penn, *Problems of Cancer in Organ Transplantation,* Heart Transplantation 2(1):71 (November 1982).
65. In the National Heart Transplantation Study, it was determined that overall, living heart transplant recipients ($N = 150$) experienced an average of 2.03 infectious episodes, deceased patients ($N = 256$) experienced 2.81 episodes prior to their death, and all patients combined ($N = 406$) experienced 2.50 episodes.
66. Sheil, *Transplantation and Cancer,* in Kidney Transplant (P. J. Morris, ed.) (Grune & Stratten, New York, N.Y.) (1979). The mechanisms leading to

cancer in the recipient include altered immune surveillance and immunoregulation of oncogenic virus, genetic factors, chronic antigenic stimulation, and the neoplastic actions of immunosuppressive drugs. Rose, *supra* note 6, at 97.

67. However, there is no obligation to inform the patient of risks that flow from an improperly executed medical procedure, and simply informing the patient that negligent acts may occur would not excuse the negligence. *See, e.g.,* McPhee v. Bay City Samaritan Hospital, 159 N.W.2d 880, 882 (Mich. App. 1968) (when the result is unexpected and caused by alleged malpractice, the lack of informed consent cannot be proximately related to the plaintiff's injuries).

68. Peters, *et al., Transmission of Tuberculosis by Kidney Transplantation,* TRANSPLANTATION 38(5):514, 515–16 (November 1984).

69. Kaufman, *et al., Post-transplant Hypersplenism,* TRANSPLANTATION PROCEEDINGS 11(1):96, 96–99 (March 1979).

70. Bush, *et al., Variant Forms of Arthritis in Human Allografts,* TRANSPLANTATION PROCEEDINGS 11(1):100, 100–103 (March 1979).

71. Ruderman, *et al., Orthotropic Complications of Renal Transplant in Children,* TRANSPLANTATION PROCEEDINGS 11(1):104, 104–106 (March 1979).

72. Pricontt, *et al., A Virological Study of Interstitial Pneumonia in Patients with Acute Lymphoid Leukemia Treated with a Combination of Methotrexate and 6-Mercaptopurine,* EUROPEAN JOURNAL OF CANCER 13:479, 479–82 (March 1977).

73. Capron, *supra* note 51, at 371–72. Use of new drug regimens will also involve FDA approval and Institutional Review Board procedures.

74. Of the patients who participated in the National Heart Transplantation Study, 79.5 percent were described as being employed prior to their transplants. Following transplant, 31.6 percent of the living patients were employed, and 66.3 percent were described as "normal; no complaints; no evidence of disease" by transplant center staff. EVANS, *supra* note 56.

75. Obviously, newer programs will have to rely upon information gleaned from other centers. However, it may be more accurate, if enough data have been generated, to use the transplant center–specific information, since centers may vary considerably in their success rates. A problem with this approach, however, is that the figures may not reflect information about the center's "real" rate of success, because there are no controls for the sickness of the patients when they receive the transplants.

76. Legal liability for overstating the odds of successful results could be argued on the basis of breach of contract as well as on the basis of informed consent. A physician who "guarantees" results can be sued for breach of contract for failure to produce what was promised. Damages in such cases are not based upon the pain the patient suffers, but instead are based upon the difference in value between the result promised and that actually delivered.

The breach of contract theory is best illustrated by the classic case of Hawkins v. McGee, 146 A. 641 (N.H. 1929). In *Hawkins,* a surgeon promised that he could perform a skin graft to replace scar tissue in a boy's palm that would leave the boy with a "100 percent good hand." The surgeon took the graft tissue from the boy's chest. A short time later, of course, the palm began to grow dense, matted hair. The trial court denied any recovery, since the boy had not shown that the surgeon had been negligent or that having hair on one's palm was any worse than having scar tissue. The appeals court reversed and explained that the proper question was whether the physician had made good on his promise. The measure of damages, the court announced, was the difference in values between the promised "perfect" hand and the hairy one delivered.

The key to *Hawkins* was the unconditional nature of the promise of good results. In general, however, courts are reluctant to use contract theory in medical treatment cases.

77. *See, e.g.,* ROSOFF, *supra* note 50, at 51. In the National Heart Transplantation Study, 66.4 percent of the patients indicated that they received assistance from private insurance in paying for their heart transplant operation. Despite this, however, 40.8 percent of the patients indicated that they had out-of-pocket expenses. J. W. EVANS, *et al.,* THE NATIONAL HEART TRANSPLANTATION STUDY: FINAL REPORT (Battelle Human Affairs Research Centers, Seattle, Wash.) (1984).

78. *Id.* at 53.

79. *See, e.g.,* Karp v. Cooley, 493 F.2d 408, 422 (1974) (no proof that heart transplantation and mechanical heart recipient would not have consented had certain materials been disclosed).

80. J. KATZ, A. CAPRON, CATASTROPHIC DISEASES: WHO DECIDES WHAT? (Russell Sage Foundation, New York, N.Y.) (1975), 82–90.

81. For a general discussion of the issue of informed consent, *see* PRESIDENT'S COMMISSION FOR THE STUDY OF ETHICAL PROBLEMS IN MEDICINE AND BEHAVIORAL RESEARCH, MAKING HEALTH CARE DECISIONS, VOL. 1 (U.S. Government Printing Office, Washington, D.C.) (1982) at ch. 1.

82. This article was previously published in the AMERICAN JOURNAL OF LAW AND MEDICINE 10:363–95 (1985).

6

Practitioner and Hospital Liability in Organ Transplantation

Nathan Hershey

This chapter is limited to a discussion of the liability of practitioners and institutions in suits brought by or on behalf of a donee, a donor, or a family member on the negligence or malpractice theory. Thus, this chapter does not discuss informed consent theory (except possibly in a peripheral sense), determination of death for transplant purposes, or processes for selecting donees involving such nonmedical factors as individual or personal merit, social considerations, or effects on other family members.

To begin, it is useful to define the term "organ." A standard medical reference work defines an organ as "a somewhat independent part of the body that performs a special function or functions."[1] This distinguishes organs from various types of manufactured devices placed in patients for therapeutic purposes. Since very few court decisions have dealt directly with liability for negligence or malpractice in the context of organ transplantation, some of the court decisions used to develop the issues discussed herein will not be limited solely to organ transplantation.

NEGLIGENCE THEORY AND ORGAN TRANSPLANTATION

To impose liability for negligence or malpractice, four elements of a tort cause of action must be established: (1) the existence of a duty to the person claiming injury, (2) a breach of that duty, (3) harm or injury, and (4) a causal relationship between the breach of duty and the harm.[2] Various tests are used by courts to establish those persons to whom a duty is owed. Crucial to duty determinations are considerations of public policy and applications of the concept of foreseeability.

Two cases have explored duty in the context of organ transplantation. The first, *Sirianni* v. *Anna*,[3] involved a suit brought by a donor—a woman who had donated one of her kidneys to her son. Previously, surgeons had operated on the young man and, it was alleged, had negligently removed all of his kidney tissue; the patient was then kept alive by a mechanical device substituting for the missing natural kidneys. As death became imminent, the only way to preserve the young man's life was to perform a kidney transplant. The mother possessed healthy, compatible kidneys, and a transplant of one kidney from the mother to the son was performed. At the time of the litigation, the son had survived four years with the donated kidney.

The mother's suit was against the surgeons who had committed the earlier alleged malpractice. The theory of the suit was that their malpractice—removing both kidneys from her son—necessitated that she agree to donate one of her two kidneys. As the result of giving up the kidney, she was now subject to a life-long threat that would not have existed had there not been malpractice in her son's original treatment.[4]

The New York appellate court was faced with the problem of determining whether the malpractice in performing the original procedure on the son constituted a wrong to the mother. The court found that the surgeons performing the procedure on the son owed no duty to the mother, and that the mother's donation of the kidney to preserve the life of her son constituted an independent act by her, done by her with full knowledge of the consequences.[5] The court said that she was well aware of the risks of living with only one kidney, and that she had accepted those risks.[6] The court specifically rejected the rescue doctrine, holding that the doctrine was limited to circumstances where an emergency brings the rescuer into action unmindful and unaware of the risks present.[7]

In 1982, another New York appellate court dealt with a similar set of facts involving a son who had agreed to a kidney transplant to save his father's life. In *Moore* v. *Shah*,[8] the court reached the same conclusion as did the *Sirianni* court. The *Moore* court rejected the notion that a physician has the responsibility to foresee each and every person related to the patient as one who might conceivably be affected by that physician's malpractice.[9] The plaintiff-son had asserted that negligence in the treatment of the father had created the situation requiring the kidney transplant. The court said: "There are serious policy considerations which militate against the recovery sought here."[10] Thus, it appears that a donor has no cause of action against the physician whose malpractice in previously caring for the donee creates the need for the transplant, even when the donor is a close relative of the donee. Of course, a duty is owed to the donor by those who evaluate and perform procedures upon the person of the donor.

The second element of liability for negligence is the breach of a duty, and, in the performance of an organ transplant, depending on the circumstances, the duty may be owed to either the donor or the donee. Simply stated, a breach of duty is a departure from the accepted standard of care. Ordinarily, in medical malpractice litigation, the standard of care requires the exercise of that degree of skill, judgment, and care exercised by competent physicians in carrying out the professional services.[11]

In *Ravenis* v. *Detroit General Hospital*,[12] the Michigan Court of Appeals was faced with a situation involving two corneal transplants that had been performed on patients who later developed ophthalmitis, resulting in total loss of vision in the eyes that had received the corneas. The plaintiffs claimed that the two corneas had been removed from a cadaver by a resident in ophthalmology at the hospital, and that the hospital had failed to establish adequate procedures to determine the suitability of a prospective donor.[13] Complicating the situation was the fact that the deceased patient's file was incomplete. While there was nothing in the deceased patient's chart that contraindicated removing the corneas for transplantation, various test results and charts covering previous admissions of the donor were missing from the hospital files when the resident reviewed the chart before removing the corneas.[14]

At the trial, the resident testified that it was not clear that anyone had specific responsibility for determining whether corneas removed from deceased patients were suitable for transplantation, and that no written guideline was available to assist in making such determinations. Testimony from the physician who had placed the corneas in the eyes of the two patients who suffered the loss of vision indicated that the operations were performed in an aseptic condition, thus leaving the donated corneas as the apparent source of the infections. The jury also heard expert testimony that cadavers with certain illnesses were generally not good choices for cornea donation.

The appellate court, in affirming the judgment of the trial court after the jury verdict in favor of the plaintiffs, stated that there was adequate evidence to support a finding of negligence on the part of the hospital because it lacked procedures that would minimize risks to corneal transplant recipients.[15]

While corneal transplants technically do not involve an organ, the principles of this case seem particularly applicable. The need to determine the suitability of a donor is made abundantly clear in the court's opinion, and it is certain that there are standards that can be employed to determine not only the basic suitability of donors, but also the relative suitability when more than one potential donor is available.

The third element necessary for imposing liability is harm. In the *Ravenis* case, the harm suffered was of a physicial nature—the patients lost total sight in the eyes which received the corneal transplants. With regard to this element, the *Ravenis* plaintiffs were probably in a situation different than that faced by most transplant recipients. In many instances, the prognosis for a transplant recipient is very poor, and it would be difficult to prove that the injured plaintiff was worse off than he or she would have been without the transplant. In the corneal transplant case, however, the donees were not in a life-threatening situation, and the hospital could have resolved doubts about the source of the corneas without further endangering the patients.

The final element necessary for imposing liability is a link between the breach of duty—the departure from the standard of care—and the harm suffered. Ordinarily, in a malpractice case, medical testimony is needed to establish this link. Courts differ about the test employed and the nature of the evidence necessary to establish causation. In some jurisdictions, the test is essentially whether it was more probable than not that the harm suffered was a result of the malpractice.[16] In others, the test is less strict; it only requires that a preponderance of the evidence support a finding that the malpractice was a substantial factor in bringing about the harm.[17] An increasing number of states are recognizing this less strict test.

Potential liability exists for both the practitioner (or practitioners) and the institution in which services connected with organ transplantation take place. The extent of institutional liability for the substandard performance of those individuals involved with transplant procedures is an important consideration. If the personnel are viewed as employees or servants of the institution, then the doctrine of *respondeat superior* will apply, and the institution as well as the individuals may be subject to liability.[18] The nature of a transplant team may complicate the determination of the status of the personnel. Even if some physician team members are independent contractors and not employees of the institution, the courts may allow the introduction of evidence indicating that the recipient of the transplant could have reasonably assumed that the physicians are the agents or servants of the institution (because of the circumstances of the transplant procedure—that is, the manner in which it is organized and conducted within the institution). Thus, some courts may be inclined to find the hospital liable under an apparent or ostensible agent theory.

Hospital liability may also exist on a corporate or institutional liability theory, as was the situation in the *Ravenis* case discussed earlier.[19] Hospitals are expected to have procedures that minimize the possible risks involved in the performance of various tasks and functions preliminary to, during, and subsequent to the transplant procedure. Even if established procedures are adequate and are found by experts to be consistent with generally accepted standards in the field, a basis for liability may exist. For example, the hospital may not have adhered to one or more of the specific steps in the procedures, and evidence may indicate that the failure to do so had a causal relationship to the harm suffered by the donee, or perhaps even the donor.

SPECIAL PROBLEM AREAS OF ORGAN TRANSPLANTS

In observing organ transplant procedures generally, one may anticipate problems in several areas that can result in liability for the individual practitioners, the institutions in which the procedures are performed, or both.

The first consideration in this connection is the need for or appropriateness of the transplant versus other procedures. Some of the questions raised with regard to the transplant of the baboon's heart in Baby Fae concerned whether such a transplant was in the best interest of the infant, since certain cardiac procedures available elsewhere in the country might have been at least as promising, if not more so, than the transplant.[20] A variation of this issue was raised with regard to the temporary use of a mechanical heart substitute by Dr. Denton Cooley. In a suit brought by the wife of a heart transplant patient, it was intimated that decisions in the patient's case were influenced by a desire for human experimentation, since all previous testing had involved animals.[21]

The second area concerns the selection of the donor and, in particular, the suitability of the donor's organ. The potential for liability in this context has characteristics similar to those in laboratory work—for example, studies to provide data for genetic counseling.[22] If a laboratory test is negligently performed or its results are erroneously reported, a potential for liability is present. Suppose, for example, that a laboratory error resulted in the use of an organ from an inappropriately matched donor, causing rejection and death; since harm resulted from the original negligence, there would appear to be a basis for a successful suit.

The third area concerns actual transplant procedure. The potential for liability at this stage appears small, unless some glaring error occurs. The potential liability would appear to be greatest for those procedures that have already been performed relatively frequently, and least for those performed only a very few times. The more common a procedure, the more likely a more patterned or structured standard for its performance has developed. This standard can be employed in court to measure the adequacy of a specific procedure performed on a particular patient.

The fourth problem area relates to the monitoring of the donee, that is, the continuation of care once the transplant procedure has been completed. As they are in an extremely debilitated condition for a lengthy period after the transplant procedure, many donees require extensive medical care.

A number of techniques are utilized to minimize risks of infection and other problems that are more likely to cause serious harm or even death to an organ recipient than to a more typical surgery patient. Since heavy reliance on equipment to sustain the patient during convalescence is required, the possibility of machine miscalibration or failure cannot be ignored. Regular performance tests must be conducted to minimize problems that can be caused by equipment malfunction.

The fifth area concerns the monitoring of a live donor; that individual also requires continuing care. This concern exists for some kidney donors, and for other procedures, such as the transfer of bone marrow from a sibling or other close relative to a recipient patient.

Another source of uncertainty is the immunity provision contained in the Uniform Anatomical Gift Act,[23] which exists in every state. The question raised in *Williams* v. *Hofman*,[24] a Wisconsin case, concerned the scope of the immunity provision. The suit was brought by the husband of the deceased patient, suing on his own behalf and on behalf of his wife's estate, based on allegedly wrongful conduct in the removal of his deceased wife's kidneys for transplantation. The complaint alleged that the wife was placed on a respirator after she suffered respiratory arrest, and that subsequently the husband was informed that the wife was dead. The husband signed a form consenting to the removal of the wife's kidneys. The complaint also stated that the wife was then kept alive by a variety of life-support techniques and devices for two days before she was pronounced dead.[25]

The court decision does not deal primarily with the facts as such, but with the scope of the immunity provision in the statute. The provision states: "A person who acts in good faith in accord with the terms of this section or with anatomical gift laws of another state (or foreign country) is not liable for damages in any civil action or subject to prosecution in any criminal proceeding for his act."[26] The court reviewed this provision in light of the other sections of the statute and concluded that the limitation on liability did not extend to treatment of the donor prior to death nor to treatment of a live transplant donee.[27] Therefore, the court rejected the claim that the defendants could rely on the Act's liability limitation provision. However, the court ruled that the part of the suit brought against the defendants alleging mutilation of the corpse was covered by the provision limiting liability.[28] The section containing this provision concerns the mechanics of giving and receiving anatomical gifts, determination of the time of death, and procedures following death.[29] The court not only found that this provision applied to the plaintiff's claim of mutilation but, further, sustained it in the face of constitutional challenges on due process and equal protection grounds put forward by the husband of the deceased.[30]

CONCLUSION

Several points should be remembered. Only a small amount of litigation has occurred concerning transplantation and malpractice or negligence theories. Most likely, the reason is the relatively small number of organ transplants performed. As the volume of such procedures increases, the ratio of good outcomes to poor ones will improve. This, in turn, will raise expectations of success. When anticipation of a good outcome is higher, dissatisfaction with poor results is likely to stimulate litigation, because disappointed patients or relatives will attribute some poor outcomes to malpractice rather than to the inherent difficulty of the procedure.

Given that the prognoses for most transplant patients are relatively poor compared to the prognoses for patients receiving more routine and less invasive surgery, one needs to consider the extent of damages that can be recovered. Even when the transplant procedure is successful, there may not be a great potential for resumption of regular work and other activities generally consistent with ordinary living; thus, recoverable damages in a malpractice action by or on behalf of a transplant recipient may be relatively small. Of course, each recipient would be evaluated in terms of his or her individual prospects, and these would differ substantially, based on the procedure itself and the conditions of the recipient's other bodily systems.

A greater concern may be consent-related issues. As organ transplantation becomes a more efficacious option, and as the number of practitioners and institutions involved in transplantation increases, one may anticipate that more issues will arise regarding the adequacy of the information provided to patients who have some degree of realistic choice between organ transplantation and other procedures. For example, some patients are faced with the choice between continuing renal dialysis and receiving a kidney transplant. It would appear that many elements in the explanation of an organ transplant and the risks associated with it could be somewhat standardized. Other aspects, however, such as the relative risk for the particular patient of not having the procedure at a particular time and the relative risk of organ transplant versus other procedures currently available, must be keyed to each individual patient's situation.

NOTES

1. DORLAND'S ILLUSTRATED MEDICAL DICTIONARY (26th ed. 1981) at 933.
2. W. PROSSER, W. P. KEETON, THE LAW OF TORTS (West Publishing Co., St. Paul, Minn.) (5th ed. 1984) at 164–65.
3. Sirianni v. Anna, 285 N.Y.S.2d 709 (1967).
4. *Id.* at 711.
5. *Id.* at 712.
6. *Id.*
7. *Id.*
8. Moore v. Shah, 458 N.Y.S.2d 33 (1982).
9. *Id.* at 34–35.
10. *Id.* at 35.
11. PROSSER, *supra* note 2, at 187.
12. Ravenis v. Detroit General Hospital, 234 N.W.2d 411 (Mich. App. 1975).
13. *Id.* at 413.
14. *Id.*
15. *Id.* at 414.
16. PROSSER, *supra* note 2, at 269.
17. *Cf.* Herskovitz v. Group Health Cooperative of Puget Sound, 664 P.2d 474 (Wash. 1983). (A 14 percent reduction, from 39 percent to 25 percent, in decedent's chance for survival was sufficient evidence of causation to allow jury to consider the possibility that physician's failure in timely diagnosis of illness was the proximate cause of his death.)
18. PROSSER, *supra* note 2, at 501–03.
19. Ravenis, *supra* note 12, at 414.
20. *Grandstand Medicine,* NATURE 312:88 (November 8, 1984).
21. *See* Karp v. Cooley, 493 F.2d 408, 418–19 (1974).
22. *See* Gildiner v. Thomas Jefferson University Hospital, 451 F.Supp. 692 (E.D. Pa. 1978); Naccash v. Burger, 290 S.E.2d 824 (Va. 1982).
23. Uniform Anatomical Gift Act, §7(c)(1968). The text of the immunity section, which exists in all fifty states and the District of Columbia in some form, is: "(c) A person who acts in good faith in accord with the terms of this section or with the anatomical gift laws of another state (or a foreign

country) is not liable for damages in any civil action or subject to prosecution in any criminal proceeding for his act."

24. Williams v. Hofman, 233 N.W.2d 844 (Wisc. 1974).
25. *Id.* at 845.
26. Wisc. Stat. Ann. §155.06(7)(c) (1974).
27. Williams, *supra* note 24, at 846.
28. *Id.* at 847.
29. *Id.* at 846.
30. *Id.* at 847–49.

7

The Role of the Institutional Review Board in Research Relating to Human Organ Transplantation

Charles R. McCarthy

Recent years have witnessed a remarkable acceleration in the number of human organ transplantations. New surgical techniques, improved blood matching and tissue typing, the 1983 Food and Drug Administration (FDA) approval of new drug applications for cyclosporin and other immunosuppressive drugs, advanced methods for preserving organs, and attention on the part of the President, the Congress, and the media have all contributed to this marked increase. These factors have also heightened the demand for blood and blood products, kidneys, hearts, livers, lungs, skin, bone marrow, corneas, and pancreases—all needed in transplant procedures.

Most of the literature addressing ethical aspects of organ transplantation has focused attention on four principal areas: (1) education and identification of potential donors, (2) equitable selection of recipients, (3) systems for organ procurement and distribution, and (4) financial aspects of organ donation and transplantation.

For the purposes of this chapter, these will be referred to as the "macro" issues of organ transplantation. They have been addressed by the Congress, the Massachusetts Task Force on Organ Transplantation, third-party insurance carriers, the Health Care Financing Administration (HCFA), the Federal Task Force on Organ Transplantation, and other bodies that formulate public policy.

It is appropriate that attention be directed to these four areas since they continue to pose puzzling problems for the public, the medical profession, and public officials. This chapter, however, will address a related area of concern, a "micro" issue associated with organ transplantation, specifically, the role of the Institutional Review Board (IRB) in reviewing research involving organ transplantation. This topic was chosen because it has not received as much attention as the other topics and because it involves an area in which this author has some experience. It is hoped that a discussion of IRB duties and responsibilities will shed light on each of the macro issues.

To begin, some facts about IRBs. These boards are created by research institutions to review proposed and ongoing research. The Department of Health and Human Services (HHS) Regulations for the Protection of Human Subjects require that before human subjects may be involved in research supported by the Department, the institution must set forth its policies and procedures for protecting human research subjects in a document called an Assurance of Compliance with HHS regulations, and the research must be reviewed and approved by a properly constituted IRB.[1] The IRB must determine, among other factors, that risks are reasonable in relation to expected benefits, and that legally effective informed consent is obtained from research subjects or from their lawful representatives.

Furthermore, if the research involves an article regulated by the FDA, such as an experimental drug, device, or biologic, then FDA regulations require IRB review and approval of the investigational procedure.[2] Because regulations promulgated by HHS pertaining to IRB review are similar to those of the FDA, this chapter's explanations concerning HHS-supported research apply also to FDA-regulated research.

While some transplantation procedures, especially those involving kidneys, have reached a point where they are not considered research, many, if not most, of the other transplant procedures continue to fall within the definitions of research contained in federal regulations. That definition, found in 45 CFR 46.102, is as follows:

> "Research" means a systematic investigation designed to develop or contribute to generalizable knowledge. Activities which meet this definition constitute "research" for purposes of these regulations, whether or not they are supported or funded under a program which is considered research for other purposes. For example, some "demonstration" and "service" programs may include research activities.[3]

Virtually all procedures that meet this definition are subject to both initial and continuing IRB review. It should be stressed that the term "research" in this context has one function—it triggers IRB review. The term is not to be confused with "experimental," a term associated with reimbursement decisions. A procedure may be research but not experimental, and vice versa. Under federal regulations the Health Care Financing Administration cannot reimburse for "experimental" procedures.[4]

In 1982, the National Institutes of Health (NIH) alone supported research on 293 projects relating to organ transplantation totaling $36.5 million.[5] The 1982 expenditures serve as a reasonable forecast for future federal efforts in organ transplantation. Transplantation research is a fixture in the HHS portfolio and will remain so. As long as any transplantation procedure is considered "research" (whether or not it is funded by NIH or another HHS component), it will, in nearly every case, require IRB review and approval.

Let us explore some of the questions an IRB may face in considering prospective transplant projects. Both the questions raised and the answers offered constitute one person's understanding of the subject and his personal views concerning how an IRB might address the questions—they are not intended as an official commentary.

Question 1. Does the procedure constitute "research" subject to federal Regulations for the Protection of Human Subjects, and, therefore, does the procedure require IRB review?

Answer. If the procedure is funded by NIH, it is research because NIH is not permitted by law to fund health services that do not involve research.[6] If the procedure is not funded by NIH, the institution must consult the definition of research contained in federal regulations, and cited above. That definition, with its key phrases, "systematic investigation" and "generalizable knowledge," provides the institution with criteria for determining the need for IRB review. Generally, if the procedure is to be reported in a medical journal, it is research. If the procedure departs from the standard practice of medicine, it is research. If the procedure requires new or seldom-tried medical or surgical techniques, it is research. If the procedure involves investigational drugs, devices, or biologics, it is research.

The determination of a procedure as research means that it must undergo initial and continuing IRB review. Again, a determination that a procedure is a research procedure does not necessarily mean that it does—or does not—qualify for reimbursement under Medicare or Medicaid. That is a separate issue considered under Health Care Financing Administration regulations. Reimbursement regulations are unrelated to IRB review regarding the protection of human subjects.

Question 2. If the donor is deceased, does the IRB have any responsibility to the donor's heirs?

Answer. Federal regulations pertain to living persons who participate in research. Consequently, federal regulations do not require an IRB to concern itself with the deceased donor or the donor's heirs.

Nevertheless, the institution in which the research is conducted has an obligation to comply with the Uniform Anatomical Gift Act operative in the jurisdiction where the transplant occurs. It must also comply with all other pertinent state or local laws. The institution may direct its IRB to ensure that these laws are enforced. In practice, therefore, although not required to do so by federal regulations, most IRBs will be required by their institutions to concern themselves with the rights of the heirs of deceased donors. For example, the IRB may be asked to review the process used by a shock and trauma unit to approach the parents of a young person killed in a motorcycle accident. Clearly, in such a situation, delicacy, tact, respect for the wishes of the parents, as well as knowledge of the laws of the state must be considered.

Question 3. If the donor is living, must the IRB concern itself with the rights and welfare of the living donor?

Answer. The IRB must concern itself with the rights and welfare of all living subjects who participate in research. There can be no question that living donors participate in the research, and are entitled to protections under federal regulations under institutional policies set forth in institutional Assurances of Compliance negotiated with HHS in accord with the regulations,[7] and, in some instances, in accord with state and local laws.

The IRB should address the following issues with respect to the living donor.

Alternative procedures, if any, should be explored and explained to donors. Donors should be told if the potential recipient's condition can be treated in any way other than transplantation.

Risks and benefits associated with each alternative should be identified and carefully explained. Clearly, the risks associated with replaceable tissues are lower than risks associated with solid organ transplants. The risks of anesthesia and surgery, including pain and discomfort, must be accurately set forth.

Coercion of the potential donor must be minimized. The IRB may regard payment of large sums of money as coercive. If the potential recipient does not know the potential donor, then a third party should approach the donor. Potential recipients must not be allowed to harass potential donors.

An example of this occurred in *Head* v. *Colloton,*[8] the Iowa case in which the appeals court refused to provide a potential bone marrow recipient with the name and address of a potential donor who had declined to donate. The appeals court rendered the correct decision. Perhaps the best method of approaching a potential donor is through the donor's physician.

If the potential donor is a *minor,* then permission must be obtained from both parents, if both are reasonably available, or from the single parent or guardian who has responsibility for the minor donor. If the minor donor is able to comprehend the situation, then the minor donor must also provide assent. Children of consenting parents who refuse to assent must not be coerced. The IRB must be very cautious in protecting minors from coercion. Since federal regulations restrict placing a minor at risks considerably greater than minimal unless the minor is likely to benefit directly,[9] most transplants are ruled out between minor donors and unknown recipients. However, in the case of *Strunk* v. *Strunk* in Kentucky, the court held that it was in the best interest of an incompetent donor to donate a kidney to his sibling.[10] An IRB, following this line of reasoning, could at least consider allowing a transplant from a minor donor or an incompetent person to a sibling. Needless to say, IRBs must be cautious in attributing benefits to persons who donate solid organs (clearly a physical deficit) on the basis of possible psychological or social benefits to the donor. It is common practice in such cases to ask the courts to appoint a guardian *ad litem* to represent the interests of the minor or incompetent donor. If the IRB does not conclude that the minor or incompetent donor will benefit directly, then it may be necessary to obtain approval from a federally constituted Ethics Advisory Board before the procedure may be approved.[11]

Not only should the IRB concern itself with the rights and the welfare of the organ transplant donor, but it must also, in an even-handed way, concern itself with the rights and welfare of potential recipients. Questions addressed by the IRB should include the following.

Question 1. Do the expected benefits to the recipient provide sufficient justification to permit the risks to both the donor and the recipient?

Answer. In considering benefits, the IRB should keep in mind the recipient's condition. The IRB must be aware of the best available medical criteria for judging the condition of the recipient and whether the recipient meets these criteria. A recipient who, except for the need of the replacement organ, is otherwise in good health is a good transplant candidate. However, it is rarely the case that candidates for solid organ transplants are devoid of concomitant health problems. The IRB must, therefore, consult with the physician and surgeon investigators to evaluate each potential transplant protocol with careful attention to the specific potential recipient's condition. It is sad, but true, that some persons who are in need of replacement organs are such poor candidates for transplantation because of their general condition, that the IRB, in consultation with the transplant team, may determine that potential benefits do not justify the risks of the procedure.

With respect to informed consent, the IRB must not only ensure that the documentation is appropriate, but also, and more important, must ensure that the process of obtaining consent is suited to the particular situation of both donor and recipient. The IRB must make sure that privacy and confidentiality issues are addressed. The degree of confidentiality that can be achieved under the protocol must be explained. This is important in cases where intrusion by the public and the media may be expected.

Question 2. What other factors should IRBs consider?

Answer. The IRB should have evidence that blood typing and tissue matching offer sufficient hope of a successful transplant and that, in light of the expected benefits, the risks are reasonable.

Question 3. Should the IRB concern itself with the distribution of scarce resources?

Answer. Because solid organs suitable for transplants are chronically in short supply, the question of the distribution of scarce resources is extraordinarily sensitive. This question is better addressed outside the IRB. The primary concern of the IRB must lie with the rights and welfare of the donors and the recipients. Other agencies, such as the Federal Task Force on Organ Transplantation, must address these macro issues.[12]

In conclusion, this chapter suggests that physicians and surgeons should work closely with their IRBs in reaching organ transplantation decisions. The ability of the IRB to consider the rights and welfare of both donors and recipients, to introduce a variety of points of view, and to maintain a necessary degree of objectivity in dealing with emotionally charged cases allows it to make a valuable contribution to organ transplantation research.

NOTES

1. 45 C.F.R. §46.103(b) (1985).
2. 21 C.F.R. §56.109(a) (1985).
3. 45 C.F.R. §46.102(e) (1985).
4. 42 C.F.R. §405.402(c)(2) (1985); 42 C.F.R. §405.422 (1985).
5. National Institutes of Health budget.
6. 42 U.S.C. §2891-1 (1982).
7. 45 C.F.R. §46.103 (1985).
8. Head v. Colloton, 331 N.W.2d 870 (Iowa 1983).
9. 45 C.F.R. §46.407 (1985).
10. Strunk v. Strunk, 445 S.W.2d 145, 146, 149 (Ky. App. 1969).
11. 45 C.F.R. §46.204 (1985).
12. An executive summary of the REPORT OF THE FEDERAL TASK FORCE ON ORGAN TRANSPLANTATION appears in Appendix A of this volume.

8

The Role
of the Nursing Professional
in Organ Transplantation

Betty C. Irwin

Defining the role of the nursing professional in organ transplantation is difficult because no one role is practiced uniformly. Rather, there are various potential roles that nurses can fulfill in all aspects of the transplantation process. For purposes of this chapter, nursing roles have been categorized into three major groups: (1) the care of potential cadaver donors, (2) the organ recovery and sharing process, and (3) the care of organ transplant recipients. The involvement and responsibilities of nurses fulfilling roles within these categories vary greatly even in transplantation centers within a given geographic area.

There is scant documentation in the nursing literature of current organ transplantation practice. Most nursing literature related to organ transplantation concerns the actual nursing care which transplant recipients receive. Currently published literature substantiating the ways in which nurses do, could, or should participate as active transplant team members is seriously lacking. This chapter analyzes more completely the practice of nursing in organ transplantation.

THE CARE OF CADAVER ORGAN DONORS

Nurses serve as a vital link in the system for identifying potential cadaveric organ donors. Nurses who practice in intensive care units, trauma centers, and emergency rooms are in a position to identify patients who have suffered irreversible brain damage and who potentially meet the brain death criteria. By discussing organ donation as an option with the physicians caring for these patients, nurses can remind physicians that they do have something to offer the families of patients for whom they can do no more. That something is, of course, organ donation. By helping the physician educate the family about the concept of brain death and by helping the family accept the death of a loved one, nurses may encourage families to be amenable to a discussion of organ donation. Most organ procurement coordinators would testify that nurses practicing in such settings are their greatest allies. This is because nurses have generally established a rapport with the family. In addition, the turnover of nurses tends to be slower than the rapid rotation of house staff through intensive care units. Thus, there is less of a need for reeducating these nurses than there is for the physicians.

The role of the critical care nurse in identifying potential organ donors causes internal conflicts. Nurses must deal with peers, other professionals, and families who may view this role as predatory. Some physicians may occasionally view a nurse's suggestion of organ donation as a threat, as an indication that the physician has failed to cure or save the patient involved. The nurse may also have his or her own inner conflicts with regard to organ donation. Among these may be conflicts about the allocation of nursing resources, death itself, and informed consent.

Once a potential organ donor has been identified, nurses may play an equally important role in providing physical care to ensure the viability of the organs. Persons who are brain dead are frequently unstable and exhibit great fluctuations in vital signs and vital organ function. Close monitoring and appropriate intervention are essential to maintenance of circulation and oxygenation to vital organs so that they remain viable for transplantation. Prevention and early detection of infections are also necessary for organ viability. Nurses are the professionals at the bedside who must make the appropriate observations, intervene as necessary, and inform the physician of changes in the patient's condition so that he or she may order appropriate therapy. And in providing such intensive nursing care to a patient who cannot survive, nurses may have an inner conflict about the allocation of nursing resources. For example, would the nurse's efforts be more appropriately directed to the care of patients who have some chance of survival and recovery?

Although the physical nursing care required of a potential cadaveric organ donor is often time-consuming, the support and emotional care of the donor family can be even more demanding. Helping families grieve and accept the patient's death, and supporting their decision about organ donation (whatever that decision is), are extremely important nursing roles. Conflict within the family about organ donation or other arrangements surrounding the death may surface. The nurse caring for the patient must be aware of such conflicts and must assist in their resolution.

What do nurses in such settings need? How can the transplant team assist? Perhaps the greatest need is information. These nurses need to have accurate, up-to-date information regarding the progress of brain death declaration, the attainment of family consent for donation, and the logistics of organ recovery. This is particularly crucial in cases of multiple organ recovery when several teams may be involved and time delays are common. Nurses need the facts to keep the family informed as well as to plan unit activities such as admissions and staffing.

Second, nurses need support, encouragement, and feedback from the attending physicians. Nurses need to feel that they are an important part of the organ recovery effort. Nurses involved in the care of cadaveric organ donors need to hear about the results of their efforts once organ recovery has been completed and the organs transplanted. Nurses need to hear that their work did make a difference to patients who await organ transplants. This final step of the process accomplishes much to ensure the continued cooperation of nurses in the identification and care of potential cadaver donors.

NURSING ROLES IN THE ORGAN RECOVERY AND SHARING PROCESS

Many transplant coordinators responsible for the organization and coordination of organ recovery efforts and organ sharing among transplant centers are nurses. Nurses are ideally suited for this role, especially if they have critical-care experience. They are familiar with the intensive care setting and its equipment. They are comfortable providing direct patient care, and their patient assessment skills have been fine-tuned. Such nurses are experienced in working with families in crisis and can educate and provide them with the necessary support. Finally, the nurse as transplant coordinator can rapidly develop collegial relationships with nurses in other units where cadaver donors are identified.

Nurses who fulfill the role of transplant coordinator are involved in identifying, evaluating, and managing potential donors. It is often their responsibility to obtain the family's consent. Once consent has been obtained, the transplant nurse coordinator assists with organ recovery efforts in the operating room. Finally, this nurse is responsible for organ preservation and sharing so that the most suitable recipient for each donated organ is located.

If organ donation is to increase to meet the current and future needs for transplantation, both professional and public education are essential. This task most often falls to the transplant coordinator charged with organ recovery and sharing. Nurses are well suited to fulfill this role. Education is a nursing forte; much emphasis in the nursing curriculum is placed on the principles of adult education, and nurses spend a great deal of their professional careers educating patients and their families. Who would be better suited to educate professionals and the public about organ donation?

Nursing Roles in Providing Care to Transplant Recipients

In providing care to transplant recipients, nurses may play many roles in various settings. They may be staff nurses in an intensive care area, on a transplant unit, or in a clinic responsible for providing direct care to the organ transplantation recipients. They may be head nurses, supervisors, or other nursing administrators responsible for directing the recipient's overall care. Or they may be highly specialized nurses prepared as clinical nurse specialists, nurse practitioners, or transplant clinical coordinators whose specific responsibilities in a particular institution are to coordinate and ensure the continuity of transplant recipient care. Nurses may work in the operating room and assist in the actual transplant. Increasingly, home care nurses also have a role in providing care to transplant recipients.

Despite the differences in the clinical settings and job functions of these various nurses, several common threads may be identified which run through all practice settings. These include: surveillance and patient assessment, patient and family education, provision of support to the patient and family, assurance of quality care, reduction of costs, preparation for discharge, and documentation. For ease of analysis, nursing roles will be examined in three categories: in-hospital care, outpatient care, and the expanded roles for nurses.

Nursing care during the immediate phase of posttransplantation involves carrying out physicians' orders, monitoring the function of the grafted organ, preventing infections and other complications, and documenting findings and interventions. Patients and their physicians rely heavily upon nurses for correct interpretation and carrying out of medical orders. During this critical time, it is vital that the nurse continually monitor the patient to assess the functioning of the transplanted organ as well as the patient's response to surgery and the administration of anesthetic agents. The patient's immune status must also be evaluated continuously and interventions planned to prevent infectious complications, rejection of the organ, and complications resulting from the administration of potent immunosuppressive agents. The nurse must have a good scientific background and understanding of both end-stage organ failure and immunology. Finally, the nurse must make appropriate notations in the record of the findings, interventions, and the patient's responses. Changes in therapy are based upon the nurse's documentation.

As the patient recovers from surgery, much of the nurse's attention focuses on patient and family education and preparation for discharge. Patients need to understand their disease and the reasons why transplantation was chosen as the treatment. A clear understanding of medications—how they are to be administered, their actions, and potential adverse effects—is crucial. Patients must comprehend the importance of continued immunosuppression for the viability of the transplanted organ as well as the need for continued medical supervision. They need to understand the signs and symptoms of rejection and other complications which may occur. Transplant recipients are not cured, only treated. Successful treatment requires that the prescribed regimen be strictly followed. Education will not ensure compliance; however, compliance must begin with education and understanding. Most of the patient education is a nursing responsibility. Patient teaching lays the foundation for patient compliance and, thus, for long-term graft function.

Nurses involved with the in-hospital phase of posttransplant care must provide support to the patient and his or her family. During this time, many uncertainties exist. Life-and-death crises are common, and the fear of rejection is an ever-present reality. The monitoring and care required at this time force the patient to be somewhat dependent. And yet, to be successfully rehabilitated, the transplant recipient must achieve some measure of independence. Nurses must assist patients in gaining the knowledge and confidence to become as independent and in charge of their own care as possible. This process must also take into consideration family members, as they may be either a great help or a hindrance in the patient's attempts to achieve independence.

With the current emphasis on cost containment and reductions in health care costs, nurses are faced with shortened hospital stays for transplant recipients. Improved methods of immunosuppression and fewer rejection episodes have further shortened hospital stays. Nurses, therefore, must prepare patients, at an accelerated pace, for discharge and self-care at home. In this process, nurses must ensure that the quality of care does not suffer and that after discharge, patients and their families remain fully prepared to assume their responsibilities. If they are not yet ready to do so, appropriate arrangements for home or out-patient care must be made. The challenge for nurses is to assure quality of care while reducing transplantation costs.

After discharge, nurses in clinics and home care agencies continue the work. Continued patient assessment and monitoring for evidence of any deterioration in graft function or complication of immunosuppression are absolutely essential. Continued support for the patient and family remains necessary, because many uncertainties and crises will arise. The importance of ongoing patient and family education cannot be overemphasized. The successful transplant recipient is one who is a knowledgeable partner in his or her own care.

The highly specialized field of transplantation is one that has encouraged the development of so-called expanded roles for nurses. Nurses can fulfill the need to have someone coordinate the movement of patients through the system, thereby assuming responsibility for the continuity of care and for preventing the fragmentation that can so easily occur when many specialists become involved in the care of one patient. Similarly, nurses can interpret the system for patients and assure that individual attention is not lost. Since transplantation is generally performed at major teaching hospitals, patients frequently travel great distances. They become involved in a complex health care system far from home. The nurses providing direct care to these patients must be educated so that the nurses may provide appropriate care. Patient follow-up after discharge must be coordinated.

Many transplant centers employ nurses to perform these and similar functions. Titles vary greatly, as does the formal preparation of the nurses fulfilling these roles. These nurses may include nurse practitioners, clinical nurse specialists, and transplant clinical nurse coordinators. The specific duties depend on the qualifications of the person filling the position as well as on the needs of the transplant institution. Many such nurses are directly involved in ongoing research, data collection and analysis, and the publication and presentation of transplantation outcomes.

Nursing professionals currently fulfill many diverse roles in the organ transplantation field. The involvement of nurses in this field will probably increase as the number of transplants performed increases, as patients are released from in-hospital care more quickly following transplantation, and as the need expands for the long-term follow-up care of these patients. We need to assess more clearly and comprehensively the ways in which nurses can provide patient care in this field. We can begin by increasing the amount of literature that examines and documents the efficacy of current nursing roles.

BACKGROUND READING

Buszta, *Patient Evaluation Pre and Post-Transplant,* NEPHROLOGY NURSE 3(3):38–42 (May–June 1981).

Irwin, *An Expanded Role for Nurses: Systematic Assessment of Renal Transplant Recipients,* JOURNAL OF THE AMERICAN ASSOCIATION OF NEPHROLOGY NURSES AND TECHNICIANS 6(2):109–19 (1979).

Irwin, *Renal Transplantation: Advances in Immunology—A Nursing Perspective,* JOURNAL OF THE AMERICAN ASSOCIATION OF NEPHROLOGY NURSES AND TECHNICIANS 10(4):11–15, 22 (1983).

Masur, *Renal Transplant: Your Role in Patient Education,* JOURNAL OF PRACTICAL NURSING 30(7):12–15, 43 (July 1980).

Section 3

Regulatory Issues

9

Regulation of Medical Practice

Dale H. Cowan

The transplantation of human organs is one of the most dramatic examples of the emerging medical technologies that are transforming
medical practice. The development of this technology, like that of all
new methods for diagnosing and treating human diseases, raises numerous issues affecting the availability, use, and financing of such practices. One of the most important and difficult issues is determining when
and under what circumstances new technologies, such as organ transplantation, evolve from experimental status to accepted standard medical practice. Some questions deserving consideration are: how are new
practices developed; by what criteria should they be judged; who has
the burden of conducting these assessments; and what are the standards
that should govern the entry of new practices into standard medical
practice?

A related question is whether organ transplantation differs from
other complex technologies and practices and whether its acceptance
into standard practice—both medically and for purposes of payment—
should be different from other complex and expensive practices.

This last question can be illustrated with an example from the
hematology-oncology field. The treatment of acute leukemia in adults
commonly involves an initial hospital stay often lasting three, four, or
more weeks; the performance of numerous diagnostic tests on a repeated basis; the administration of numerous drugs, including chemo-
therapeutic agents and antibiotics; the use of large quantities of blood
and blood products; and the personal attention of a vast array of medical
specialists and allied health professionals.

This initial treatment, or induction therapy, costs anywhere from
$30,000 to $50,000 or more, depending on the ease with which the
patient enters remission and the number, type, and severity of disease-

related or treatment-related complications. If the patient enters a complete remission, additional therapy is provided that may, over the balance of a year, cost an additional $30,000 to $50,000 or more. Despite this intense treatment, and allowing for the substantial improvement that has occurred in the treatment of acute leukemia, the rate of complete remission is 60 percent to 80 percent, and the rate of survival at one year is about 50 percent—a rate lower than that for heart transplantation.

Yet we do not hear debate about whether to pay for the treatment of acute leukemia or about the effect the use of the resources consumed in its treatment has on the availability of resources for treating other conditions. Similarly, little is said about the standards and criteria by which to determine whether the treatment of leukemia is experimental or standard practice, the manner in which criteria are applied, and the individuals or institutions that make these decisions.

Why? What accounts for the special concern accorded organ transplantation? Is it the involvement of a donor, the problems of procurement, or the extent of the technological infrastructure that must be assembled to provide the therapy? Or is it the wonderment that accompanies a dramatic surgical procedure—the media attention sought by anguished patients and their families as well as by publicity-seeking physicians and institutions interested in attracting attention and enlisting support?

There is really no clear answer. Perhaps, if one looks at the basic medical, ethical, social, and economic issues, there is no fundamental difference between transplantation and other extreme and expensive technologies. And perhaps it is more useful and appropriate to consider how medical practice is regulated in general and how new technologies are assessed, rather than beginning a discussion of whether and how transplantation as a medical practice should be regulated by treating it as a special case.

This chapter defines standard medical practice and reviews the means by which such practice is regulated. It then considers the status of innovative therapies or practices and distinguishes these from standard practice and research. There follows a discussion of criteria that are or may be used to determine when experimental and innovative activities become acceptable "therapeutic" approaches in patient treatment. Finally, this chapter discusses whether and how the movement of practices from the experimental to the therapeutic setting can or might be regulated, with particular focus on the unique problems presented by organ transplantation, and concludes with a proposal for undertaking such regulation.

STANDARD PRACTICE

DEFINITION

Although judicial decisions and scholarly writings repeatedly use the terms "standard medical practice" and "accepted medical practice," a precise definition of standard medical practice is elusive. In *The Belmont Report*,[1] the National Commission for the Protection of Human Subjects of Biomedical and Behavioral Research[2] stated:

> The term "practice" refers to interventions that are designed solely to enhance the well-being of an individual patient or client and that have a reasonable expectation of success. The purpose of medical or behavioral practice is to provide diagnosis, preventive treatment, or therapy to particular individuals.[3]

This definition focuses on the intent of the practitioner in undertaking a particular intervention. It presupposes and is predicated upon the existence of a physician-patient relationship wherein the physician assumes and accepts the responsibility to act with good faith toward the patient.[4] To this definition should be added the concept that standard medical practice is that practice which has been "sufficiently tested to meet peer group or regulatory agency standards for acceptance or approval."[5]

The type of testing that underlies the acceptance or approval of a practice may range from anecdotal, uncontrolled "experiences" of numerous clinicians to highly organized, rigorously conducted randomized clinical trials. The key consideration is that the potential benefits and risks of the practice and the ability to control them are approaching a level of predictability that therapists and patients find acceptable. Although all the risks may not be known, the degree of ignorance of these risks has been sufficiently reduced in relation to the anticipated benefits to justify the practice in a setting where the sole intent is to promote the patient's well-being.

REGULATION

Medical practice is regulated by the legal constraints imposed by the tort liability system and by professional peer review based on professional ethics, codes, and norms.

Tort Liability

Tort liability is based on negligence—the failure to exercise ordinary care—and on the lack of disclosure—the failure adequately to disclose information about a procedure to ensure informed consent.

A physician will be liable for damages if he or she fails to possess a reasonable degree of skill and fails to exercise this skill with ordinary care and diligence. Establishing a cause of action based on negligence requires four elements: a duty to conform to a certain standard of conduct to protect others against unreasonable risks; a failure to conform to the standard required; an injury; and a causal connection between the conduct and the injury.[6]

The key element in the legal requirements for negligence is establishing the accepted standard of medical care. The accepted standard of care is usually determined by the practice of other physicians under similar circumstances. For example, the court in *Owens* v. *McCleary*[7] stated:

> Conformity with the established mode of treatment is the test ordinarily applied in determining whether a physician or surgeon, in a given case, has brought to the treatment of his patient the requisite knowledge and skill. A failure to employ the methods followed or approved by his school of practice, evidences either ignorance or experimentation on his part. The law tolerates neither. If he wishes to avoid civil liability, he must employ in the treatment of his patients methods which are recognized and approved by his profession as most likely to produce favorable results.[8]

Although the accepted standard of care is determined by the established practice of the profession, there is often little inquiry into whether an established practice is based on scientifically validated data or on nonvalidated conventional wisdom or experience. An example of a practice formerly considered standard on the basis of experience is performing a mastectomy immediately after a breast biopsy on the basis of a frozen section analysis of the biopsied tissue. The rationale for this practice was a desire to lessen the risk of spilling cancer cells in the biopsy incision and, hence, to lessen the risk of spreading any cancer that might be present. A consequence of this practice was the occasional removal of a nonmalignant breast. Only after the question of this risk was subject to critical analysis by undertaking a clinical trial was it determined that no such risk existed. Rather, delaying proposed mastectomies until the biopsy specimens could be adequately studied allowed for a more accurate diagnosis of malignancy and reduced the possibility of unnecessary surgery.

On occasion, courts have imposed a standard of care that exceeded the accepted professional standard. The most notable case is that of *Helling* v. *Carey and Laughlin*.[9] In *Helling*, the court found the defendant ophthalmologists liable for failing to administer a test for glaucoma to a thirty-two-year-old patient. The accepted practice of the profession was that the test for glaucoma was not routinely administered to patients under forty years of age because the incidence of glaucoma in persons under forty was 1 in 25,000.

In rejecting the defendant's evidence, the court found the entire profession at fault for failing to exercise reasonable care in not routinely administering the test for ocular pressure. It described the following reasons for imposing a standard greater than that of professional practice:

1. The technology in question was highly accurate.
2. The procedure was painless and not dangerous to the patient.
3. The procedure was relatively inexpensive.
4. The disease the procedure was designed to detect was potentially serious.

In the words of Justice Holmes:

> What usually is done may be evidence of what ought to be done, but what ought to be done is fixed by a standard of reasonable prudence, whether it usually is complied with or not.[10]

In addition to liability for failing to conform with accepted standards of care, physicians may be liable for failing to disclose adequate information to patients in order to obtain consent. The duty to disclose, like the duty to act in patients' best interests, derives from the physician-patient relationship. This is based on the ethical principle of autonomy or respect for persons and reflects the concept that the autonomous person can ascertain his or her best interests more competently than one who would substitute a judgment about that person's best interests.[11] The legal formulation of the ethical principle of autonomy was most succinctly stated by Judge (later Justice) Cardozo:

> Every human being of adult years has a right to determine what shall be done with his own body.[12]

In general, except in an emergency, a physician may not treat a patient without consent. The duty of the physician is to disclose the diagnosis and proposed treatment, the anticipated benefits and risks, and, in some jurisdictions, alternative treatments and their anticipated benefits and risks. This duty was stated by the court in *Cobbs* v. *Grant*:[13]

> A medical doctor, being the expert, appreciates the risks inherent in the procedure he is prescribing, the risks of a decision not to undergo the treatment, and the probability of a successful outcome of the treatment . . . once this information has been disclosed, that aspect of the doctor's function has been performed. The weighing of these risks against the individual subjective fears and hopes of the patient is not an expert skill.

Such evaluation and decision is a nonmedical judgment reserved to the patient alone.[14]

Two standards are used to measure the disclosure duty. The standard held in the majority of states is that the duty to disclose is based upon that which reasonable medical practitioners in a similar situation would find medically necessary to disclose. This standard was expressed by the court in *Natanson* v. *Kline*:[15]

> The duty of the physician to disclose . . . is limited to those disclosures which a reasonable medical practitioner would make under the same or similar circumstances. How the physician may best discharge his obligation to the patient . . . involves primarily a question of medical judgment.[16]

By this standard, the medical community determines the nature and scope of information a physician must disclose.

The other standard for disclosure, adopted in a minority of jurisdictions, holds that the duty to disclose is determined by the informational needs of the patient, not the medical community. This standard, termed the "materiality" standard, was first articulated by the court in *Canterbury* v. *Spence.*[17] The court stated:

> In our view, the patient's right of self-decision shapes the boundaries of the duty to reveal. That right can be effectively exercised only if the patient possesses enough information to enable an intelligent choice. The scope of the physician's communications to the patient, then, must be measured by the patient's need, and that need is the information material to the decision. Thus the test for determining whether a particular peril must be divulged is its materiality to the patient's decision: all risks potentially affecting the decision must be unmasked.[18]

In addition to disclosing information concerning the proposed procedure, the duty to disclose also includes informing the patient of alternative procedures that could be equally effective. The physician, therefore, has an overall duty of "reasonable disclosure of the available choices with respect to the proposed therapy and of the dangers inherently and potentially involved in each."[19] Both failure to conform with prevailing standards of care and failure to disclose may lead to an award of money damages if the patient can show that he or she was injured as a result of the physician's error.

The problem with the tort liability system as an effective regulator of medical practice is that it is retrospective. Additionally, the tort liability system applies only if an injured patient chooses to bring an action against a physician, and the system places the burden of proof of an alleged error on the person bringing the charge. Even if these criteria are met, the system is still fraught with numerous procedural rules that may affect the outcome without addressing the substantive merits of the claim.

Peer Review

To some extent, medical practice is regulated by professional ethics and codes and peer review. Codes of professional ethics are generally hortatory and carry no specific sanctions. Although most physicians subscribe to and comply with these ethical precepts, there is insufficient evidence to indicate that the presence of professional codes and norms alone adequately regulates medical practice.

A more formal method of regulating medical practice is professional peer review. Peer review is primarily a hospital-based activity and consequently is only concerned with professional activities in the hospital setting. Peer review is mandated for all hospitals that seek accreditation by the Joint Commission on Accreditation of Hospitals (JCAH).[20] Since many third party insurers, including Medicare, only reimburse hospitals accredited by the JCAH, the JCAH standards are universally adopted.

The recommended standards for hospitals seeking accreditation are listed in the Accreditation Manual for Hospitals. A series of standards is established for the hospital medical staff of which Standard VI states:

> As part of the hospital's quality assurance program, the medical staff strives to assure the provision of high-quality patient care through the monitoring and evaluation of the quality and appropriateness of patient care.[21]

The required characteristics of this review include departmental or medical staff monitoring of the clinical performance of its members; surgical case review; and reviews of drug therapy practice and drug utilization, medical records, blood usage, antibiotic usage, and other relevant clinical activities.

The peer review mechanism serves two functions. First, it establishes standards of medical practice and sensitizes members of the medical staff to these standards. Second, it monitors adherence to the standards. The limitations of the peer review mechanism are that the monitoring function is necessarily retrospective and that it is applied only to activities occurring within hospitals. Peer review of professional activities occurring within physicians' private offices is virtually nonexistent. Notwithstanding these limitations, and in part as a result of lawsuits brought against hospitals and their medical staffs alleging failure to monitor and control physicians' activities, peer review is seen as an increasingly effective means of regulating medical practice.

INNOVATIVE THERAPY AND RESEARCH

DEFINITION OF INNOVATIVE THERAPY

Several definitions of innovative therapy have been proposed. The National Commission for the Protection of Human Subjects identified innovative therapies as a class of procedures that were "designed solely to enhance the well-being of an individual patient or client" but had not been tested sufficiently to meet the standard of having "a reasonable expectation of success."[22] Levine defined innovative therapies as activities "ordinarily conducted by . . . physician[s] with either pure practice intent or with varying degrees of mixed research and practice intent" that have been insufficiently tested to meet standards for acceptance or approval.[23]

INNOVATIVE THERAPY DISTINGUISHED
FROM STANDARD PRACTICE

Several characteristics of innovative therapies have been identified that distinguish them from standard medical practice.

Claude Bernard, who may be considered the father of clinical research, suggested that the difference between standard practice and innovative therapy is merely the difference between a beginning and an advanced level of medical practice.[24] He defined the standard practitioner as an "empirical physician" who "contents himself with noting facts solely on the basis of medical tradition." Although the practitioner may participate in experimental medicine to the extent of prescribing active medications, as opposed to mere observation, there is no attempt to discover new facts that would advance medical science.

Levine observed that innovative therapies are defined by the "lack of suitable validation of [their] safety and efficacy" rather than their "novelty."[25] A practice might not be validated due to insufficient testing needed to certify its safety and efficacy for an intended class of patients or because of evidence from its use that previously held assumptions about its safety and efficacy should be questioned.

In general, practices or therapies that are standard have known risks and benefits, and some basis exists for thinking that the benefits outweigh the risks. By contrast, the potential benefits and risks of innovative therapies are less well known or predictable. Consequently, their use exposes patients to a greater likelihood that the balance of benefits and risks may be unfavorable due either to the therapies being ineffective or entailing greater, possibly unknown, risks.

A factor contributing to the risk of innovative therapies, apart from the actual harm that might occur, relates to the issue of intent—the reason physicians seek to undertake the new procedure. In the traditional practice setting, the primary, if not sole, interest of physicians is promoting the patient's well-being. In contrast, physicians planning to undertake innovative therapies may have personal goals in addition to the patient's interests. Such goals may include a desire for career advancement or a desire to gain recognition by pioneering a new procedure. The existence of these personal goals may affect a physician's ability to calculate the risk-benefit ratio, willingness to expose patients to the innovative therapy, and/or disclosure to patients of salient informed consent factors.

DEFINITION OF RESEARCH

Before attempting to distinguish innovative therapies from experimentation or research, it is necessary to define what is meant by the term "research." In *The Belmont Report,* the National Commission stated:

> [T]he term "research" designates an activity designed to test a hypothesis, permit conclusions to be drawn, and thereby to develop or contribute to generalizable knowledge (expressed, for example, in theories, principles, and statements of relationships). Research is usually described in a formal protocol that sets forth an objective and a set of procedures designed to reach that objective.[26]

Levine defined research involving humans as

> any manipulation, observation, or other study of a human being—or of anything related to that human being that might subsequently result in manipulation of that human being—done with the intent of developing new knowledge and which differs in any way from customary medical (or other professional) practice.[27]

Norton describes experimental procedures to be those

> that are untested or unproved with respect to clinical efficacy, or are by their very nature not related to the therapy of the patient but rather performed solely for the purpose of obtaining scientific data.[28]

These definitions refer to several elements that characterize research, including: (1) a departure from standard medical practice, (2) having untested or unproved efficacy or no therapeutic intent, (3) designed to test a hypothesis, and/or (4) an intent to develop new knowledge. Additionally, research is conducted according to a defined plan. Another characteristic of research, and one that distinguishes it from practice, is the use of the human as a subject rather than as a patient.[29] This latter distinction becomes blurred in clinical research settings in which studies designed to test diagnostic or therapeutic procedures may have a direct "beneficial" effect on the subject-patient in addition to contributing to general medical knowledge.

INNOVATIVE THERAPY DISTINGUISHED FROM RESEARCH

The distinction between innovative therapy and experimentation can be drawn by focusing on the forementioned four elements characteristic of research. Like research, innovative therapy generally represents a departure from standard medical practice. Whereas research is generally (it is hoped) based on a sound hypothesis, innovative therapy may or may not be so grounded. Innovative therapy may, therefore, differ from research in the degree to which the planned departure from standard practice is rationally based.

Given the variety of research activities and proposed innovative therapies, it is difficult to distinguish these activities based solely on their untested or unproved efficacy. Research activities and innovative therapies have been proposed that have both little known or proved efficacy and substantial potential benefit. This criterion is not, therefore, useful in distinguishing these activities.

By contrast, innovative therapy can be distinguished from research by whether it is designed to test a hypothesis or to develop new knowledge. Innovative therapies generally represent uncontrolled, often single, interventions intended to manage or to solve particular clinical problems. They are not ordinarily designed to test hypotheses. Additionally, they are not undertaken to gain new knowledge beyond the patient's needs. Although the use of innovative therapies may lead to the development of new knowledge, this consequence is secondary to the primary purpose—benefiting patients.

CRITERIA FOR DETERMINING WHEN EXPERIMENTAL OR INNOVATIVE PRACTICES BECOME ACCEPTED PRACTICES

EXISTING CRITERIA

Except for drugs and devices that are regulated by the Food and Drug Administration (FDA),[30] it is difficult to define specific criteria according to which experimental or innovative practices become accepted standard medical practice. To be accepted into standard medical practice, new drugs and devices must be shown by controlled clinical testing to be both safe and effective.[31] In contrast, no regulatory standard applies to such activities as surgery, invasive diagnostic techniques, diagnostic imaging techniques, the use of radioisotopes, radiation therapy, other physical forms of therapy, or behavioral approaches to psychotherapy. Thus, no formal regulatory criteria currently exist by which to determine when, for example, liver or heart transplantation ceases to be experimental and becomes standard medical practice. Rather, "[t]he introduction of new medical technologies in the United States tends to take on a life of its own, and the impact of governmental policy on its diffusion has been very limited."[32]

Despite the lack of formal criteria, it is possible to discern criteria that appear to apply in determining when unregulated practices evolve from the experimental stage to the level of accepted practice. One set of criteria is that utilized by the FDA in assessing drugs and devices, namely, safety and efficacy. Evidence for the safety and efficacy of experimental or innovative practices may be gathered from formal clinical studies conducted in accordance with established research procedures previously defined. The data from such studies are susceptible to rigorous analysis and the conclusions may be highly probative for determining that the specific procedure merits standard practice status.

It is possible, however, that evidence regarding the safety and efficacy of procedures may be determined by examining the results of the procedures in ad hoc or uncontrolled circumstances. Two factors may affect the validity of the conclusions drawn from the uncontrolled use of experimental or innovative practices. One factor is the setting in which the practice is employed. The other is the scientific and medical qualifications of the individuals undertaking the particular activity.

The successful use of an innovative therapy in individuals with a serious or life-threatening illness for which no therapy exists may indicate to other practitioners that the therapy is worth pursuing even if the initial use was undertaken on an ad hoc basis without a formal research protocol. In other settings, the reason for using an innovative therapy may be less apparent and its safety and efficacy might not be so clear-cut. The key determination is whether the balance of benefits and risks of the therapy is favorable in relation to the anticipated outcome without the therapy. Presumably, therapies for which the balance of benefits and risks is not favorable are not accepted as standard medical practice.

Regrettably, despite the apparent logic of this approach, in most settings it is an unreliable basis for accepting the proposed new therapies. The history of medicine is replete with examples of treatments resulting from uncontrolled practices that were found, after formal studies, not to have the anticipated benefit or relative lack of risk. Thus, although the criteria of safety and efficacy might be appropriate, the "data" from such uncontrolled practices upon which determinations of safety and efficacy are made may be flawed.

The second factor that may affect the validity of conclusions drawn from the use of uncontrolled experimental or innovative practices is the qualifications of the individuals undertaking and promoting the practices. Like other professions, medicine is hierarchical. Great credence is given to statements and opinions of individuals who occupy positions of leadership, such as chairmen of major clinical departments in hospitals and medical schools. Assertions by such individuals that a particular therapy is effective tend to be accepted by many practitioners and patients without critical regard for the scientific basis on which the assertions are purportedly grounded. A leading example of this is the assertion by one Nobel prize laureate of the value of high doses of vitamin C in preventing cancer, despite the lack of credible supporting evidence and in the face of credible evidence to the contrary. Therefore, the prestige of the individuals promoting the value of experimental or innovative practices cannot substitute for the controlled observations needed to determine their safety and efficacy.

Another criterion commonly used as evidence that experimental or innovative practices have become accepted into standard practice is the frequency with which such practices are undertaken. It is perhaps the norm in medical practice for new therapies to be adopted on an ad hoc trial basis in response to both expected and unexpected clinical situations. The sheer repetition of such therapies lends a legitimacy to them that results in widespread adoption. These practices are usually never subjected to critical safety and efficacy analyses.

Examples of surgical practices that were widely used without such critical analyses are the radical mastectomy and tonsillectomy. The widespread use of such practices waned only after controlled studies were published demonstrating that the procedures were not as efficacious as previously believed or contained unnecessary risks previously unknown or unrecognized. Thus, the sheer frequency with which a practice or therapy is undertaken is not an adequate criterion by which to determine that its use should become or remain standard medical practice.

PROPOSED CRITERIA

The criteria used by the FDA in assessing the acceptability of new drugs and devices, that is, their safety and efficacy, are reasonable and could be appropriately utilized to determine when experimental or innovative therapies should become standard medical practice. The determination of safety and efficacy basically focuses on the relative benefits and harms of the proposed practices in relation to the conditions under which they are applied.

The key inquiry is the nature of the evidence upon which the assertions of safety and efficacy are based and the type and extent of oversight that need be exercised in evaluating the evidence and its resulting conclusions.

REGULATION OF THE PASSAGE OF AN ACTIVITY FROM RESEARCH TO ACCEPTED PRACTICE

It is generally agreed that no mechanism exists at this time to regulate the passage of an activity from the realm of research or innovation to the status of accepted medical practice. Moskowitz et al. note that the Department of Health and Human Services (HHS) has not "developed a coherent strategy for evaluating the origins, development, transfer, and early dissemination of new medical practices."[33] Most of HHS's assessment begins after the practice has been widely accepted. This lack of procedures for assessing innovation has led to problems in the evaluation and adoption of new medical practices. "Some efficacious medical practices have been adopted too slowly; some practices have been displaced too slowly; and others, though clinically valuable, have been too costly." [34]

This section will consider several approaches for monitoring the movement of practices from an unproved status to acceptance. In doing so, it is necessary to consider that the types of practices and activities in question vary greatly with respect to the setting or environment in which they are to be used, the impetus underlying their development and adoption, the intent of the investigators and practitioners seeking to establish them as part of medical practice, the extent of departure from existing practice, their cost and complexity, their use of resources, their anticipated availability, and the ethical and social consequences of their being adopted. Thus, the practices may range from using an approved drug for nonapproved purposes, an act an individual physician may undertake solely to benefit his or her patients, to transplantation of human organs, an activity that is highly complex, very costly, uses considerable resources, has limited availability, and raises major ethical and social policy issues.

Because of the diversity of practices potentially subject to any regulatory scheme, it is probable that no single approach will suit all practices. For this reason, this chapter will consider five types of controls that may contribute to a regulatory framework for the passage of new practices into standard medical practice. These are: (1) the tort liability system, (2) the peer review system, (3) the research-IRB model, (4) the FDA model, and (5) the creation of a special review board.

THE TORT LIABILITY SYSTEM

Reference was previously made to the general proposition that the use of innovative therapies has been relatively disfavored in medical jurisprudence. The court, in the early English case of *Slater* v. *Baker*,[35] stated:

> For any thing that appears to the Court, this was the first experiment made with this new instrument; and if it was, it was a rash action, and he who acts rashly acts ignorantly . . . contrary to the known rule and usage of surgeons.[36]

This sentiment was expressed by the court in *Carpenter* v. *Blake*[37] in which the defendant physician was held liable for harm arising from the treatment of a dislocated arm without a sling. In *Carpenter,* however, the court appeared to sanction new practices when it stated:

> [I]t is incumbent on surgeons called to treat . . . an injury, to conform to the system of treatment thus established; and if they depart from it, they do it at their peril. . . . If, however, it is shown that surgeons have applied a different system to treatment, and found it to succeed as well or better than the one prescribed, it is not negligence to resort to the system thus practically tested.[38]

The court here is suggesting that physicians are potentially liable for departing from standard medical practice, but that no liability will be found for departures that are shown to be effective. Additional bases given by courts for sanctioning departures from standard medical practice include the extent of departure from the accepted practice[39] and the lack of a suitable alternative to the innovative practice.[40]

As with cases involving standard medical practices, practitioners utilizing innovative therapies may be liable if they fail to disclose information required for legally effective consent.[41]

It may be questioned, however, whether the tort liability system will deter physicians from using innovative therapies except when they may be reasonably expected to benefit patients and when patients consent. As Robertson has observed:

> The tort system is not calibrated to deal with every deviation from ethical conduct. First it operates only after an injury occurs. . . . Second, where

the risk does materialize, a number of factors may operate to prevent a successful suit. . . . Finally, if a suit is filed, the chances for recovery are slim. . . . For all these reasons, the threat of a law suit and legal liability may not prevent physicians from using innovative therapy in situations that ignore patient interests, if use otherwise seems justified.[42]

On the basis of these considerations, the tort liability system is not likely to be an effective means to regulate the passage of therapies from the realm of research and innovation to accepted practice.

THE PEER REVIEW SYSTEM

The standards promulgated by the JCAH for hospital medical staffs require that the practices of members of the medical staff be reviewed, evaluated, and monitored on a regular basis.[43] The standards specify that reviews be undertaken of surgical cases, drug therapy practice and drug utilization, blood usage, and the use of antibiotics.

Although the precise manner by which these standards are judged is left to the hospitals, committees usually perform the reviews. For example, the review of surgical cases is generally conducted by a Tissue Committee. The JCAH standards indicate that surgical case review is conducted for each case and that all cases are evaluated in which a major discrepancy exists between the preoperative and postoperative diagnoses. No review of surgical technique is prescribed or suggested. Such review, however, can be undertaken at the discretion of the hospital and its medical staff.

Similarly, the pharmacy and therapeutics function includes:

1. Review of the appropriateness of empiric and therapeutic use of drugs through an analysis of individual or aggregate patterns of drug practice
2. Development or approval of policies and procedures relating to the selection, distribution, handling, use, and administration of drugs and diagnostic testing materials

   . . .

5. Evaluation and, if appropriate, the approval of protocols concerned with the use of investigational or experimental drugs.[44]

The JCAH standards provide an overall quality assurance program for important aspects of patient care designed to enhance that care through ongoing objective assessment. Additionally, the standards mandate the development, adoption, and periodic review of medical staff bylaws—by which the medical staff can establish a framework of self-government—and a means of accountability to the governing body.

The standards promulgated by the JCAH and the precise manner in which hospitals arrange their internal governance in response thereto creates a formal system of internal control over all activities for which hospitals are responsible. This system, largely through the medical staff and its committees, constitutes a regulatory framework for directing and overseeing all medical practices. One consequence of this highly ordered and statutorily mandated system of internal regulation is that accreditation standards create a duty on the part of hospitals to review innovative therapies.[45]

Several factors may influence the effectiveness of medical staff peer review as a regulatory mechanism for controlling innovative practices and their adoption as standard medical practice. To the extent that the reviews are conducted by peers, physicians may be induced to make appropriate decisions regarding benefit-risk ratios and consent procedures. Failure to do so may lead to both formal and informal sanctions (such as loss of referrals). And since the review committees generally include members of the hospital administration in addition to members of the medical staff, the opportunity exists to discuss concerns for organizational integrity and risk management as well as professional concerns regarding creative activity and expanding knowledge.

However, the peer review activities may be limited by the fact that not all practices that should be reviewed will come to the review committees' attention. Further, the criteria and standards applied may not coincide with those of the general medical community or society.

Despite these limitations, and given the fact that many innovative practices are undertaken by individual physicians solely for the benefit of their patients and represent relatively insubstantial departures from prevailing practices, hospital peer review committees can exercise a useful regulatory function without unduly burdening the creativity of well-meaning physicians. Such reviews, appropriately conducted, can safeguard the well-being of patients and minimize the risks of the innovative practices.

THE IRB MODEL

Federal regulations require that all research involving human subjects conducted by HHS or funded in whole or in part by a grant, contract, cooperative agreement, or fellowship from HHS be reviewed by an Institutional Review Board (IRB) established at each institution in which the research is conducted.[46] The regulations define research as "a systematic investigation designed to develop or contribute to generalizable knowledge."[47] The regulations further specify minimum requirements for the composition of IRBs[48] and require that each institution engaged in research covered by the regulations must file a written assurance to the secretary of HHS that "it will comply with the requirements set forth in [the] regulations."[49]

In order to approve research covered by the regulations, IRBs must determine that a number of requirements are satisfied.

1. Risks to subjects are minimized.
2. Risks to subjects are reasonable in relation to anticipated benefits, if any, to subjects, and the importance of the knowledge that may reasonably be expected to result.
3. Selection of subjects is equitable.
4. Informed consent will be sought from each prospective subject or the subject's legally authorized representative.

    . . .

6. Where appropriate, the research plan makes adequate provision for monitoring the data collected to insure the safety of subjects.[50]

Other sections of the regulations specify, in detail, the requirements for informed consent and the manner in which informed consent must be documented.[51]

In addition to the regulations issued by HHS, the FDA issued a parallel set of regulations.[52] The FDA regulations require review and approval by an IRB for any experiment that involves a test article, that needs one or more human subjects (either patients or healthy persons), and that is subject to the requirements for prior submission to the FDA.[53] Such review is also required for any experiments whose results will be submitted later to, or held for inspection by, the FDA. A few differences exist between the FDA and HHS regulations arising from the differences in the underlying legislative mandates. However, the procedures and criteria set out in the FDA and HHS regulations are substantially similar.

Although the HHS regulations apply only to research conducted or funded by HHS, they are viewed as the norm for reviewing human research proposals in the United States. Therefore, they have been adopted by most, if not all, private granting agencies. Additionally, all or nearly all institutions in which research is conducted use the standards and procedures set forth in the HHS regulations as the basis for reviewing all human research proposals regardless of funding. In effect, then, the HHS regulations define the accepted standards and norms for reviewing and approving research involving human subjects.

The question arises whether all intentional deviations from standard practice should be subject to the review requirements that are applied to activities formally labeled "research." Authorities differ. Levine states that innovative therapy should be reviewed and conducted as if it were research.[54] He asserts that innovative therapy is similar to "therapeutic" research, that is, research in which some patient benefit is intended together with the enhancement of knowledge. He further argues that the systematic evaluation of innovative practices during the innovation process is likely to result in fewer ineffective practices established as customary practice.

Robertson agrees in theory with Levine—that treating innovative practices as research for the purposes of prior review will probably improve the reliability of data from which judgments of their safety and efficacy can be made.[55] However, Robertson cites a number of problems that arise in requiring prior IRB approval for all innovative practices. These problems relate to the constitutionality, scope, administrative cost, and implementation of such a requirement.

Robertson would not treat all innovative practices as research. For many innovative practices, patient benefit is the sole intent. Others are undertaken primarily to benefit patients and secondarily to develop new knowledge. Provided that decisions to undertake innovative practices are not influenced by interests contrary to patients' needs, they need not be treated as research. Rather, only those activities in which the primary intent is to generate new knowledge beyond the patients' needs should be identified as research for which IRB approval would be required.

An additional issue raised by Robertson is the assumption that IRB review would lead to tighter control over the uses of innovative therapies without more evidence that individual uses of innovative therapy can be developed through controlled clinical trials.[56] On a practical basis, this would appear to be unlikely.

The National Commission observed:

> Radically new procedures . . . should . . . be made the object of formal research at an early stage in order to determine whether they are safe and effective. Thus, it is the responsibility of medical practice committees, for example, to insist that a major innovation be incorporated into a formal research project.[57]

This observation was not, however, incorporated into the HHS regulations. Therefore, there is presently no federal regulation that classifies innovative therapies as research nor is there any regulation that requires that such practices be conducted according to the norms of research unless they are included in a formal research protocol.

Is the IRB model a useful model for regulating whether and when innovative practices should become accepted practices? No simple answer can be given. Rather, it would appear that the use of the IRB model would depend on the nature, scope, complexity, and potential risks of the proposed practices.

Innovative practices undertaken for the sole benefit of particular patients, although perhaps deserving of some control, should not be subject to a formal IRB approval procedure. To do so would create an impossible case load for IRBs and would be administratively burdensome as well as very costly. To the detriment of the patient, it might also delay needed therapy.

By contrast, innovative therapies that represent major departures from standard practice, utilize substantial resources, raise issues of resource allocation, and are associated with significant risks should be subject to review using an IRB model. It is doubtful that such activities would be conducted by individual practitioners on a case-by-case basis. It is further doubtful that they would be undertaken without at least some intent to generate new knowledge beyond that needed for the care of the particular patients involved.

THE FDA MODEL

The process by which new drugs are approved for general use involves an orderly progression of experiments beginning with *in vitro* and animal studies. Testing in human beings occurs after review of animal (preclinical) studies indicates a particular agent may be useful in the diagnosis or treatment of a particular disorder. The stages of testing in human beings include studies of toxicology, pharmacology, and the spectrum of clinical activity, and assessments of efficacy (benefits) and safety (risks). The information required for the studies and assessments are generated from formal research activities designed to yield statistically valid data. As noted previously, the use of human subjects in these studies must follow the procedures specified in formal FDA regulations.

As stated by Levine: "The FDA model demands that certain criteria be met before a potential therapeutic innovation might even be considered an acceptable research activity."[58] These include the determination from animal studies of the appropriateness of the drug for use in humans, the initial determination of toxicity in humans, and the controlled administration of the drug to individuals having the disease for which the drug is intended.

With certain limitations, these criteria could be applied to innovative practices other than the use of new drugs, such as proposed new surgical techniques, innovative diagnostic procedures, and imaging studies. The limitations include the practical inability or inappropriateness of subjecting certain practices to preclinical testing or to the type of incremental dose-toxicity studies that characterize initial clinical testing. One cannot incrementally increase a dose of surgery. The limitations do not, however, diminish the usefulness of the model for assessing a variety of medical innovations and their acceptance as standard practice.

The problem that arises concerns the process by which the model can be implemented. Possibilities range from the establishment of a new national organization to review all innovative practices to the creation of review groups in all institutions where such activities occur. Either alternative, and others that might come about, create administrative problems and generate substantial costs.

The FDA model is useful for defining criteria and standards according to which innovative practices may be reviewed and approved. The implementation of the model does not appear to be practical except for major activities such as organ transplantation.

THE SPECIAL REVIEW BOARD—
REGULATION OF ORGAN TRANSPLANTATION

Certain innovative practices by their very nature involve expensive technologies and raise issues of societal values, ethics, financing, and availability. Of these, the most dramatic is organ transplantation. Because of the range of issues involved, the regulation of organ transplantation—and similar complex and expensive new practices—should differ significantly from proposed regulatory processes that might be applied to other innovative practices.

Since organ transplantation is undertaken not solely for the benefit of a patient, but also with the intent to generate new knowledge beyond that needed for the care of a particular patient, it should be regulated as research. Thus, organ transplantation should be subject to the review procedures mandated for all research involving human subjects. In addition, because of the social, ethical, financial, and resource allocation issues involved, it is appropriate that organ transplantation be subject to a special review process. A group composed of respected authorities representing a spectrum of disciplines, as well as the community at large, should perform this review process. A proposal of this type has been put forth by the Massachusetts Task Force on Organ Transplantation.[59]

A major question with respect to implementing a review process of this type is whether it should be done on a local, state, or national level. The scope of the issues extends beyond the political boundaries of individual institutions and communities. Thus, local review is not appropriate. Review on a statewide level—the current procedure—provides for greater participation of interested and affected parties. However, since the societal and ethical issues, as well as those relating to resource allocation, are national in scope, a review process at a national level would be most appropriate. Review at a national level would allow for the widest possible discussion of the issues, and would offer the best chance that the clinical, social, ethical, and economic consequences of organ transplantation would be fully studied and reviewed, resulting in a national consensus.

PROPOSAL

Depending on the activity involved, this author proposes that the assessment of innovative practices and their acceptance as standard medical practice be accomplished at either of two levels: one level is the local hospital level and uses the peer review system that currently exists in all hospitals; the other level is national.

Regardless of the level at which the assessment is undertaken, several considerations must be addressed:

1. Are there standards for the assessment that can be generally agreed upon and that are appropriate for the determination?
2. Who undertakes the assessment?
3. Where do the data for assessment come from, and who has the burden of supplying the data?
4. Is the burden of the assessment reasonable in relation to the practice being scrutinized? That is, what is the cost-benefit ratio of subjecting a practice to such an assessment?
5. Is the assessment prospective or retrospective?
6. Is the assessment realistic, and will it be credible to the medical community?

How, on a practical basis, can the hospital peer review system work to regulate innovative practice and assess its acceptability as standard practice? This can be answered by referring back to the considerations listed above.

1. The standards or criteria for the assessment could be adopted from those used by the FDA—safety and efficacy.

    Physicians seeking to undertake new practices would have to justify their use on some basis—animal studies, clinical observations, etc.

Physicians proposing that new practices be considered acceptable would be expected to produce data attesting to the benefits and harms in relation to the disease for which they are to be used.

2. The assessment would be done by members of the medical staffs in the course of their staff committee work. This chapter neither proposes creating a new committee specifically for this purpose nor recommends that it be the role of the IRBs. IRBs are not constituted or equipped to handle this type of assessment.

Is it burdensome to the medical staffs? Of course it is. But whether or not medical staffs have watched over their colleagues in the past is not a reason for not doing so now. The environment surrounding medical practice would appear almost to require that physicians assume this responsibility.

3. The responsibility for providing the data would be that of the physician seeking to pursue the particular practice.

4. To the extent that the purpose of peer regulation is to protect patients and, incidentally, to promote more rational medical practice, the cost-benefit ratio of subjecting a practice to such an assessment would appear always to be favorable.

5. Where possible, the reviews would be prospective. Recognizing that many practices currently exist that are of marginal or questionable utility, over time these could eventually be assessed. It would be analogous to the FDA having to go back and assess the efficacy of drugs approved before the 1962 amendments. It would not be inappropriate for physicians to have to justify and be accountable for their practices. They will grumble, but they should not object violently if this is being conducted by their own peers in their local institutions.

6. A local regulatory process of this type would in time gain the support of physicians and be viewed as credible and useful. Given all the pressures physicians are now facing, they are more receptive to the need for accountability and have a greater willingness to undertake critical peer review.

The process would be enhanced measurably by the development of a national reporting system so that physicians throughout the country could expand their data base both in relation to the scope of existing practices and as possible bases for accepting new practices.

Would local peer review be adequate to regulate technology-intensive practices—such as organ transplantation or treatment of acute leukemia—that are costly, extreme, life-saving, and for which there may be no existing alternative therapies? This author thinks not because innovative therapies of this type represent major departures from standard practice, utilize substantial resources, raise issues of resource allocations, and are associated with significant risks.

The conduct of these practices should be reviewed as research activities subject to all IRB safeguards. Most important, for purposes of assessing whether such practices merit acceptability into standard medical practice, data from studies and activities around the country should be submitted to a national review group established by HHS and comprised of government, private sector, and public representatives.

The responsibility for generating and providing the data for the review belongs to the proponents of the practice—be it organ transplantation or some other activity.

The criteria for assessment would be the benefits and harms of the practice in relation to the disease to which the practice is being applied.

The reviews should always be prospective.

In essence, this chapter proposes a single review process applicable to *all* innovative practices, utilizing substantially similar criteria.

The major decision is whether a particular practice merits review at a national or a local level. It would seem that very few practices need an extensive national network.

The burdens of such a review would be the necessary cost and administrative support. The benefits would be a more orderly and rational process for bringing new technologies and practices into standard medical practice. This would influence a number of key areas, including:

1. Tort liability—by providing better standards for accepted medical practice
2. Reimbursement—by providing a rational basis for payers to authorize payment
3. Most important, protection of patients while promoting their interest.

Notes

1. National Commission for the Protection of Human Subjects of Biomedical and Behavioral Research, The Belmont Report: Ethical Principles and Guidelines for the Protection of Human Subjects of Research (DHEW Pub. No. (OS) 78-0012) (1978) [hereinafter referred to as The Belmont Report].

2. The Commission was established by Congress in Title II, Part A, §201(A) of the National Service Award Act of 1974, Pub. L. No. 93-348, 88 Stat. 142. The purpose of the Commission was to conduct a comprehensive investigation and study to identify the basic ethical principles that should underlie the conduct of biomedical and behavioral research, evaluate existing guidelines for the protection of human subjects, and make appropriate recommendations to the secretary of Health, Education, and Welfare concerning further steps, if any, to be taken. *Id.* at §202(a)(1)(A).

3. THE BELMONT REPORT, *supra* note 1, at 2–3.

4. Tvedt v. Haugen, 70 N.D. 338, 294 N.W. 183, 187 (1940).

5. Levine, *The Boundaries Between Biomedical or Behavioral Research and the Accepted and Routine Practice of Medicine,* THE BELMONT REPORT, Appendix I, Paper No. 1 (DHEW Pub. No. (OS) 78-0013) (1978).

6. W. L. PROSSER, THE LAW OF TORTS (West Publishing Co., St. Paul, Minn.) (4th ed. 1982) at 143.

7. 313 Mo. 213, 281 S.W. 682 (1926). Defendant physician treated his patient for rectal ulcerations by injecting "a weak solution of iodine echinacea and also genlose," a method of treatment that had been distinctly disapproved by the medical profession.

8. 281 S.W. at 685.

9. 83 Wash. 2d 514, 519 P.2d 981 (1974).

10. Texas & Pacific Railway v. Behymer, 189 U.S. 468, 470, 23 S.Ct. 622, 623, 47 L.Ed. 905 (1903).

11. T. L. BEAUCHAMP, J. E. CHILDRESS, PRINCIPLES OF BIOMEDICAL ETHICS (Oxford University Press, New York, N.Y.) (2d ed. 1983) at 169.

12. Schloendorff v. Society of New York Hospital, 211 N.Y. 125, 106 N.E. 92, 93 (1914).

13. 8 Cal.3d 229, 502 P.2d 1, 104 Cal. Rptr. 505 (1972). Defendant surgeon operated on a patient for a duodenal ulcer without explaining the risks of surgery. When injuries occurred, the patient brought suit claiming negligence for the physician's failure to disclose the risks, such disclosure being a necessary prerequisite to the patient's informed decision.

14. *Id.* at 10.

15. 186 Kan. 393, 350 P.2d 1093 (1960). Plaintiff charged negligence against the defendant physician for excessive irradiation treatments, the risks of which had not been adequately disclosed.

16. *Id.* at 1106.

17. 464 F.2d 772 (D.C. Cir. 1972). Patient fell after what appeared to be a successful laminectomy, and thereafter suffered from bowel paralysis and urinary incontinence. The patient charged, among other things, that the physician did not inform him of the risks of serious disability inherent in a laminectomy.

18. *Id.* at 786–87.

19. *Supra* note 13, at 10.

20. The Joint Commission on Accreditation of Hospitals (JCAH) was founded

in 1951 by the American College of Surgeons, the American College of Physicians, the American Hospital Association, the American Medical Association, and the Canadian Medical Association. Since then, the Canadian Medical Association has left JCAH and the American Dental Association has joined. JCAH's tasks include reviewing hospital survey reports, granting accreditation based on these reports, and continuously reviewing the standards. Revisions in standards are based on input from specialty organizations and experts, feedback from surveyors, and information from health care professionals.

21. AMH/85: ACCREDITATION MANUAL FOR HOSPITALS (Joint Commission on Accreditation of Hospitals, Chicago, Ill.) (1985) at 84.

22. NATIONAL COMMISSION FOR THE PROTECTION OF HUMAN SUBJECTS OF BIOMEDICAL AND BEHAVIORAL RESEARCH, REPORT AND RECOMMENDATIONS: RESEARCH INVOLVING CHILDREN (DHEW Pub. No. (OS) 77-0004) (1977); REPORT AND RECOMMENDATIONS: RESEARCH INVOLVING THOSE INSTITUTIONALIZED AS MENTALLY INFIRM (DHEW Pub. No. (OS) 77-0006) (1978).

23. Levine, *supra* note 5, at 14.

24. C. BERNARD, AN INTRODUCTION TO THE STUDY OF EXPERIMENTAL MEDICINE (Dover Publications, Inc., New York, N.Y.) (Reprinted 1957).

25. Levine, *Clarifying the Concepts of Research Ethics,* HASTINGS CENTER REPORT 9 (6):21, 22 (June 1979).

26. THE BELMONT REPORT, *supra* note 1, at 3.

27. Levine, *supra* note 5, at 6–7.

28. Norton, *When Does an Experimental Innovative Procedure Become an Accepted Procedure?* in MEDICAL EXPERIMENTATION: ITS LEGAL AND ETHICAL ASPECTS (A. Carni, ed.) (Turtledove Publishing, Ramat Gan, Israel) 105 (1978) at 107.

29. Ladimer, *Ethical and Legal Aspects of Medical Research on Human Beings,* JOURNAL OF PUBLIC LAW 3:467 (1954).

30. Food, Drug, and Cosmetic Act, Pub. L. 75-717, 52 Stat. 1040 (1938) *as amended, codified* at 21 U.S.C. §301 *et seq.*

31. 21 C.F.R. §312.1(a)(2) (1977).

32. REPORT OF THE MASSACHUSETTS TASK FORCE ON ORGAN TRANSPLANTATION, reprinted in part in LAW, MEDICINE & HEALTH CARE 13:8–26 (February 1985); reprinted in Part II of this volume.

33. Moskowitz, *et al. Biomedical Innovation: The Challenge and the Process,* in BIOMEDICAL INNOVATION (R. B. Roberts, *et al.*, eds.) (MIT Press, Cambridge, Mass.) (1981) at 2.

34. *Id.*

35. 95 Eng. Rep. 860 (1767). Defendant physician was found liable for harm sustained by the patient resulting from the use of a novel device to treat a broken leg.

36. *Id.* at 862–63.

37. 60 Barb. 488 (N.Y. Sup. Ct. 1871), *rev'd on other grounds,* 50 N.Y. 696 (1872).

38. *Id.* at 514.

39. Fortner v. Koch, 272 Mich. 273, 261 N.W. 762 (1935). Defendant physician injected his syphilitic patient with an antitoxin solution instead of pursuing normally used treatments.

40. Miller v. Toles, 183 Mich. 252, 150 N.W. 118 (1914). Defendant physician attempted to save the plaintiff's foot from amputation by injections of an experimental solution.

41. Fiorentino v. Wenger, 19 N.Y.2d 407, 280 N.Y.S.2d 373 (1967). Plaintiff was injured from a private physician's use of a "spinal jack" operation to correct a curvature of the spine.

42. Robertson, *Legal Implications of the Boundaries Between Biomedical Research Involving Human Subjects and the Accepted or Routine Practice of Medicine*, THE BELMONT REPORT, Appendix II, Paper No. 16 (DHEW Pub. No. (OS) 78-0014) (1978) at 20.

43. *Supra* note 21.

44. *Id.* at 86.

45. Cowan, Bertsch, *Innovative Therapy: The Responsibility of Hospitals*, JOURNAL OF LEGAL MEDICINE 5:219 (1984) at 246.

46. 45 C.F.R. §46.101 *et seq.*

47. 45 C.F.R. §46.102(e).

48. 45 C.F.R. §46.107.

49. 45 C.F.R. §46.103(e).

50. 45 C.F.R. §46.111.

51. 45 C.F.R. §§46.116, 46.117.

52. 21 U.S.C. §301 *et seq.*

53. 21 C.F.R. §§50.3, 56.103.

54. Levine, *supra* note 5.

55. Robertson, *supra* note 42.

56. *Id.*

57. THE BELMONT REPORT, *supra* note 1, at 3–4.

58. Levine, *supra* note 5, at 37.

59. *Supra* note 32.

10

The Food and Drug Administration's Perspective on Organ Transplantation

Frank E. Young

The perspective of the Food and Drug Administration (FDA) can best be described as that of an onlooker, albeit a fascinated one, when it comes to the legal and ethical issues surrounding live organ transplantation. Although the FDA regulates most of the products associated with organ transplants, it does not regulate the organ itself—its quality and integrity—or the transplantation procedures.

Organ transplantation is a remarkable product of science and technology. The technologies associated with transplantation are undergoing a phenomenal evolution and growth. These technologies are developing from—and combining with—the innovations flowing from biotechnology and other high technologies that include organ-controlling and microprocessor-assisted devices. The technologies are being furthered by the discoveries of new immunosuppressants and new surgical techniques.

WHAT THE FDA DOES AND DOES NOT REGULATE

Organ transplantation covers a complex of entities: (1) artificial devices; (2) devices made in part with treated, nonliving tissues or organs; (3) devices made in part of living tissues, which, for lack of a better term, one might call hybrids; and (4) whole, living organs.

As mentioned earlier, although the FDA does not regulate live organs for transplantation, it does regulate almost everything else connected with the organ transplantation procedure. This includes the human leucocyte antigen (HLA) reagents used in tissue typing the organs for the major histocompatibility complex antigens, as well as for the experimental use of monoclonal antilymphocyte globulin (ALG), used to fight the graft rejection phenomenon. The FDA also regulates most radiological, medical-device, biological, and drug products associated with transplants, including:

—Oxygen gas cylinders
—Anesthetics and anesthesia machines
—Antibiotics and anticoagulants
—Immunosuppressants
—Saline and dextrose intravenous solutions
—Gauzes, bandages, sutures, etc.
—Catheter trays
—Irrigation trays and syringes.

Perhaps one area in which the FDA approaches organ regulation is in its regulation of blood—but there are some major differences between the regulation of blood, which is a tissue, and live organs. Modern blood transfusion procedures date back to World War II—over forty years ago. The passage of that much time has permitted the evolution of widely accepted and precise standards. In addition, scientific advances have permitted an extension of the allowable storage time for the red cells and platelets to forty-two and seven days, respectively. This allows an opportunity for quality control, including testing, that is not now possible with living whole organs.

The FDA has also been directly involved in the regulation of other tissues since the early 1970s when it exercised jurisdiction over the review and approval of investigational new drug applications for human umbilical cord arteries and veins intended as vascular grafts. Since those vessels were treated chemically, they were not considered living tissues. For this reason, the FDA re-evaluated the status of those products after the medical device amendments became law and the Bureau of Medical Devices was established.[1] Those investigational applications were transferred to the Bureau in 1978 following agreement within the FDA that they fit the definition of a device, and that they should be regulated under the device amendments.

"Traditional" commercial manufacturers who are investigating processed tissues or intend to market processed tissues have also been regulated by the FDA; however, no tissue bank making tissues available for clinical use has been regulated. Tissue banks have been informed that, while the transport media they prepare for their own use are devices as defined in the Food, Drug, and Cosmetic Act and are subject to the misbranding and adulteration provisions of the Act,[2] the banks themselves are not subject to active regulation unless they make the transport solutions available to other users.[3]

The FDA must currently focus on the issue of what types of processing bring a product under FDA jurisdiction. The Agency must also apply consistent logic to the regulation of those entities for transplantation that it does regulate.

The recent incident involving what is called the "Phoenix Artificial Heart"[4] raised some striking issues. In this incident, a clinically untested artificial heart was implanted in a patient as an emergency interim measure following an unsuccessful transplant procedure. In the context of that situation, the procedures followed in the decision-making process appear to have been carefully and properly evaluated. However, the FDA has concluded that it has a responsibility to address the possibility that similar incidents will occur in the future and to provide guidance to facilitate decision making under such conditions.

Extensive study of the decision-making process is needed, and the FDA is doing just that. First, it has concluded that the emergency decision process most appropriately begins with the physician, based on his or her familiarity and empathy with the patient. Thus, the physician and the hospital administration, in consonance with the family and appropriate institutional officials, are best able to make an emergency decision. In an emergency, the FDA will not intervene.

Before the crisis arises, however, the FDA does need to be involved to provide guidance that can be routinely followed, sparing participants wasted time figuring out what steps to take. The Agency, therefore, is working to develop—for clinicians, hospital administrators, Institutional Review Boards, and other appropriate individuals—an explanation of the considerations that go into deciding that an emergency situation exists and what to do when one occurs. We cannot evade this problem simply because it raises difficult questions. A policy will be developed to meet this new challenge.[4]

THE FDA'S APPROACH TO REGULATION

An explanation of the FDA's position regarding organ transplantation requires some background about the nature of the field as well as about the FDA's philosophy and strategy in the areas that it does regulate, including those affected by technological advancement. The basic responsibility of the Food and Drug Administration has always been to ensure the safety and efficacy of the products it regulates. This regulation involves several specific steps that are briefly reviewed here to demonstrate the difficulties the FDA would encounter were it to attempt to regulate organs—at best, a hypothetical case. It should be re-emphasized that the FDA currently does not regulate organs for transplant, nor does it have any immediate plans to do so.

One extremely useful approach to the regulation of new technology has been to conduct intramural research programs related to the development, manufacture, testing, and use of new products. Such studies often provide the basis for safety and efficacy standards of new products. At present, the FDA has ongoing research directly related to transplantation problems, specifically in the areas of biotechnology and cytomegalovirus (CMV) research. Although such research can be extremely useful, at this time the FDA is not able to contemplate large research programs related to organ transplantation. Without an extensive intramural research program, how would the FDA conduct the development of safety and efficacy standards for organ transplants?

A related problem is quality control. A standard procedure used for many regulated products is the testing of samples. Some biological products—polio vaccine, for example—are released on a lot-by-lot basis after testing. The application of this procedure to organ and tissue transplantation would have significant limitations. How would one randomly sample an organ for transplant?

Another aspect of the FDA's traditional regulatory approach—licensing and inspecting the physical facility where a product is manufactured—is problematic when applied to organ transplantation. It is clear that for organ transplants the source facility and the transplantation facility are almost inevitably hospitals or medical centers. It is clear that live organ transplants simply would not fit readily or easily into the regulatory scheme the Agency utilizes to regulate a wide range of products.

Much more important, perhaps, is the fact that transplantation as it is currently practiced is adequately regulated on a voluntary basis by the parties involved; there has been no need for the FDA to do what is already effectively accomplished in the private sector. Put another way, there is no need for the FDA figuratively to appear at the door with the message, "I'm from the federal government, and I'm here to help you."

Instead, by taking the initiative, industry and the medical community have helped the science of transplantation, the practice of medicine, and the transplant patient. So far, in the field of organ transplantation, this author believes that the public, the industry, and the biomedical community have created and maintained a good course in optimizing safety and benefits. This course can continue. Certainly, the FDA is more than willing to provide support by helping in the development of guidelines or in any other appropriate way. However, the FDA will avoid heavy-handed regulation.

Already thousands of kidneys and corneas are transplanted each year, not to mention the more publicly visible but smaller numbers of hearts and livers. The individual health providers are in a much better position than the FDA to assess how well equipped the current system is for handling the anticipated increased volume and stress. It is critically important that health professionals and health specialty organization professionals make every effort to continue to establish and support voluntary guidelines and standards as the numbers of transplantation centers and procedures increase.

Congressional Action

Congress recognizes the advances made in recent years as well as the problems related to the short time that organs can be preserved, the shortage of organs, and the need for help in increasing organ donations.

The Organ Procurement and Transplantation Act, signed into law by President Reagan on October 19, 1984, includes a provision requiring the secretary of Health and Human Services to consult with the commissioner of the Food and Drug Administration in preparing an evaluation of the scientific and clinical status of transplantation. Nothing in the Act deals directly with aspects of quality assurance, that is, with regulating the way in which organs are treated from the time of harvesting to the time of transplantation.

The impending "explosion" in the demand for human tissues and organs for transplantation will no doubt result in the need for greater concentration on the quality control aspects of harvesting, processing, preserving, and transporting human tissues and organs. These are formidable and interesting tasks, and the determination and ingenuity already demonstrated by the medical community will no doubt continue. Certainly, those efforts will have the support of the FDA and the Department of Health and Human Services.

Critical elements affecting future work in this field are information, quality, and support. Authoritative information is needed on exactly what tissues and organs are being transplanted, with what frequency, and what quality assurance difficulties are associated with their procurement, processing, storage, and transportation. Also needed is a thorough understanding of the quality control deficiencies that can impair the success of organ or tissue transplantation. In addition, industry and trade organization support for voluntary compliance with guidelines and standards will be an important influence.

Organ transplantation is an imperfect replacement technique. If it were within our capability to reset the genetic forces that drive regeneration, we would have the ideal organ replacement solution. Every basic biology textbook poses for us tantalizing examples of regeneration in the primitive planaria and the starfish. However, organ regeneration in higher animals is beyond our reach. We have opted for the next best solution: surgical removal of the crippled organ and replacement of it with a living organ from another human body. In this process we are indebted to others for the "donated organ." Accordingly, we must be ever mindful of the ethical considerations that relate to organ transplants.

Biomedical science has worked with the transplantation process and has steadily improved it. There is always the hope of mastering the phenomena of rejection, immune tolerance, histocompatibility, and immune suppression. Perhaps today's fantasies will be tomorrow's realities. Perhaps someone will inject monoclonal "silver bullets" that will find and destroy unseen target cells that orchestrate the rejection phenomenon in transplant patients, leaving everything unscathed except the target cells. Perhaps someone will develop a high-technology fourth generation wonder drug—an immunosuppressant that selectively suppresses the histocompatibility immune function, leaving the other body defense systems intact. Maybe someone will develop a transplant growth factor or hormone to ensure the fusion of the transplant graft to the host tissues. Alternatively, we may be able to repopulate cells or organelles in existing tissue. Even multicellular structures such as islets of Langerhans may be transplanted routinely in the not-too-distant future.

Whatever the future brings, the continuing cross-fertilization of health care professionals, educators, and government will surely provide a sound basic germ plasm on which to build the future of organ transplantation.

Notes

1. Medical Device Amendments of 1976, Pub. L. No. 94-295, 90 Stat. 539 (1976).
2. 21 U.S.C.A §321(h), 351, 352 (1982 and West Supp. 1986).
3. 21 U.S.C. §331(a) (1982).
4. *Notice of Availability of Guidance for the Emergency Use of Unapproved Medical Devices*, FEDERAL REGISTER 50(204):42866 (October 27, 1986).

11

Products Liability and Artificial and Human Organ Transplantation— A Legal Overview

Richard E. Nolan
Whitney L. Schmidt

> The dying heart was an ugly yellowish color when Dr. William DeVries finally cut it loose, tore it out of the mercurochrome-stained chest cavity, and put it to one side. For the next three hours, while a nearby heart-lung bypass machine kept the unconscious patient alive—and while a tape in the background eerily played Mendelssohn and Vivaldi—DeVries' sure hands carefully stitched into place a grapefruit-size gadget made of aluminum and polyurethane. At 12:50 P.M. . . . the Jarvik-7 artificial heart newly sewn inside William J. Schroeder began beating steadily, 70 beats to the minute. When Schroeder opened his eyes 3½ hours later in the intensive-care unit, DeVries bent over his patient and whispered assurances, "The operation is all through. You did really well. Everything is perfect."[1]

This miraculous extension of life by organ transplantation represents the very frontier of medicine, science, and technology. Organ transplantation, not only of human organs but also of mechanical substitutes, represents an awesome and tangible product of the powers of science and technology.[2]

Developing concurrently with the remarkable achievements of modern science and technology has been a similarly profound legal revolution in the body of law commonly known as products liability. The legal developments surrounding organ transplantation have their origins in established legal concepts from which the search for solutions to problems arising from technological improvement is rooted. Organ transplantation represents a new medical frontier, while it presages new and continued refinements to established products liability concepts developed in recent decades.[3]

This chapter reviews the theories available to an individual who alleges an injury caused by a defective product and sets forth the elements necessary to establish a cause of action on any of the principal products liability theories. After examining these theories of recovery, the focus shifts to the potential liability of the manufacturer of an artificial organ. The liability of a physician and hospital with respect to human and artificial organ transplants is then examined. This chapter then reviews the various products liability defenses available in the organ transplant setting. An analysis and comment on the future of products liability and organ transplantation concludes this legal overview.

THEORIES OF PRODUCTS LIABILITY

A person who alleges an injury caused by a defective product may elect to base his legal cause of action on any of the three principal products liability theories: negligence, warranty, or strict liability.[4] These bases of liability are governed by state, rather than federal, law and there are variations, in some instances significant, in their application by the courts of the various states.

The legal doctrine of negligence may be defined in terms of the duty of the person of "ordinary sense" to recognize that he must use "ordinary care and skill."[5] Elaborating upon this basic definition, the *Restatement (Second) of Torts* defines negligence as "conduct which falls below the standard established by law for the protection of others against unreasonable risk of harm."[6] Proceeding on a negligence theory in a products liability case requires an injured party to show that a specific defendant failed to exercise proper care in designing, testing, manufacturing, or marketing the allegedly defective product and that, as a reasonably foreseeable and proximate result of such negligence, the plaintiff suffered injury.[7]

Historically, a purchaser of goods has also been able to claim a breach of warranty against the immediate seller on the grounds that the goods were not as they were contracted to be. If a buyer could show that a seller made representations either expressly or impliedly about the quality of the goods that turned out to be inaccurate, the buyer would be allowed to recover appropriate damages without establishing any negligence by the seller. In early common law, the rule of *caveat emptor,* or "buyer beware," prevailed. Changing social and economic considerations resulted in warranties, but only in situations where there had been an actual sale contract.[8] Given the contractual underpinnings of this cause of action, courts were reluctant to expand recovery for breach of warranty against anyone with whom the plaintiff had not directly contracted. The term "privity" was given to the requirement that the parties have had actual dealings among themselves.[9] As the common law developed, however, certain aspects of tort law were grafted onto warranty law. As a result of this commingling of tort and contract law with breach of warranty actions, the privity requirement gradually eroded.[10] Today, most states allow a suit for breach of warranty against a seller by the ultimate consumer—any individual, other than the immediate purchaser, who logically would have been expected to use the product.[11]

An injured party proceeding on a warranty theory of liability need not prove negligence. Instead, it must be shown that the manufacturer or seller breached an express or implied promise that the product was both free from defects and fit for the ordinary purposes in which such products are customarily used.

The principles of the breach of warranty cause of action, as a separate and independent products liability theory, are well illustrated by the leading case of *Crocker* v. *Winthrop Laboratories* decided by the Texas Supreme Court.[12] The defendant in *Crocker*, a drug company, manufactured a pain-killing drug called Talwin. At the time of the initial sales of the product, the company believed that the drug was nonaddictive, and mentioned this nonaddictive quality in the accompanying medical literature. A doctor prescribed Talwin to the plaintiff, who developed an addiction which ultimately led to his death. The court held the defendant drug company liable, stating:

> Whatever the danger and state of medical knowledge, and however rare the susceptibility of the user, when the drug company positively and specifically represents its product to be free and safe from all dangers of addiction, and when the treating physician relies upon that representation, the drug company is liable when the representation proves to be false and harm results.[13]

Many states have evolved a further basis for liability on the part of the manufacturer of a defective product. This is known as "strict liability in tort."[14] The theory behind strict liability is that it is better social policy for manufacturers, rather than injured consumers, to bear the economic burdens, through products liability insurance or otherwise, for any injuries caused by defective products.

In essence, strict liability is the trial of a product rather than of a defendant.[15] If a product is not reasonably safe when it leaves the control or custody of the manufacturer or distributor, liability follows.[16] The *Restatement (Second) of Torts* §402A defines strict liability as follows:

Special Liability of Seller of Product for Physical Harm to User or Consumer

(1) One who sells any product in a defective condition unreasonably dangerous to the user or consumer or to his property is subject to liability for physical harm thereby caused to the ultimate user or consumer, or to his property, if
  (a) the seller is engaged in the business of selling such a product, and
  (b) it is expected to and does reach the user or consumer without substantial change in the condition in which it is sold.

(2) The rule stated in Subsection (1) applies although
  (a) the seller has exercised all possible care in the preparation and sale of his product, and
  (b) the user or consumer has not bought the product from or entered into any contractual relation with the seller.[17]

Today, §402A has "literally swept the country." A substantial majority of American jurisdictions adopted the general theory of strict tort liability, if not the precise language of §402A, for defective products.[18] However, as discussed in detail subsequently, there is a significant limitation on the scope of §402A with regard to products such as prescription drugs, which by their very nature are unavoidably dangerous.

Under the strict liability theory, an injured party need not prove negligence or any breach of warranty, but rather must establish only that the product causing the injury was defective when it left the control of the manufacturer or the seller.[19] Generally, there are four fundamental types of product defects.[20] The first may be considered the "manufacturing defect." An improperly manufactured product is one that has been incorrectly manufactured or assembled and is thereby different from similar products manufactured. The second category of defective products is the defectively designed product. Such a product is identical to similar products manufactured by the defendant, all of which bear a common design flaw that renders the product unreasonably dangerous. The third category is a product that is defective because it has been inadequately tested. The fourth category is a product that is considered defective because the manufacturer has failed to provide the user with proper warnings or instructions regarding the product's use. This type of claimed defect occurs frequently in cases involving pharmaceutical and medical products. Under the strict liability theory, potential liability attaches not only to the product's manufacturer, but also to its retailer and to any other person in the distribution chain who is "in the business of selling such a product."[21]

However, one who sells *services,* rather than goods, will not be held liable under a strict liability theory or under a theory of implied warranty because those bases of liability are dependent on selling goods, rather than rendering services. In the leading case of *Magrine* v. *Krasnica*,[22] the issue confronting the New Jersey court was whether a dentist could be held strictly liable for the use of a defective product that injured his patient. In *Magrine*, the defendant dentist inserted a defectively manufactured hypodermic needle into the plaintiff's gum, where it broke. There was no evidence that the dentist knew, or even should have known, of the needle's latent defect. Therefore, the plaintiff was not able to establish a negligence cause of action against the dentist. The court denied the plaintiff's attempt to assert a strict liability theory against the dentist, since he was in no way responsible for manufacturing the needle, and "did not put the needle in the stream of commerce or promote its purchase."[23]

Each development in products liability theories, from negligence through strict liability, has made it easier for an injured party to establish a viable theory of recovery. Each new theory has expanded the law rather than merely replaced its predecessor.[24] This broadening of recovery theories, however, has added new complexities to the products liability field. Depending on the facts of the case and upon the theories advanced, each products liability cause of action will have separate elements, varying burdens of proof, and different potential defenses. The central theme, however—which runs throughout all products liability causes of action—is the existence or nonexistence of a product defect at the time the product left the defendant's control. This theme is essential to products liability and distinguishes it as a separate and unique field of law.[25]

LIABILITY OF THE MANUFACTURER

A manufacturer's liability for its products may be established under the three theories discussed above—negligence, warranty, and strict liability. For an injured-party plaintiff to establish a successful cause of action in negligence it must be proved that the defendant-manufacturer departed from reasonable standards of due care with respect to the design, testing, manufacture, assembly, inspection, packaging, or advertising of the product or failed to warn or give adequate instructions with respect to its use. The manufacturer owes this duty of due care to the ultimate user and not just to the immediate purchaser.[26]

A manufacturer's liability on the theory of breach of warranty is often more closely linked with the contract of sale between the parties involved, specifically the manufacturer and the injured buyer. Privity of contract has been the principal hurdle in breach of warranty actions.[27]

Even if privity can be established, traditional warranty theory also requires the plaintiff's reliance, to his detriment, on an express or implied assertion by the defendant about the nature of the defective product.[28] Without all of these elements, which are often difficult to establish, a warranty action will fail.

Strict liability is a more attractive theory for a plaintiff because it eliminates the key requirement of a negligence cause of action—the need for the plaintiff to show that the defendant failed to exercise proper care in the manufacturing or marketing of the product. It also avoids the need for any contractual obligations between the manufacturer and the injured party as a requirement for recovery.[29] Under the strict liability theory, a plaintiff needs only to establish that the product in question was so defective as to be unreasonably dangerous and that, as a result, injury was suffered.

An examination of the potential liability of the manufacturer of an artificial organ appropriately begins with an analysis of the liability concepts already developed regarding prescription drugs. This liability analogy is particularly appropriate. Pursuant to the Medical Device Amendments of 1976 to the federal Food, Drug, and Cosmetic Act,[30] any device that has the potential for harmful effect or involves special collateral measures requiring expertise is given a special classification; it subsequently may be restricted by regulation as a device subject to performance standards[31] or may be even further restricted by limiting its availability "upon such other conditions as the Secretary [of Health, Education, and Welfare] may prescribe," in order to assure its safe and effective use.[32] Any medical product that is to be implanted internally, such as an artificial organ, is necessarily hazardous because its operation in the human body and its effects upon the body are generally unknown. Therefore, this type of device is usually included in the most stringent category as a Class III device established by the Medical Device Amendments of 1976.[33] Class III devices are defined as those "whose safety and effectiveness are sufficiently uncertain that they cannot be determined without additional testing."[34]

In developing drug liability theories, the courts have expressly recognized and taken into account the fact that some products are "unavoidably unsafe" given current scientific knowledge. While there are very few decided cases, it would seem that this previously developed liability jurisprudence is directly applicable to artificial organs, given the embryonic nature of scientific understanding and experience in this field.

The federal Food, Drug, and Cosmetic Act has long required that a manufacturer test prescription drugs for safety and efficacy.[35] The

Medical Device Amendments impose a similarly rigorous series of testing requirements upon the manufacturer with respect to extraordinary medical devices, especially artificial organs.[36] Even though FDA approval has never been regarded as legally conclusive evidence of adequate testing, the requirements of the Medical Device Amendment Act for artificial organs would appear to present significant obstacles to a claim based on a negligence theory unless the plaintiff is able to establish that the manufacturer falsified test results, manipulated data reported to the FDA, or failed to provide warnings of known risks.[37]

To support the analogy of artificial organ liability concepts in terms of established drug liability theories, greater detail of a manufacturer's duty deserves review. The manufacturer has the duty to warn of complications, side effects, and any potential hazards associated with its products.[38] This duty requires a manufacturer to warn of known hazards as well as those hazards that it has a reasonable basis to suspect might occur.[39] The courts have expressly recognized that prescription drugs are "unavoidably unsafe products" that can be dispensed only under a physician's authorization. This is expressly recognized by Comment k to §402A of the *Restatement (Second) of Torts* (1965) which provides as follows:

> *Unavoidably unsafe products.* There are some products which, in the present state of human knowledge, are quite incapable of being made safe for their intended and ordinary use. These are especially common in the field of drugs. An outstanding example is the vaccine for the Pasteur treatment of rabies, which not uncommonly leads to very serious and damaging consequences when it is injected. Since the disease itself invariably leads to a dreadful death, both the marketing and the use of the vaccine are fully justified, notwithstanding the unavoidable high degree of risk which they involve. Such a product, properly prepared, and accompanied by proper directions and warning, is not defective, nor is it *unreasonably* dangerous. The same is true of many other drugs, vaccines, and the like, many of which for this very reason cannot legally be sold except to physicians, or under the prescription of a physician. It is also true in particular of many new or experimental drugs as to which, because of lack of time and opportunity for sufficient medical experience, there can be no assurance of safety, or perhaps even of purity of ingredients, but such experience as there is justifies the marketing and use of the drug notwithstanding a medically recognizable risk. The seller of such products, again with the qualification that they are properly prepared and marketed, and proper warning is given, where the situation calls for it, is not to be held to strict liability for unfortunate consequences attending their use, merely because he has undertaken to supply the public with an apparently useful and desirable product, attended with a known but apparently reasonable risk.

Comment k adopts an ordinary negligence concept through its "qualification" concerning the manufacturer's duty to properly prepare and to warn about an unavoidably unsafe product. Although the focus of the drafters of Comment k was on prescription drug products, its reasoning should apply *a fortiori* to prescription devices such as artificial organs. Therefore, when a plaintiff in an artificial organ case asserts a strict liability theory of recovery, pursuant to Comment k, the standard to be applied should remain a negligence one.

With prescription drugs, it is generally held that the manufacturer's duty to warn extends solely to the medical community, including both treating and prescribing physicians.[40] These physicians are regarded as "learned intermediaries" between the manufacturer and the patient.[41] This rule is based on an awareness of the fact that prescription drugs differ from ordinary consumer products in that consumers would find it difficult, if not impossible, to comprehend fully the medical literature that must accompany most prescription medications. Over-the-counter drugs, however, place a different duty on the manufacturer— the duty to warn the patient directly.[42]

With extraordinary medical devices, there is no question that the manufacturer has the duty to furnish full and complete warnings to any physician considering implanting such a device. The question which logically and necessarily follows is whether the manufacturer's duty to warn also extends to the patient-consumer. Although in the prescription drug context a manufacturer's duty to warn generally extends only to the medical community, it is unclear at present whether, with respect to extraordinary medical devices, the manufacturer's duty to warn should also extend to the patient-consumer.[43]

LIABILITY OF THE PHYSICIAN

A patient's suit against a physician for an injury resulting from the physician's treatment is predicated on professional negligence or malpractice. Malpractice may be defined as "bad or unskillful practice on the part of a physician or a surgeon resulting in injury to a patient."[44] The "failure of a physician to exercise the required degree of care, skill, and diligence," or "the treatment by a surgeon or a physician in a manner contrary to accepted rules and with injuries resulting to the patient," are all bases upon which malpractice claims may be founded.[45]

To present a cause of action for malpractice successfully against a professional practitioner, the patient-plaintiff must establish four essential elements.[46] First, a cause of action must show that the physician in question owed the patient-plaintiff a particular duty or obligation. This legal duty derives from the physician-patient relationship which requires the physician to act in accordance with specific standards of care established by the profession for the protection of the patient against unreasonable risks.

Second, the patient-plaintiff must establish that the physician failed to act in accordance with these standards. An act or omission (failure to act when required to do so) violating the standard of care owed to the patient is required.

Third, the patient-plaintiff must establish that a causal and reasonably foreseeable connection exists between the acts or omissions of the physician and the resulting injury.

Fourth, the patient-plaintiff must prove that the physician's acts or omissions caused some actual loss or damage. The failure to establish any one of these four elements may defeat a malpractice claim.

Claims for breach of warranty provide an alternative approach for actions by patients against medical practitioners resulting from injuries suffered from medical instruments, drugs, or devices used in treatment. The determinative issue in this instance is whether a sale existed upon which a warranty action could be based. A sale of goods, independent of the medical services provided, is generally the touchstone for warranty recovery.

In most jurisdictions, warranty claims are governed by statutes incorporating the Uniform Commercial Code (UCC). Thus, the provisions of the UCC tend to guide claims based upon express warranties, implied warranties of merchantability, and implied warranties of fitness for a particular medical purpose.[47] In order to establish a claim for a breach of warranty, it is necessary to establish that the furnishing of the product or device during the course of treatment constituted a sale to which a warranty could be said to have attached. Guided by the UCC, most courts have required a specific sale of goods, although some courts have found the relationship between patient and physician sufficient to support a warranty action.[48]

Strict liability, as established by the *Restatement (Second) of Torts* §402A, has become a frequent theory upon which attempts to establish a physician's liability are often premised by a patient injured through the use of any medical instrument or device. However, courts have been hesitant to apply strict liability against physicians. Courts analyzing the physician-patient relationship have noted that the primary purpose of this relationship is the performance or rendition of professional medical services, distinguishing this from the sale of medical products.[49] Accordingly, most courts have rejected the application of the strict liability theory to the medical treatment provided by physicians.

LIABILITY OF THE HOSPITAL

After addressing the scope of a physician's potential liability in the organ transplant context, the corollary issue of the hospital's liability necessarily emerges.

The law in this area has undergone a dramatic evolution. A perspective on the historical developments may be helpful in understanding the current state of the law. Traditionally, the hospital was viewed as an "innkeeper," simply providing the facilities in which a patient's privately retained doctor would practice his profession.[50] A hospital could not direct the course of treatment for a patient—that remained solely within the doctor's professional judgment. Since the doctor, and not the hospital, was directly responsible for the patient's ultimate care, it was often difficult to establish any legal basis of liability against a hospital for a physician's error, even one occurring within the hospital. Although it was once widely accepted that a doctor was not a hospital's "employee," this view has recently undergone dramatic changes, increasing the potential liability attributable to a hospital or medical center. The legal principle of *respondeat superior* provides the basis for attaching liability to the hospital for services provided therein.

Respondeat superior is a common law doctrine that imputes responsibility for an employee's acts, carried out during the course of his employment, to the employer as the one who derives advantage from the act and, therefore, must answer for any resultant injury.[51] The two requirements for application of this doctrine are specific.[52] The person charged with liability must be an employer, or someone in direct control of the party who allegedly caused the injury. Further, the person charged with causing the injury must have been acting within the "scope of his employment" at the time the injury resulted. These two requirements have restricted application of this doctrine in the health care context. A doctor is a professional and traditionally was not classified as a hospital employee. Rather, the doctor was viewed as an independent contractor—retained at the expense and will of the patient, not the hospital.[53]

Although development in this area has been slow, some jurisdictions have changed the legal status accorded hospitals. Hospitals have an integral role in the patient's overall treatment, and patients assume that if an error is committed, the hospital will take responsibility. This is based on the "apparent authority" of the hospital to supervise the treatment given, and has become another basis for attributing liability to hospitals.[54]

This changing attitude is illustrated by the New York Court of Appeals case of *Bing* v. *Thunig*.[55] The decision in this case directly overruled prior decisions, and held applicable the *respondeat superior* theory. In *Bing*, the court stated forcefully:

> The conception that the hospital does not undertake to treat the patient, does not undertake to act through its doctors and nurses, but undertakes instead simply to procure them to act upon their own responsibility, no longer reflects the fact. Present-day hospitals, as their manner of operation plainly demonstrates, do far more than furnish facilities for treatment. They regularly employ on a salary basis a large staff of physicians, nurses and interns, as well as administrative and manual workers, and they charge patients for medical care and treatment, collecting for such services, if necessary, by legal action. Certainly, the person who avails himself of "hospital facilities" expects that the hospital will attempt to cure him, not that its nurses or other employees will act on their own responsibility.
>
> Hospitals should, in short, shoulder the responsibilities borne by everybody else. There is no reason to continue their exemption from the universal rule of *respondeat superior*. The test should be, for these institutions, whether charitable or profit-making, as it is for every other employer, was the person who committed the negligent injury-producing act one of its employees and, if he was, was he acting within the scope of his employment.[56]

This view reflects the law accepted in a majority of jurisdictions.[57] A hospital's potential liability has been extended to encompass most, if not all, of the hospital's physicians, specialists, and staff.

Another basis adopted by some jurisdictions for hospital liability for negligent treatment is termed corporate negligence. Under this doctrine, established by the Illinois Supreme Court in the leading case of *Darling v. Charleston Community Memorial Hospital*, a hospital has a duty to provide adequate medical care to its patients.[58] This duty charges the hospital with responsibility for all treatment which takes place within its boundaries, extending liability beyond activities traditionally considered under their direct control and governed by principles of *respondeat superior* and, thus, includes liability for acts or omissions of persons, such as physicians, who are not hospital employees.

These broad principles of negligence liability on the part of the hospital would seem to be equally applicable in the specialized area of organ transplantation, although it must be recognized that proof of negligence in this evolving scientific area may often be difficult.

STATUTORY DEVELOPMENTS

In the organ transplant field, the Organ Procurement and Transplantation Act,[59] signed into law by President Reagan on October 19, 1984, deserves examination. One important section of this Act prohibits the sale, for valuable consideration, of human organs for use in human transplantation, providing as follows:

(a) It shall be unlawful for any person to knowingly acquire, receive, or otherwise transfer any human organ for valuable consideration for use in human transplantation if the transfer affects interstate commerce.

(b) Any person who violates subsection (a) shall be fined not more than $50,000 or imprisoned not more than five years, or both.

(c) For purposes of subsection (a):
(1) The term "human organ" means the human kidney, liver, heart, lung, pancreas, bone marrow, cornea, eye, bone, and skin, and any other human organ specified by the Secretary of Health and Human Services by regulation.
(2) The term "valuable consideration" does not include the reasonable payments associated with the removal, transportation, implantation, processing, preservation, quality control, and storage of a human organ or the expenses of travel, housing, and lost wages incurred by the donor of a human organ in connection with the donation of the organ.
(3) The term "interstate commerce" has the meaning prescribed for it by section 321(b) of Title 21.[60]

Although the terms of subsection (a) appear to prohibit the sale of any human organ, the critical term in the act is "valuable consideration" as defined in subsection (b). Pursuant to this subsection, valuable consideration does not include any reasonable payment associated with removal, transportation, implantation, processing, preservation, quality control, and storage of a human organ with regard to the donation of the organ.

For products liability purposes, the Act's prohibition on the sale of human organs prevents the development of any commercial harvesting and sale of human organs for transplantation. Moreover, the Act's definition of "valuable consideration" appears to classify any transaction with respect to the transplant of a human organ as a service rather than a sale. This classification, coupled with the Act's prohibition of the sale of any human organ, suggests that warranty and strict liability theories will remain inapplicable to human organ transplantation.

Additional protection for physicians and hospitals against products liability claims by human organ transplant plaintiffs may be found in various state statutes. A majority of state statutes expressly limit a physician's liability by providing that certain medical care and use of certain human products are deemed services rather than sales of any product, thereby generally restricting the viability of warranty and strict liability claims. A compendium of these statutes is set forth in Appendix E of this volume.[61] The legislative impetus for the majority of these statutes arose as a result of claims made by patients who had received blood transfusions containing the hepatitis virus. Most of these statutes, however, are not limited to blood or blood products, but extend to include other human tissues and, in one instance, even include artificial organs.

In evaluating the degree of protection afforded a physician undertaking the responsibility of transplanting a human organ by one of these state statutes, it is important to examine carefully the relevant statute. The following questions deserve consideration and close examination under the statute of the jurisdiction involved. Does the statute address claims founded on merely one or on all of the three principal liability theories available—negligence, warranty, and strict liability? Is the statute limited to blood or blood products, or does it also include human organs and tissues? Does the statute declare that an organ transplant procedure is a medical service rather than a sale, thus barring the application of a strict liability theory?

The range and variety of statutorily created or prohibited liability is dramatic. At one extreme are statutes which limit warranty liability only. In Massachusetts, an example of such coverage provides as follows:

> The implied warranties of merchantability and fitness shall not be applicable to a contract for the sale of human blood, blood plasma or other human tissue or organs from a blood bank or reservoir of such other tissues or organs. Such blood, blood plasma or tissue or organs *shall not for the purpose of this Article* be considered commodities subject to sale or barter, but shall be considered as medical services. [Emphasis added.][62]

As is readily apparent, a statute such as this limits only the implied warranties of merchantability and fitness. Express contractual warranties as well as tort liability remain unaffected.

In Minnesota, on the other hand, a more comprehensive statute provides as follows:

> The use of any part of a body for the purpose of transplantation in the human body shall be construed for all purposes whatsoever, as a rendition of a service by each and every person participating therein and shall not be construed as a sale of such part for any purpose whatsoever.[63]

The extensive coverage of this statute ("any part of a body") and the flat classification of any human transplant as a service and not a sale for any purpose serves to eliminate many otherwise available theories for potential recovery.

A third type of statute covering not only blood and blood products but also other human tissues and even artificial organs is the Michigan statute providing as follows:

> (2) The procurement, processing, distribution, and use of *whole blood*, plasma, blood products, blood derivatives, *and human or artificial tissues such as corneas, bones or organs for the purpose of injection, transfusing, or transplanting into a human body,* is declared to be, for all purposes, *the rendition of a service* by a person participating therein and, whether or not any remuneration is paid therefor, is declared not to be a sale thereof for any purpose.

> (3) An express, implied, or other warranty does not attach to these services. A person involved in the rendition of any such service is not liable as a result thereof, except for the person's own negligence or wilful misconduct. [Emphasis added.][64]

This statute is unique in that it expressly includes artificial as well as natural human tissues or organs. Moreover, this statute expressly provides that a transplant has no warranty whatsoever. Additionally, the transplanting physician is expressly protected from claims based on strict liability.

These statutes help to codify and establish the generally recognized rule that a physician is not strictly liable for providing services, including the furnishing of a human or artificial organ. The physician's exposure to liability in the organ transplant setting, therefore, is predominantly based on negligence or malpractice principles, the standards of which are already well developed.

Applicable Products Liability Defenses

The defenses generally available in a products liability case may be divided into four broad categories: (1) defenses which are related to the plaintiff's conduct—contributory negligence, assumption of the risk, comparative fault, and obviousness of the defect; (2) defenses which relate to conduct of the purchaser or user of the product who may or may not be the plaintiff—misuse, alteration, and compliance with the purchaser's specifications; (3) product related defenses—compliance with the state of the art, government regulations, and industry custom; and (4) those related to the passage of time—useful life and statutes of limitation.[65]

Within these broad areas of potential defenses to a products liability claim, three specific defenses have the greatest applicability to products liability claims concerning organ transplants. These are: (1) the patient's assumption of the risk; (2) the state-of-the-art defense; and (3) special applications of statutes of limitation.

A plaintiff may assume the risk of certain types of possible injury if he voluntarily consents to take his chances, risking the possibility that such harm may occur. Accordingly, a plaintiff may either expressly or impliedly assume a known risk and, therefore, may not have a right to recover for injuries thereby incurred.[66]

It is well established that the risk of harm from a service rendered or a product supplied may be assumed by an express agreement between the parties.[67] In addition to an express agreement between the parties, a disclaimer may also serve to protect a manufacturer or physician by creating the situation where the purchaser or the patient in an organ transplant procedure has assumed the risk.

The general rule concerning disclaimers is that they remain valid only between the actual parties to the contract.[68] Moreover, a disclaimer must fulfill other requirements to be an enforceable waiver of liability. It must be conspicuous, agreed to at the time of contract, unambiguous, and not "unconscionable" (so harsh as to be grossly unfair against the disclaimed party).[69] A manufacturer's disclaimer of liability for its product, if valid, generally bars recovery on any products liability theory. The New York Court of Appeals recognized this principle in *Velez* v. *Craine & Clark Lumber Co.,*[70] stating:

> Although strict products liability sounds in tort rather than in contract, we see no reason why in the absence of some consideration of public policy parties cannot by contract restrict or modify what would otherwise be a liability between them grounded in tort.[71]

Specifically addressing artificial organ transplants, the preferable approach would be for both the manufacturer and physician to enter into an express agreement with the prospective patient after each had carefully reviewed the proposed procedures. This would allow for agreement recognizing that, given the present state of human skill and knowledge, the operation may still remain unavoidably dangerous. In the situation where the operation is unavoidably dangerous, perhaps more than any other, the utility and social value of the procedure may outweigh the risks. Therefore, provided the proper warning and directions are given, it would appear that an express agreement between all concerned parties is clearly the most prudent course of action.

Intertwined with the unavoidably unsafe product concept is the equally important "state-of-the-art" defense.[72] In essence, the state-of-the-art defense requires that the manufacturer apply the leading edge of scientific knowledge in the development, design, or manufacture of a product or the warnings issued therewith.[73] The state-of-the-art defense is generally applicable in two specific situations. First, if the existence of a potentially dangerous condition in a product is not discoverable by modern scientific technology, this defense may be viable.[74] Second, when the technology necessary to make a product safe is unavailable at the time of manufacture although the danger is known, this defense is even more appropriate.[75] Since artificial organ implantation is clearly on the cutting edge of medical developments and technology, courts should readily accept the state-of-the-art defense. Society would risk medical and scientific stagnation if liability was based on injuries that could not be prevented given current knowledge and expertise.

A statute of limitation is the time period within which a lawsuit must be commenced.[76] If the claim is not made within the appropriate statutorily defined time period, it will be dismissed outright by the court upon a defendant's proper request. The goal of statutes of limitation is to prevent stale claims, which are difficult to defend against, from being raised long after they should have been. The period of limitation will vary from jurisdiction to jurisdiction, as does the method for determining when the statute of limitation begins. Usually the time of accident or injury is the starting point, but when the injury does not manifest itself for many years after contact with a product, many states now apply a different rule. The time of discovery rule, most common in the medical area, holds that the statute of limitations begins "when the patient discovers, or in the exercise of reasonable care and diligence for his own health and welfare, should have discovered the resulting injury."[77]

Of particular interest with respect to the statute of limitation period concerning a manufacturer's liability for an artificial organ malfunction is the recent New York Court of Appeals case of *Martin* v. *Edwards Laboratories.*[78] The New York statute of limitations is normally calculated from the date of the malpractice or other negligent act or omission, even though its effect may not be manifested until later. In the *Martin* case, the court considered the issue of when the statute of limitations began for personal injury caused by the malfunctioning of a prosthetic device implanted in the human body. In *Martin,* an artificial aortic valve was implanted in the plaintiff's decedent. The plaintiff alleged that Teflon particles originating in the artificial heart valve lodged in the decedent's brain causing his death. The Court of Appeals held that the proper rule for products implanted or inserted in the human body was neither the time of implantation or insertion nor the time of discovery of the defect, but rather a date of injury rule—the date when the product malfunctioned.[79]

Thus, the broad spectrum of defenses available today against a claim asserted by an injured organ transplant patient decreases significantly the chance of his recovery.

CONCLUSION

The foregoing overview of products liability theories in the rapidly developing field of organ transplantation highlights several aspects of established legal doctrine as well as the uncertainty that surrounds the future. This uncertainty is best typified by the recent and ongoing legislative activity at both the state and federal level.[80] For example, the effect of the Organ Procurement and Transplantation Act of 1984 has yet to be determined. Although the Act's elimination of the commercial sale of human organs for transplantation was immediate, a major portion of the legislation focused upon the establishment of a Task Force on Organ Transplantation.[81] The Task Force's final report was submitted in April 1986.[82]

The legal concepts of products liability suggest that traditional negligence principles will probably continue to be augmented by statutory and case law refinements resulting in even more clearly delineated standards. Until such developments occur, established legal concepts suggest that traditional negligence principles will continue to guide most cases litigated in this field. To this end, the appendixes to this chapter provide a list of helpful references in this evolving area of the law.

ACKNOWLEDGMENTS

The authors gratefully acknowledge the valuable assistance provided by Charles Victor Lang, Columbia University School of Law, J.D. 1987, in the preparation of this chapter.

NOTES

1. Friedrich, O., *One Miracle, Many Doubts,* TIME 124(24):70 (December 10, 1984).
2. Address by Commissioner Frank E. Young, M.D., PH.D., before the Conference on Legal and Ethical Issues Surrounding Organ Transplantation. (*See* ch. 10 of this volume).
3. Set forth as a selected bibliography hereto is a list of references concerning the issues of products liability and organ transplantation which the authors have relied upon in preparing this chapter. With respect to the topic at hand, the authors direct interested readers to two leading articles in this field: Berg, Kosseff, *The Life and Death of Barney Clark: A Manufacturer's Liability for Extraordinary Medical Devices,* FOR THE DEFENSE 25(6):22 (June 1983);

Noblett, *An Overview of Litigation Concerning Products Liability and Medical Devices,* AMERICAN JOURNAL OF TRIAL ADVOCACY 5(2):309 (1981).

4. *See generally,* W. PROSSER, W. P. KEETON, THE LAW OF TORTS (West Publishing Co., St. Paul, Minn.) (5th ed. 1984) at 677–79 [hereinafter cited as PROSSER].

5. Heaven v. Pender, 11 Q.B.D. 503, 509 (1883). For a good discussion of negligence standards, *see Towards a Jurisprudence of Injury: The Continuing Creation of a System of Substantive Justice in American Tort Law,* Report to the American Bar Association (1984) at 5-20 to 5-24.

6. RESTATEMENT (SECOND) OF TORTS §282 (1965).

7. PROSSER, *supra* note 4, at 685–89. For a good discussion of products liability in the medical-legal area, *see also* K. FINEBERG, *et al.,* OBSTETRICS/GYNECOLOGY AND THE LAW (Health Administration Press, Ann Arbor, Mich.) (1984) at 111 [hereinafter cited as FINEBERG].

8. PROSSER, *supra* note 4, at 679.

9. *Id.* at 681.

10. *See* Prosser, *The Assault upon the Citadel,* YALE LAW JOURNAL 69(7):1099–1148 (1960).

11. PROSSER, *supra* note 4, at 682.

12. 514 S.W.2d 429 (Tex. 1974).

13. *Id.* at 433.

14. PROSSER, *supra* note 4, at 690–92.

15. Julien, *Products Liability—Strict Liability's Basis,* NEW YORK LAW JOURNAL (October 28, 1983) at 1 [hereinafter cited as Julien].

16. *Id.*

17. RESTATEMENT (SECOND) OF TORTS §402A (1965).

18. W. PROSSER, J. WADE, V. SCHWARTZ, CASES AND MATERIALS ON TORTS (7th Ed. 1982) at 762. Most states have adopted, either by judicial decision or by statute, §402A of the RESTATEMENT (SECOND) OF TORTS. A handful of states have adopted the RESTATEMENT position but have eliminated the requirement of proving that the product is unreasonably dangerous. *See, e.g.,* Cronin v. J. B. E. Olson Corp. 501 P.2d 1153 (Cal. Sup. Ct. *en banc,* 1972); Suter v. San Angelo Foundry and Machine Co., 406 A.2d 140 (N.J. Sup. Ct. 1979); Berkebile v. Brantly Helicopter Corp., 337 A.2d 893 (Pa. Sup. Ct. 1975). *See also* J. ALLEE, PRODUCT LIABILITY (Law Journals Seminars-Press) (1984) at §§2.01, 2.05, 2.05 n.63.

19. FINEBERG, *supra* note 7 §2.71 at 112.

20. Julien, *supra* note 15, at 2, col. 1 (this article considers and analyzes the four fundamental categories of product defects).

21. RESTATEMENT (SECOND) OF TORTS §402A (1)(a) (1965).

22. Magrine v. Krasnica, 227 A.2d 539 (1967), *aff'd* 250 A.2d 129 (N.J. Sup. Ct. 1969).

23. *Id.* at 227 A.2d 543.

24. FINEBERG, *supra* note 7 §2.71 at 112.

25. 1 M. WEINBERGER, NEW YORK PRODUCTS LIABILITY (Callaghan and Company, New York, N.Y.) (1982) at §1.05.

26. *See, e.g.,* MacPherson v. Buick Motor Co., 111 N.E. 1050 (N.Y. Ct. App. 1916).

27. *See supra* note 9 and accompanying text.
28. *Cf.* PROSSER, *supra* note 4, at 680.
29. FINEBERG, *supra* note 7 §2.71 at 118.
30. 21 U.S.C. §360–k (1982). For a good overview of these amendments, *see* Foote, *Loops and Loopholes: Hazardous Device Regulation Under the 1976 Medical Device Amendments to the Food, Drug and Cosmetic Act,* ECOLOGY LAW QUARTERLY 7:101–35 (1978).
31. 21 U.S.C. §360d (1982).
32. 21 U.S.C. §360j (e)(1)(B) (1982).
33. 21 U.S.C. §360c (1982) defines the Device Classifications generally as follows:
    Class I devices are those which have reasonable assurance of the safety and effectiveness of the device, or do not present a potential for, or unreasonable risk of, illness or injury.
    Class II devices are those which have insufficient data to provide reasonable assurances of safety and effectiveness, but for which a performance standard can be established to provide the necessary assurances of safety.
    Class III devices are those which do not have either the needed assurances of safety and effectiveness, or the information necessary to establish Class II performance standards. Devices, however, which serve a valuable life supporting or sustaining role will receive Class III Premarket Approval on this basis, despite the potential of unreasonable risk of illness or injury, because of their social utility.
34. *Id.*
35. 21 U.S.C. §§301–92 (1982).
36. 21 U.S.C. §360j (1982).
37. Berg and Kosseff, *supra* note 3, at 24.
38. PROSSER, *supra* note 4, at 685–86.
39. *Id.* at 697.
40. See, *e.g.,* Lindsay v. Ortho Pharm. Corp., 637 F.2d 87 (2d Cir. 1980); Reyes v. Wyeth Laboratories, 498 F.2d 1264 (5th Cir.), *cert. denied,* 419 U.S. 1096 (1974). For a good review of case law in the area of drug liability litigation, *see* Birnbaum, *Liability of Drug Manufacturers, Government, Druggists, Physicians and Others,* printed in materials accompanying the Law Journal Seminar-Press program, Drug Liability Litigation—An Advanced Workshop, 1980.
41. *Reyes, supra* note 40, at 1276.
42. *See, e.g.,* Torsiello v. Whitehall Laboratories, 398 A.2d 132, *cert. denied,* 404 A.2d 1150 (N.J., 1979).
43. Berg and Kosseff suggest that with respect to extraordinary medical devices, the manufacturer's warnings should be given not only to the physician but also to the patient. *Supra* note 3, at 25–26.
44. C. KRAMER, D. KRAMER, MEDICAL MALPRACTICE (Practicing Law Institute, New York, N.Y.) (5th Ed. 1983) at 5.
45. *Id.* at 6. *See also* 70 C.J.S. Physicians and Surgeons §40 (1951).
46. PROSSER, *supra* note 4, at 164. *See also,* M. McCAFFERTY, S. MEYER, MEDICAL MALPRACTICE: BASES OF LIABILITY (Shepard's/McGraw-Hill, New York, N.Y.) (1985) at §2.01.

47. U.C.C. §2-313 addresses express warranties. U.C.C. §2-314 covers implied warranties of merchantability. U.C.C. §2-315 covers implied warranties of fitness for a particular purpose.

48. McCafferty, Meyer, *supra* note 46, at §15.10 (1985).

49. *Id.* at §9.05. *See also,* Perlmutter v. Beth David Hospital, 308 N.Y. 100, 123 N.E.2d 792 (N.Y. 1954), *reh. den.,* 125 N.E.2d 869 (1955). *Contra* Cheshire v. Southampton Hosp. Ass'n, 53 Misc.2d 355, 278 N.Y.S.2d 531 (Sup. Ct. Suffolk Co. 1967). *See generally,* 1 Weinberger, *supra* note 25, at §§3.06– 3.15.

50. 1 D. Louisell, H. Williams, *Medical Malpractice* §16.08 (1985), and authorities cited therein.

51. *See* 37A: Words and Phrases 22 (1950 and Supp. 1984).

52. Prosser, *supra* note 4, at 499–508.

53. 1 Louisell, Williams, *supra* note 50, at §16.08.

54. *See, e.g.,* Mehlman v. Powell, 378 A.2d 1121 (Md. Ct. Spec. App. 1977). *See also,* McCafferty, Meyer, *supra* note 46, at §13.06.

55. 143 N.E.2d 3 (N.Y. 1957).

56. *Id.* at 8.

57. *See* 1 Louisell, Williams, *supra* note 50, §16.08 at note 4, 16–36.

58. 211 N.E.2d 253 (Ill. 1965), *cert. denied,* 383 U.S. 946 (1966). *See also* McCafferty, Meyer, *supra* note 46 at §13.02.

59. 42 U.S.C.A. §§273–74 (West Supp. 1985) (originally enacted as Pub. L. No. 98–507, 98 Stat. 2339).

60. 42 U.S.C.A. §274e (West Supp. 1985).

61. Appendix E of this volume is a comprehensive listing of text and citations for state statutes concerning blood transfusions and organ transplantation. In the compilation of the statutory appendix, the authors acknowledge the assistance provided by the following sources: 2 *Product Liab. Rep.* (CCH); M. McCafferty, S. Meyer, Medical Malpractice: Bases of Liability, Appendixes A and B (1985); *Comment: Blood Transfusions and the Transmission of Serum Hepatitis: The Need for Statutory Reform,* American University Law Review 24:367, 404 n.143 (1975).

62. Mass. Ann. Laws ch. 106, §2-316(5) (West Supp. 1986).

63. Minn. Stat. Ann. §525.928 (West 1975).

64. Mich. Stat. Ann. §14.15(9121) (Callaghan 1980).

65. Allee, *supra* note 18, at §8.01.

66. *See, e.g.,* Brown v. Link Belt Corp., 565 F.2d 1107 (9th Cir. 1977).

67. *See* Restatement (Second) of Torts §496B (1965).

68. 1 Weinberger, *supra* note 25, at §23.18.

69. *Id.*

70. 305 N.E.2d 750 (N.Y. 1973).

71. *Id.* at 754, 350 N.Y.S.2d at 623.

72. P. Sherman, Products Liability for the General Practitioner (Shepard's/McGraw-Hill, New York, N.Y.) (1981) at §9.14.

73. *See, e.g.,* Schenebeck v. Sterling Drug, Inc., 423 F.2d 919 (8th Cir. 1970). *But see,* Beshada v. Johns-Manville Products Corp., 447 A.2d 539 (N.J. 1982).

The availability and application of this defense varies greatly from jurisdiction to jurisdiction. For an excellent analysis of this defense, *see* ALLEE, *supra* note 18, at §8.08.

74. *See e.g.,* Heritage v. Pioneer Brokerage and Sales, Inc., 604 P.2d 1059 (Alaska 1979).
75. *See generally,* Bruce v. Martin-Marietta Corp., 544 F.2d 442 (10th Cir. 1976).
76. *See* ALLEE, *supra* note 18, at §8.13.
77. Teeters v. Currey, 518 S.W.2d 512, 517 (Tenn. 1974).
78. 457 N.E.2d 1150 (N.Y. 1983).
79. *Id.* at 1155–56.
80. At the state level, a number of states have adopted comprehensive product liability statutes or other statutes which address product liability issues. For a compilation and discussion of such statutes, *see* ALLEE, *supra* note 18. On the federal level, a number of legislative proposals have been introduced in recent years which would supersede state standards of product liability law in favor of national standards. The ultimate outcome of such legislation is uncertain.
81. 42 U.S.C.A., §273 (West Supp. 1985).
82. A copy of the EXECUTIVE SUMMARY of the REPORT OF THE TASK FORCE ON ORGAN TRANSPLANTATION appears in Appendix A in this volume. If further information is required, contact: Task Force on Organ Transplantation, Secretary of Health and Human Services, Office of Organ Transplantation, Parklawn Building—Room 17-60, 5600 Fishers Lane, Rockville, Maryland 20857, Telephone No. (301) 443-5911.

SELECTED BIBLIOGRAPHY

TREATISES

J. ALLEE, PRODUCT LIABILITY (Law Journal Seminars-Press) (1984).

M. BERTOLET, L. GOLDSMITH, HOSPITAL LIABILITY: LAW AND TACTICS (Practicing Law Institute, New York, N.Y.) (4th ed. 1980).

DRUGS IN LITIGATION: DAMAGE AWARDS INVOLVING PRESCRIPTION AND NON-PRESCRIPTION DRUGS (The Allen Smith Company) (2d ed. 1982).

K. FINEBERG, *et al.,* OBSTETRICS/GYNECOLOGY AND THE LAW (Health Administration Press, Ann Arbor, Mich.) (1984).

L. FRUMER, M. FRIEDMAN, PRODUCTS LIABILITY (Matthew Bender) (1984).

W. KIMBLE, R. LESHER, PRODUCTS LIABILITY (West's Handbook Series, St. Paul, Minn.) (1979).

N. McCAFFERTY, S. MEYER, MEDICAL MALPRACTICE: BASES OF LIABILITY (Shepard's/McGraw-Hill, New York, N.Y.) (1985).

J. O'REILLY, FOOD AND DRUG ADMINISTRATION (Shepard's/McGraw-Hill Regulatory Manual Series, New York, N.Y.) (1984).

W. PROSSER, W. KEETON, THE LAW OF TORTS (West Publishing Co., St. Paul, Minn.) (5th ed. 1984).

P. Sherman, Products Liability for the General Practitioner (Shepard's/ McGraw-Hill, New York, N.Y.) (1981).

Towards a Jurisprudence of Injury: The Continuing Creation of a System of Substantive Justice in American Tort Law, Report to the American Bar Association (1984).

U.S. Department of Commerce, Interagency Task Force on Product Liability, Final Report (1978).

M. Weinberger, New York Products Liability (Callaghan and Company, New York, N.Y.) (1982).

ARTICLES

Berg, Kosseff, *The Life and Death of Barney Clark: A Manufacturer's Liability for Extraordinary Medical Devices,* For the Defense (June 1983) at 22.

Berman, *The Legal Problems of Organ Transplantation,* Villanova Law Review 13:751 (1968).

Comment: Liability and the Heart Transplant, Houston Law Review 6:86 (1968).

Finesilver, *Organ Transplants: A Multi-Discipline Challenge,* Trial (April-May 1969) at 40.

Jennings, *Litigating Medical Device Product Liability Claims,* The Forum 20:141 (1984).

Kosanovich, *Medical Malpractice Liability and the Organ Transplant,* United States Federal Law Review 5:223 (1971).

Leavell, *Legal Problems in Organ Transplants,* Mississippi Law Journal 44:865 (1973).

Note: An Overview of Litigation Concerning Products Liability and Medical Devices, American Journal of Trial Advocacy 5:309 (1981).

Perper, *Ethical, Religious, and Legal Considerations to the Transplantation of Human Organs,* Journal of Forensic Science 15:1 (1970).

Richards, *Medical-Legal Problems of Organ Transplantation,* Hastings Law Journal 21:77 (1969).

Rose, *Medicolegal Problems Associated With Organ and Tissue Transplantations,* Medical Trial Techniques Quarterly 31:99 (Summer 1984).

Segal, *Medical Malpractice in an Organ Transplant Case,* Practice of Law 15:65 (1969).

Stieglitz, *The Law's Race to Catch Medical Technology,* The Brief 14(2):10 (Winter 1985).

Ward, *Human Organ Transplantation: Some Medico-Legal Pitfalls for Transplant Surgeons,* University of Florida Law Review 23:134 (1970).

Wasmuth, *The Medical, Legal, and Ethical Considerations of Human Organ Transplantations,* William and Mary Law Review 11:636 (1970).

12

The Role of State Health Departments in Assuring Equitable Selection and Regulation of Resources

David L. Jackson

For centuries, medical science has sought to unlock the secrets necessary to reverse the effects of major organ failure, thereby retarding death. Yet relatively little effort has been expended on developing systems that address the social and ethical dimensions of the numerous issues surrounding the introduction of new technology. In the mid-1980s, however, intense public concern has focused on such issues as they relate to transplantation.

In many ways, the interest in organ transplants appears to exceed its relative importance in the health care system, and it is important to understand why. Major solid organ transplants are viewed by the public—and by many in political life—as life saving, thus giving transplants high visibility. In addition, transplantation surgery remains limited and expensive. This has raised serious questions about the rationing of health care, and for the first time in our society, has opened this issue to professional and public discussion. We are beginning, as a society, to perceive, however dimly, the complex problems inherent in the frequent denial of transplants on strictly financial grounds. This denial of care directly challenges our society's sense that essential health care services are an intrinsic right of all people, not only the wealthy. The media are also a cause of the increased attention transplantation receives. The media have been able to identify easily those patients and families involved in transplant situations, thus using individuals' personal stories for maximum publicity impact.

In the midst of these technological and media changes and in response to the high cost of transplant services, the United States has witnessed the exploitation of the plight of individual patients and their families by the media and various political forces. Families have had to beg on television and in the newspaper for funds to place their loved ones on a transplant waiting list. This has led to the "Queen for a Day" mentality in lieu of any rational and equitable policy that responds to the difficult and complex choices we must make.

There was a case of one child in Massachusetts where the refusal by the state Medicaid program to cover the cost of the proposed transplant led to a bitter war of words in the media. The patient's father charged that the governor of Massachusetts would be responsible for the death of his daughter. Because of that public pressure, the state rescinded its denial of coverage and agreed to cover the transplantation cost. The patient's father later lamented, "After working all my life, they made a panhandler out of me." In another case, a hospital scheduled to host a transplant refused to admit the patient, even though the family pledged over $180,000 in real estate assets; the hospital insisted on $100,000 in more liquid assets before the patient could be admitted.

Over the past two years, there have been increasing numbers of politically motivated ambulance chasers. Political figures on both sides of the issue have used the media to highlight individual cases. The zenith of this theater of the absurd was the case of an eleven-month-old infant in Texas who had progressive liver failure and was an excellent candidate for a liver transplant. Never before nor since this case has the Texas Medicaid program agreed to cover transplant services; however, in the face of intense political pressure, legislation authorizing payment for that one patient was rushed through the Texas legislature. The full weight of the state and federal government was mobilized behind this one patient's situation. President Reagan announced on his weekly Saturday afternoon radio program that an Air Force jet was available to recover a donor organ for that child. Sadly, no donor organ was found in time, and the child died without receiving a transplant. Not long after this occurred, there was a case in Texas of a two-year-old child with the same disease. However, the family could not get Medicaid coverage because it did not have that sharp political focus. The applause meter is far too crude a device to make these difficult decisions.

So far, federal policy has focused on organ availability. The goals of the American Council on Transplantation and the new Office of Organ Transplantation have concentrated on increasing public and professional education, approving donor identification and referrals, and encouraging multiple organ availability. This approach minimizes concerns many of us share about the inefficiencies, problems, and gaps inherent in the development of a fragmented private sector response. Instead, our nation can and must develop effective responses to the complex ethical and social dimensions of this expensive and limited-access technology if its growth is to be proportional to the benefits society can derive.

The past two centuries of health care in America have focused on providing quality services to all in need. Until recently, health care costs have not been a significant priority in health planning, but today they are. And open discussion of the rationing of limited health care services is rare. In this author's experience as the director of an intensive care unit, every day when we had a full unit and a new patient in the emergency room, we made implicit *sub rosa* rationing decisions based on very little data, in an attempt to maximize, in the utilitarian sense, the public and the individual patient's good; yet we never discussed this rationing.

The direct challenge in transplantation is achieving the appropriate balance among three equally important considerations: quality of health care services, fairness and equity to access, and rational cost containments. The goal is to avoid pricing basic services out of the reach of the average working American. The health care professions, state government, and federal government must work together to develop a rational, equitable, and effective transplant program that includes organ procurement and reasonable and fair reimbursement policies.

A fair and rational program has already been developed in Ohio. In 1984, Ohio was in the midst of a seven-month moratorium on the certificate of need process. Included in the legislation that mandated the moratorium was a requirement that major nonrenal organ transplant services receive a certificate of need review. This gave the Ohio Department of Health and Ohio Governor Richard Celeste leverage with institutions that had already filed notices of intent to apply for certificates of need to start transplant services.

Three institutions had filed those notices of intent: the Cleveland Clinic Foundation, University Hospital of Cleveland, and Ohio State University Hospitals of Columbus. These three institutions and the Ohio Department of Health, after a series of open discussions, developed a philosophical and operational consensus on the critical issues of recipient selection, donor procurement, treatment protocols, and the sharing of results in appropriate research studies. It was felt that such an approach ensured, as close as was possible in 1985, an optimal and equitable application of transplant services for the broadest public benefit. It was agreed that the situation in Ohio presented a unique opportunity to foster the introduction of this technology in a way that would maintain the traditions of medical excellence and technological valuation of those institutions, and yet would be socially responsible. A statewide consortium was developed, facilitated by the close cooperation of three (later four) hospitals and different departments of state government, including the Department of Insurance, the Department of Human Services, the Medicaid program, and the Department of Health. Only those institutions that had previously demonstrated both a commitment toward and experience in renal transplants could be considered for membership in the consortium because we did not want to add significant costs to the system by introducing new technology. All consortium institutions agreed to follow the guidelines set forth by the Public Health Council and the Department of Health. A rough calculation determined that three to four institutions was the optimal number for a population base of eleven million during the initial three-year pilot study.

In addition, each institution had to demonstrate a commitment to transplantation by the availability of the requisite medical and administrative personnel and facilities, and an adequate physical plant; and each institution had to demonstrate that it could provide these without any additional capital costs through the certificate of need process. These institutions also agreed to share organ-specific patient management protocols and a specific patient selection process. There is a uniform data collection system, a follow-up commitment to joint research efforts, and joint funding for the long-term research projects from local foundations—the Cleveland Foundation, the Columbus Foundation, and the Cincinnati Foundation.

For several reasons, the Ohio effort was unique: not only did we work collaboratively with the five regional organ recovery service programs in Ohio, but we developed a single patient selection committee for the entire state. Cooperative efforts led to the development of medically valid criteria that were not based on social judgments but rather on uniform medical criteria. These criteria are established by the statewide task force, and the single statewide selection committee will develop more organ-specific criteria. The selection process is racially, sexually, and economically nondiscriminatory. This was possible because Governor Celeste agreed that the state Medicaid program would cover all expenses for heart, liver, and pancreas transplants for all Medicaid-eligible patients, including those who received Social Security disability payments and those who "spent down" their resources to meet Medicaid eligibility. The Governor went one step further by mandating the Department of Human Services and the Department of Health to monitor the Medicaid program to verify that the availability of resources for primary and preventive services was not decreased. This goal was possible to achieve because recent changes in the Medicaid program had created a more cost-effective health care system. We have encouraged health maintenance organizations and primary management; we are the fourth state in the nation to have prospective reimbursement for inpatient services; and we project that we can cover the Medicaid recipients' expenses for transplant services without diminishing—in fact, while increasing—the number of dollars available for more basic services.

Concomitantly, negotiations between the business community and third-party payers in the private sector yielded an agreement to cover organ transplants using the statewide patient selection committee as a gatekeeper. Three of the major Blue Cross plans in Ohio and all of the state's business coalitions agree that transplantation is no longer experimental and should be covered under the consortium process.

Another unique aspect of the Ohio plan is the commitment made by the hospitals and the doctors. They have agreed that 25 percent of all professional fees and 25 percent of institutional gifts from patients or the families of patients who have received transplant services will create a fund to cushion the impact of transplant costs on those families and patients who fall between the cracks of Medicaid eligibility and private insurance. This fund will not pay for all expenses, but it will serve as a significant buffer.

The statewide selection committee has a diverse membership. It includes transplant surgeons, an attorney with a background in medical ethics, a member of the clergy who is the director of an interprofessional studies group at Ohio State University, and the director of the Ohio Department of Health. After a patient has been recommended for a transplant by the institutional review committee, the patient is then evaluated by the statewide selection committee. For those patients who are unstable, the review is performed by conference telephone calls, and in the following monthly session, all of the evaluative processes are reviewed. Among the first fifteen patients, there was one general relief patient, six Medicaid patients, and eight private insurance patients. Because the group is so small, the statistics on gender and race are unreliable.

Nevertheless, there is at least a rough correlation between the at-risk population and its payer source of distribution among patients who have been accepted for transplants. Once the patients have been evaluated as excellent candidates, they are divided into urgent (those who are likely to die within a week) and semiurgent (those who are likely to die within six months) categories. Of course, this kind of prognosis judgment is limited. The patients who are urgent are on the first priority list; those who are semiurgent are on the next priority list; both groups are then screened by red-cell and white-cell compatibility and by size and blood types. If more than one person is an acceptable candidate for a particular donor organ and both patients are on the urgent list, the patient who has been on the list the longest would receive the organ. "First come, first served" is the way the allocation decision is made.

If, however, one patient is on the urgent list and one patient is on the less-urgent list, the patient in the urgent situation would be the first choice for the organ. Ohio has also determined how it will implement this system on a broader regional basis. Within the system, a high-priority urgent patient in Pennsylvania, Tennessee, or Minnesota, for example, would receive preference over a less urgent patient in Ohio; however, if there were an equally urgent patient in both Ohio and Pennsylvania, the Ohio patient would receive marginal preference.

Beyond the uniform systems for patient selection and reimbursement, Ohio's consortium is also unique in its development of a single collaborative research program involving all the consortium institutions. The consortium is currently establishing a nonprofit corporation that will serve as the umbrella organization for all consortium activities. The review of the data after the three-year pilot program is completed will be performed by outsiders in addition to people involved in the consortium. And an independent, broadly based statewide task force will examine Ohio's future course.

It is dangerous to be trapped in the "Mount Everest" syndrome in technology, where one tries continually to climb a mountain simply because it is there. The members of the consortium and the governor are deeply committed to an unbiased re-evaluation after the three-year pilot program to see whether we want to increase availability, decrease availability, or keep the status quo.

In considering the success of the Ohio program, we compare it with the theoretical model that the Massachusetts Task Force on Organ Transplantation devised a few months after Ohio's program was initiated. Ohio's program has many similarities to the theoretical optimum devised by the Massachusetts Task Force in its important document in October 1984. The similarities are much more striking than the differences. Within our constraints, Ohio has attempted to address some of today's social and ethical issues. The collaborative approach instituted in Ohio provides the most effective and efficient use of the collective expertise across Ohio in internationally and nationally recognized medical institutions. It is central to ensuring a system for equitable access, because we cannot have a system that sensationalizes access or that makes financial resources the single, entry-level criterion.

It is only by putting aside territorial considerations, which have frequently been the primary imperative in the introduction of new health care technologies, and by developing the kind of constructive public and

private sector interface that exists in Ohio that our nation can successfully meet the challenges presented by the continuing medical technology explosion.

13

Organ Transplants:
Are We Treating
the Modern Miracle Fairly?

George J. Annas

Discussions of organ transplantation tend to run on one of two tracks: it is a medical marvel that should be promoted by encouraging organ donation; or it is an extreme and expensive technology that society will need new assessment and allocation techniques to provide in a high-quality, equitable, cost-responsible manner.

The press has taken the lead in promoting the first view; the "life from death" drama of transplantation appears regularly in major newspapers. Those who see a medical system doing more and more to fewer and fewer people at higher and higher cost worry about issues of cost, access, and quality, and, as a means of addressing these issues more broadly, have focused on transplantation. Some believe this focus is unfair to transplantation, arguing that singling out organ transplantation "for careful scrutiny is unduly harsh . . . and narrow-minded."[1]

THE CONTEXT

Government officials, aided and abetted by the press, have shamelessly promoted themselves by promoting transplants. The president of the United States has made public appeals for livers for young children with biliary atresia, but his administration has steadfastly refused to set standards for retrieval and allocation of organs among the nation's 100-plus organ procurement agencies. Governors have been providing Medicaid funding for individuals who have successfully publicized their cases, but most of these politicians have refused to deal with the broader social issues organ transplantation raises. Dr. David Jackson, former Commissioner of Health in Ohio, properly characterizes the current state of organ transplantation as the "bipartisan political exploitation" of dying patients.

Traditionally, Medicare has provided reimbursement for "safe and effective" procedures that are medically "necessary and reasonable," and state Medicaid programs usually follow Medicare's lead. But when the question of Medicare coverage for heart transplantation was discussed in 1979, secretary of Health and Human Services (HHS) Patricia Harris decided that because the magnitude of the potential expense was unknown, she did not want to approve Medicare coverage without further study. Interpreting "necessary and reasonable" to mean far more than simply "not experimental," she commissioned a massive study to determine the social, economic, and legal consequences of Medicare transplantation coverage. The result was a private $1.6 million study by the Battelle Human Affairs Research Centers of Seattle that was released by HHS in mid-1985.[2] This study is a potential prototype for medical technology assessment. Although the authors were specifically instructed *not* to tell HHS whether or not Medicare should fund heart transplants (Medicare eligibility would be limited to those people over sixty-five or disabled for two years), the study clearly indicates that Medicare should. It argues that the total cost to HHS would be minimal because the pool of Medicare eligible patients is small. Moreover, total potential coverage is limited by the supply of human hearts (in a worst-case scenario where the federal government would cover all heart transplants), and the technology has advanced to a point where, in most cases, survival for many years with good prospects for rehabilitation can be expected.

The main point of the Battelle Report is that as long as the cost of heart transplants is similar to the costs of other expensive medical procedures currently being offered, transplants should be funded on the same basis as these other procedures. Not to do so, to use a new set of access and financing standards for transplants, seems to be unfair to potential transplant patients.[3] But perhaps it is time to challenge the assumption that all new medical technologies should be judged by comparing them to existing medical technology.

WHY TRANSPLANTS ARE DIFFERENT

The major reason HHS has treated transplants differently from any other medical technology is that they *are* different. Most of their public appeal, for example, revolves around the fact that every successful major organ transplant represents a public health tragedy: the sudden death of a healthy, young person who can become an organ "donor."

In addition, *kidney transplantation is already treated differently from any other surgical procedure.* In the early 1970s, when kidney dialysis was first made available to large numbers of patients (many waiting for kidney transplantation), a patient was dialyzed in front of a congressional committee in a dramatic demonstration of the technology. With very little debate, Congress determined that since the technology was available, and rationing methods seemed inherently unfair, "lifesaving" dialysis and kidney transplantation should be provided to all in need, regardless of economics. The result was Medicare's End-Stage Renal Disease program. Today, about 80,000 patients annually receive dialysis, and about 6,000 receive kidney transplants, at a federal cost of approximately $2 billion. There is no other surgical procedure that has this type of universal federal coverage, and because of the kidney precedent, heart and liver transplantation seem the logical next candidates.

Unlike most medical technologies that only change what we can do, transplants change our self-perceptions. Even before funding became the major issue, transplant surgeons in many states during the 1960s refused to do transplants at all unless and until their state legislatures passed laws on "brain death" that limited what they saw as potential legal liability for "harvesting" organs. This involvement of state legislatures in setting the legal and social stage for a medical procedure—by changing our very perception of death—is unique in this country's medical-legal history. Similar issues were publicly debated regarding the Uniform Anatomical Gift Act, and now some states have even adopted "required request" laws requiring hospitals to ask the relatives of all potential organ "donors" about organ donation. From the corridors of state houses to the corridors of hospitals treating patients unrelated to potential recipients, there is no other medical procedure that requires this *public* involvement.

Not only do organ transplants have a unique legal and economic history, but they also raise the issue of equity of access more dramatically than any other medical intervention. That is why individuals such as Jamie Fisk are able to command media attention. They are clearly identifiable, they will die without a transplant, and the refusal to pay for their transplant seems to place a specific price on life.

Many individual states, frustrated by the lack of federal leadership, have also singled out organ transplantation for special study and have required it to meet more rigorous standards than any other medical procedure. In Massachusetts, for example, a *public* Task Force on Organ Transplantation was appointed to make recommendations regarding the introduction of heart and liver transplantation, public funding, priorities, access, and patient selection standards.[4] The Task Force itself suggests why organ transplants were targeted for special treatment: they are extreme and expensive, potentially costing four to ten times as much as any other currently available medical procedure (based on comparative average fully allocated first-year survival costs); their introduction could distort the medical system to the detriment of higher-priority medical care; and organ transplantation has for the first time put rationing (by organ scarcity if not by ability to pay) on the public agenda. The Task Force recommended that organ transplants not be introduced at all if they could not be provided independent of ability to pay, or if they diminished "higher-priority" medical care.[5] It also recommended that patient selection criteria be public and based on objective medical criteria aimed at identifying candidates able to survive "a significant period of time with reasonable prospects for rehabilitation," and that such candidates should undergo transplantation on a first come, first served basis, after taking organ match into account.[6] The Task Force's recommendations were adopted unanimously as policy guidelines by the Massachusetts Department of Public Health, and formed the basis for two three-year demonstration projects on heart and liver transplantation currently implemented in Massachusetts.

THE FUTURE OF MEDICAL TECHNOLOGY ASSESSMENT

Transplants have not been randomly or unfairly chosen as the nation's "test case" on medical technology assessment. Transplants have a unique political, economic, and legal history, and are also unique in that they require another human being as a "donor." The opportunity they present to do reasonable public assessment work is especially important in view of the likely future development of mechanical implants that do *not* require a human donor source. There will be no natural limitation on the total number of implants, such as artificial hearts, and their total cost (and capacity to skew and distort the medical system) will be higher than all organ transplants combined. Therefore, the way we resolve issues of introduction, diffusion, access equity, cost control, and quality control in organ transplants will have an almost immediate potential payoff in evaluating the role mechanical implants should play in our future medical care system.

The fact that artificial hearts will be *the* most expensive medical technology ever introduced into the medical system on a wide scale, and that work in the area of transplants *might* give us some reasonable methods for evaluating their human usefulness and costs before artificial hearts take on a "life of their own," provides perhaps the most powerful argument for rigorously treating the introduction of heart and liver transplants. We still have an opportunity (albeit a fading one) to begin the introduction of meaningful public participation into medical technology assessment and diffusion. It seems fair and reasonable that we make the most of that opportunity.

NOTES

1. Evans, *The Socioeconomics of Organ Transplantation,* TRANSPLANTATION PROCEEDINGS 17(6, supp. 4):129–36 (December 1985).
2. R. W. EVANS, *et al.* THE NATIONAL HEART TRANSPLANTATION STUDY: FINAL REPORT (Battelle Human Affairs Research Centers, Seattle, Wash.) (1984).
3. *See Id.*, ch. 27–30.
4. REPORT OF THE MASSACHUSETTS TASK FORCE ON ORGAN TRANSPLANTATION, reprinted in part in LAW, MEDICINE AND HEALTH CARE 13:8–26 (February 1985), and in Part II of this volume.
5. Annas, *Regulating Heart and Liver Transplants in Massachusetts: An Overview of the Report of the Task Force on Organ Transplantation,* LAW, MEDICINE AND HEALTH CARE 13:4–7 (February 1985); reprinted in Part II of this volume.
6. Annas, *The Prostitute, the Playboy and the Poet: Rationing Schemes for Organ Transplantation,* AMERICAN JOURNAL OF PUBLIC HEALTH 75:187–89 (1985); reprinted in Part II of this volume.

Section 4

Reimbursement Issues

14

Ethical Implications of Reimbursement Policies

Samuel Gorovitz

Why is reimbursement policy ethically interesting? One reason is obvious: the treatment that gets paid for influences how resources are allocated and who gets access to treatment. There is also a subtler reason. When, for instance, one agrees to speak at a meeting, one is typically told that travel costs will be reimbursed; it is understood what that means. The speaker pays the cab driver, gets a receipt, tells the sponsor about it, and the sponsor reimburses him or her. But when people in the medical world discuss reimbursement, that is not necessarily what they mean. They typically just mean "getting paid." Yet when one buys a record or a book, one does not "reimburse" the clerk. One does not summon a waiter and say, "Bill, please. I'd like to reimburse the management." The use of the word "reimbursement" in the medical context can distort our perceptions of the situation.

Why has the reimbursement concept been invoked in this environment? Very simply, "reimbursement" conveys an aura of entitlement. One is getting what one is due. The idea of reimbursement makes this seem less controversial than the terms "fees," "payments for services rendered," or "bills." In the medical world, euphemism flourishes. People in hospitals never die: they pass away, transcend, fail to make it, cross over, or expire. And health care providers do not want to get paid, just reimbursed. This use of the term "reimbursement" in health care economics is a clue that we ought to beware.

The most obvious cluster of ethical issues associated with reimbursement policy—or, as this chapter will refer to it, payment policies—is that pertaining to the direct linkage between the policy and the allocation of scarce or costly resources. In the United Kingdom, for example, people over age fifty-five are rarely given dialysis because they are judged to be too old—not too old medically to survive or benefit, but too old for the health care system to afford to treat.[1] Since the criteria for eligibility for medical treatment, in the author's view, should be need-related, Britain's reimbursement or payment policy has an undesirable ethical consequence. People die because an investment in them has been judged unworthy.

Arthur Caplan has discussed various principles of exclusion that are essentially economic and result in decisions about who gets access to treatment.[2] One issue that needs further exploration is the extent to which economic factors are legitimate variables in determining health policy. When one thinks about saving lives, one is inclined to say, "Spare no expense." But none of us really believes that. Every year people are killed at railroad crossings. This is a trivial technical problem, but we do not solve it, not because of concern for the environment or the esthetics of the railroad crossing without an overpass, but because we do not want to pay for the overpass. Is this any more justifiable than the British constraints on dialysis of the elderly? Are both of these viewpoints, perhaps, justifiable after all?

Many people would argue that placing economic constraints on saving lives is just. The question is how much is too much? We avoid this question whenever possible, but the arguments are building to the point where avoiding the question is no longer possible.[3] Dr. Caplan is right in his assertion that there is nothing sacrosanct about the percentage of the gross national product devoted to health care delivery, whether the percentage is 10.5 or any other antecedently determined figure.[4] Yet the capacity of the health care industry to absorb investment is limitless, not because it is an evil empire, but because it is so very successful. Medical successes increase medical bills. Every life saved yields a health care consumer, rather than a mortician's customer.

We must, somehow, determine appropriate principles for limiting health care expenditures. These principles will have direct consequences for who has access to what; this is a fundamentally ethical issue, not an actuarial or a technical matter. The question of whether an old person's life is worth saving is very different from the question of what the probabilities are of success, given a particular patient profile and a particular contemplated intervention. We turn to physicians for an answer to the latter question, but we turn to one another for an answer to the former.

Sometimes the questions overlap. The Institute for Medical Genetics in Oslo, Norway, was authorized to perform amniocentesis five hundred times in 1985 by the government, which claimed that was as many as it could afford.[5] The Institute juggled the figures in order to perform the test seven hundred times. Nevertheless, the staff estimates that about fifteen hundred cases a year warrant amniocentesis, so in the absence of specific risk factors other than age, the tests were performed only on women aged thirty-eight and over. This is resource allocation based on a political determination of the appropriate cost for the procedure. The consequence is that some people who want access to a service—even if they are willing to pay out of their own pockets—cannot obtain it.

This constraint is different from one, for example, that states that we will not dialyze New York Yankees fans, regardless of their medical or financial circumstances, because society is better off without them. That kind of "social worth" criterion is arbitrary and unjustifiable. However, we will have to grapple with determining which criteria are appropriate. Some ethicists argue that these criteria should be explicit,[6] but I have some misgivings about the prudence of that approach.[7]

Consider a softer allocation constraint, as opposed to such a clear and crisp one as age constraint. Thomas Starzl's allusion to a "flow of gold" is a wonderful metaphor.[8] It conjures up an image of a volcanic phenomenon—but instead of lava descending from Mount St. Helens, gold flows from Washington to nephrologists everywhere. Dr. Starzl pointed out the distorting impact this flow has had on the incidence of home dialysis and kidney transplantation, as compared with institutional dialysis which is very profitable for those who operate such programs.[9] If a person on dialysis could benefit from a transplant and does not receive one because it was not recommended by the physician, that patient is denied access as much as the patient who is rejected for transplantation because of age. If one is medically eligible for a kidney transplant, but is in an environment that does not encourage transplants because of economics, that individual is denied access in an implicit but still fundamentally evil way. This chapter does not suggest that the operators of dialysis centers are self-serving evildoers. But there does seem to be, in the judgment of some physicians, reason to believe that at least a little skulduggery occurs in some dialysis centers. Roger Evans has written about "how dramatically the extension of Medicare benefits to patients with ESRD [End-Stage Renal Disease] affected the composition of the patient population."[10] This illustrates the profound consequences that payment of service has on how health care is delivered.

How can we remedy denial of access to care? One possibility would be to make payment for dialysis contingent upon a periodic affirmation of its appropriateness. This could be accomplished by an independent consultant who must also confirm that if the patient is an appropriate recipient for a transplant, he or she is on the waiting list. Such a procedure would be costly and would create some bureaucracy. Still, it is worth considering because, for many patients, transplantation is a preferred outcome to continuing dialysis.

It could be argued that the waiting lists for kidney transplantation are so long that additions to them should not be encouraged. This is an unfair response if one considers that any appropriate transplant patient who is kept on dialysis and is denied the opportunity to be put on a transplant waiting list is an abused patient; this is a profoundly immoral situation. Waiting lists should accurately reflect the need for organs, regardless of the severity of the shortage.

Thus far, this chapter has discussed the effect of payment for services on individual patients. We make an assumption, one that is typically considered valid, that any good or service that benefits its recipients is generally beneficial. If something is good for every patient who receives it, it is apparently good. Yet, it might not be so. This is the point emphasized recently by the Stanford historian, Bart Bernstein.[11] Instead of worrying about the possible failures of the artificial heart program, Bernstein asks us to consider the problems that would attend its success. He spells out some of these potential problems, not least of which is the immense social cost of developing a program that might benefit individual recipients. Regardless of whether or not Bernstein is right on that particular issue, his approach illustrates the difference between the local and the universal view. We do not ask the right question when we ask only, "Is this good for each person?" We must also ask, "How good or bad is this for all people?"; and the answer cannot be inferred from a concatenation of the answers to questions about individual recipients.

Let us sketch a possible future. Third-party payers rapidly extend coverage to all sorts of transplants, but with certain limitations. For example, heart transplants may be given to those under age fifty-five. The subscriber who is fifty-six may not want to continue paying high premiums for insurance that covers an expensive treatment for which he or she is not eligible. Instead, he or she may choose a competing insurer's policy that has lower premium rates and does not provide any coverage for heart transplants. This could lead to markedly different insurance policies that cater to different segments of the market. A person with healthy and grown children, no alcoholism in the family, and no history of congenital organ difficulty would probably not want coverage that includes liver transplantation. If other people make similar choices about insurance, we will have created a multitiered system of broad coverage for those who want to pay higher premiums and poorer coverage for those who see themselves as ineligible. These no-frills flights into the world of insurance will be attractive not only to healthy, low-risk people, but also to poor, high-risk people. What, then, of the notion of equal access? What of the notion that we provide services as a function of need rather than ability to pay?

The final point of this chapter concerns the idea, often affirmed by physicians, that the physician should never engage in controversy over how to slice a tiny pie. Instead, society should make the pie bigger. According to this view, doctors should not decide or even be concerned with allocation of resources. Yet is it always sufficient to say that the pie should be made larger? At some point, we will run out of ingredients. We must recognize that this solution—enlarge the pie so that all patients can receive all the desired medical care—is a dream. Not only is it unrealistic, it is receding further into the distance. It was tried unsuccessfully in Bahrain, a tiny oil-rich, Middle East country. Some years ago Bahrain decided on a national policy of providing the best health care available, free of cost, to everyone. Despite a small population and a huge per capita income, Bahrain has discovered that it cannot afford that policy. The country is now wrestling with the problem of backing away from such a commitment.

We, too, must anticipate these questions, and we must continue to debate the kinds of investments we are willing to make and the kinds of limitations we are willing to accept in vital health care. Such inherently ethical issues are raised by the complex of phenomena surrounding organ transplantation. Dr. Starzl thus understates the problem when he claims that the only ethical issues arising out of organ transplantation are those associated with the use of human subjects as experiments. The reality of organ transplantation challenges us to make difficult moral judgments about what is of greatest value to us, what sacrifices of resources or autonomy are justified in pursuit of that value, and how our society should respond to the changing patterns of medical care and human mortality.

NOTES

1. H. J. Aaron, W. B. Schwartz, The Painful Prescription: Rationing Hospital Care (Brookings Institution, Washington, D.C.) (1984) at 34–37.
2. See Caplan, ch. 1 of this volume.
3. See Evans, *Health Care Technology and the Inevitability of Resource Allocation and Rationing Decisions, Parts I and II*, Journal of the American Medical Association 249(15):2047; 249(16):2208 (1983); reprinted in Part II of this volume.
4. See Caplan, *supra* note 2.
5. This information comes from discussions the author had with Oslo Institute staff members in March 1985.

6. *See* Caplan, *supra* note 2.

7. *Cf.* Gorovitz, *The Artificial Heart: Questions to Ask and Questions Not to Ask,* THE HASTINGS CENTER REPORT 14(5):15–17 (October 1984); reprinted in Part II of this volume.

8. T. Starzl, in remarks made at the American Society of Law and Medicine's Conference on Human Organ Transplantation (April 1985).

9. *Id.*

10. *See* Evans, *supra* note 3, p. 2216.

11. Bernstein, *The Misguided Quest for the Artificial Heart,* TECHNOLOGY REVIEW 87(8):13–19 (November-December 1984).

15

Paying for Organ Transplants Under Medicare

Carolyne K. Davis

The subject of organ transplants is an urgent one. As evidence of this urgency, we need look no farther than our television sets where we frequently see people pleading for organ donors for their loved ones.

Granted that television is performing a service in doing this, one must still ask: can't we do more for these desperate people? Some of the answer depends on the direction public policy is headed with regard to organ transplants. And time is of the essence. Almost overnight, it seems, the science of replacing the body's organs has come of age. Future improvements will occur just as rapidly. It is important that we consider where we have stood on these issues, and even more important, where we should be going. The issues that surround the new transplant technologies are going to end up on the doorstep of the Health Care Financing Administration (HCFA)—since someday Medicare may have to decide whether to cover transplants. This chapter discusses how Medicare decides on which treatments to cover and reports on new developments that will influence how future decisions will be made.

How Decisions Are Made

The Medicare Law, which is our guidepost, states that Medicare cannot pay for any device or service that is not "reasonable or necessary" for diagnosis and treatment.[1] This translates into the question: Is it safe, effective, and generally accepted in the medical community? Normally, Medicare does not cover any procedure regarded as experimental. These are paid for, when approved for clinical trials, by the National Institutes of Health.

The Food and Drug Administration (FDA) is responsible for ruling on the safety and effectiveness of any medical devices, prior to HCFA's decision, to determine its "reasonable and necessary" status for coverage under Medicare.[2] At present, Medicare pays for kidney, cornea, and some liver transplants. Heart, heart-lung, adult liver, and pancreas transplants, which are still regarded as investigational, will be discussed later.

First, however, this chapter describes how the Department of Health and Human Services (HHS) determines whether Medicare will cover a new technology.

Most coverage issues are either local or regional and never reach Washington, since they are determined by fiscal intermediaries after consultation with one of HCFA's regional offices. But, every year about sixty coverage issues of a national nature do reach HHS's attention. The Office of Coverage Policy then reviews the relevant medical literature on the technology to see if it can resolve the issue. If not, the issue goes to a panel of physicians from HCFA and the Public Health Service's Office of Health Technology Assessment.

If this panel of physicians cannot reach a decision, the issue is referred to the Public Health Service for an assessment. A formal assessment is a public process, involving professional organizations and others in the private sector. The comments and reactions of health professionals, their organizations, and the public at large are solicited in the *Federal Register*. After the comment period, a determination is made about whether a consensus exists that the technology in question meets the tests of safety, efficacy, and general acceptability. Sometimes, if an issue is still unclear, the Public Health Service hosts a consensus conference to encourage further deliberations.

The findings of the Public Health Service on these issues, along with a formal recommendation, are sent to HCFA. Inside HCFA, the Bureau of Eligibility, Reimbursement, and Coverage (BERC) makes a final recommendation concerning coverage by Medicare and forwards it to the HCFA administration for a final decision, sometimes in consultation with the HHS secretary.

POLICY-SHAPING EVENTS

It is absolutely critical that we develop a strong capability to make these assessments. An important new element improving our capability is a provision of a law enacted last year, which authorizes the National Center for Health Services Research and Health Technology Assessment to conduct research into issues dealing with the cost-effectiveness of new medical technologies.[3]

In March 1985, then-HHS Secretary Margaret Heckler signed a

charter that created a National Advisory Council on Health Care Technology Assessment.[4] This council advises the secretary on health technology issues. It also develops criteria and methods for helping HCFA decide whether specific new technologies should be reimbursed under federally financed programs.

THE NATIONAL ORGAN TRANSPLANT ACT

Still another noteworthy development is the National Organ Transplant Act that President Reagan signed in October 1984.[5] Title I of this law established a Task Force on Organ Procurement and Transplantation. It consists of twenty-five members, eighteen of whom are experts in the field (nine physicians or scientists; three persons from the organ procurement field; two insurers; four persons with group expertise in law, theology, ethics, health care financing, and social and behavioral sciences); three of whom are members of the general public; and four of whom are government representatives, including persons who represent HCFA and the office of the surgeon general, the NIH director, and the FDA commissioner.

This Task Force had two deadlines to meet: the first, on August 14, 1985, issued a report to the secretary and to Congress on immunosuppressive drugs used to prevent organ rejection. The second report came out January 14, 1986, on the medical, ethical, social, legal, and technical aspects of organ procurement and transplantation. (The executive summaries of these two reports appear in Appendix A and Appendix B of this volume.)

The law authorizes the secretary to help set up a National Organ Procurement and Transplantation Network.[6] This network will provide a computerized registry for matching organ donors with those who need organs. The secretary is also authorized to provide seed money to help organ procurement organizations get started. HHS will also develop a scientific registry of those who receive organ transplants. This law also makes the selling of human organs a federal crime. A separate unit of the Public Health Service has been established to help implement all of these changes.

This chapter will now advance a more detailed report on where Medicare stands with regard to the different transplant technologies.

KIDNEY TRANSPLANTS

Medicare began covering kidney transplants in 1973 as part of its services to end-stage renal disease (ESRD) victims. This is an appropriate transplant to examine, for the issues it poses typify the questions that will emerge because of new transplant technologies.

The first issue that kidney transplants pose is their relative value compared to renal dialysis. Renal dialysis has been the dominant technology in Medicare's ESRD program. But we are faced with rapidly escalating costs in this program, and the search for cost-effectiveness is urgent, as is our concern for improving the quality of life for individual ESRD beneficiaries.

ESRD beneficiaries comprise only one-fourth of 1 percent of all Medicare beneficiaries; yet in 1983 they accounted for about 3.7 percent of the program's total outlay. In 1974, this program cost $229 million and served 16,000 patients. In 1985, it is expected to cost $2.4 billion and to serve up to 84,000 patients. Kidney transplants cost a mere fraction of this total—just under $200 million for 5,358 transplants in 1982— but the issue they pose is intriguing: are kidney transplants, when feasible, a less costly alternative to renal dialysis? And are they more desirable? These questions are of more than academic interest as we continue our search for ways to cap ESRD program costs, while still providing access to quality care.

Some time ago, HCFA analyzed the costs of transplants versus the costs of dialysis.[7] As predicted, it showed that, at the outset, transplants cost more. In 1983, the average cost per kidney transplant was $47,000, while the average cost of dialysis was $19,000 for a year of therapy of which Medicare pays 80 percent.[8] Researchers estimate that four years after a person receives a kidney transplant, however, a cost break-even point is reached; after that, a net savings for Medicare is achieved.[9] Kidney transplants are also favored because patient surveys show that people who have them are happier about the quality of their lives than are renal dialysis patients.

Kidney transplants illustrate the problem of comparing competing health technologies on a shifting data base. What makes that base so insecure and difficult now, however, is the revolution in payments that has brought us to an era of predetermined reimbursement.[10] This is leading to dramatic economies in the industry that may well render old cost data meaningless when we compare an older technology with a new one. Even more uncertainty is introduced as we realize that every new technology runs up higher costs at the outset, but costs less as economies of scale take hold. However difficult this may be, it is important that we try to quantify these elusive factors. Data are the raw material of public policy decisions; when they are difficult to come by, the public policy process is impeded. Government agencies that deal with health care recognize the problem and are trying to overcome it. We need to develop new methodologies that will allow us to make meaningful cost comparisons between competing technologies, and that will tell us how much less a new medical technology will cost once it has achieved general usage. Perhaps most important, we need to know that the data on which we are basing our coverage decisions reflect today's realities, not yesterday's. Cost data analyses must be balanced with the difficult assessments of the quality of life improvements a new technology offers.

We must hasten to develop expertise in all these areas. These, indeed, are HCFA's current goals. Our fiscal 1985 research budget earmarked $2.5 million for studies of coverage and technology issues. The bulk of this effort relates to heart- and kidney-related technologies, including transplants.[11] Other federal agencies that are also developing their expertise in this arena are the Public Health Service, the Prospective Payment Assessment Commission, and Congress's Office of Technology. To this we must add the effort of health insurers and universities.

OTHER CONUNDRUMS

One conundrum we may have to address is whether we should limit Medicare coverage for certain transplants to selected centers that have demonstrated the highest survival rates, and if so, by which criteria should these centers be designated? Who decides who qualifies? Answering these questions would be a first for Medicare, since it has always paid for coverage in any institution that meets the program's Conditions of Participation.

In organ transplantation, there is also the question of age as it pertains to a patient's suitability. Previous reports indicate that the most successful heart transplants result when a patient is under age fifty-five.[12] Indeed, most cost estimates of future expenditures are based on an assumption of current models of practice. Yet, an artificial heart has now been placed in a patient who is sixty-one.[13] Breaking the age barrier has implications for Medicare's decision about covering transplants. To borrow a lesson learned in the kidney transplant program, once a coverage decision is made, people of all ages will receive the service, since Medicare cannot use age discrimination in its coverage policies. Therefore, we need to view any projection of future expenditures with the realization that current practice patterns may change quickly once Medicare decides to cover a certain technology.

Another issue is the question of who should be considered as liver transplant candidates. This may conjure up the gloomy idea of rationing care, but if one looks squarely at the issue, it turns out to be no such thing. In hospitals, decisions about performing a given procedure for a patient are made every day. The medical teams involved must decide when it is inappropriate to subject a patient to a procedure that may have only a marginal impact on his or her survival prospects or on the quality of his or her life. If this is rationing—and this author does not think it is—then it is done all the time. Increasingly, physicians and families are aided in these sometimes painful, always difficult decisions by a growing body of counselors with expertise in the ethical and human areas. This is as it should be—and we should anticipate a growing need for these experts.

On a broader level, Medicare does get involved in decisions regarding patient selection. We decide, for example, who will and who will not be covered for bone marrow transplants. Currently, we limit these to people with leukemia and aplastic anemia, although we are in the process of re-examining this decision.

Experimental Organ Transplantation

There are several transplant technologies that are still experimental and for that reason we do not normally cover them. Heart transplants fall under this category.

Medicare has paid for fifteen heart transplants as part of a national study of this evolving technology.[14] This study has investigated the medical, financial, legal, and ethical aspects of heart transplants as well as the patients' posttransplant quality of life. This study is an important contribution to the literature of transplantation and will enable Medicare to consider further covering heart transplants.

Pancreas transplants are also still experimental. In October 1981, we asked the Public Health Service (PHS) to give us their view on these, especially for people in the End-Stage Renal Disease Program who are both diabetic and have transplanted kidneys. The service said then, and repeated in its September 1984 study update, that pancreas transplants are still experimental and are being conducted at only a few centers in the United States.[15] Only a few have been performed, but, the PHS noted, pancreatic transplants did seem to improve the condition of kidney transplant patients. No further recommendations were made.

Heart-lung transplants are another frontier technology where questions of coverage are nowhere near being addressed. But this whole field is alive with similar developments, such as the artificial heart and animal heart transplants. No one can say how soon we may have to confront coverage decisions. We are beginning to see our frontiers of experimental science advancing into multiple organ transplants. With these advances will come an even more difficult bioethical decision about who should receive how many different organ transplants.

TRANSPLANTS UNDER MEDICAID

Transplant coverage under state Medicaid programs presents another situation. Each state is free to do what it will in these matters; some states take their cue from Medicare. Other states are handling coverage issues in unique ways. Pennsylvania, for example, has decided to use a diagnosis-related group (DRG) system to pay for liver and bone-marrow transplants. A statewide consortium in Ohio is serving Medicaid patients who are considered good candidates for heart, heart-lung, liver, and pancreas transplants.[16] Illinois negotiates with the individual hospital and pays up to 60 percent of usual, customary, and reasonable transplant charges.

CONCLUSION

This concludes the overview of federal policy developments in transplant technology. However, here is one parting thought. Medicare coverage policy in this area cannot operate without taking into consideration budget realities. Quite plainly, we have a responsibility to keep Medicare from going broke, and that responsibility will have to be exercised as we consider coverage decisions such as those presented by transplants.

The Reagan administration has made remarkable progress in slowing down the health care cost spiral: from 1973 to 1982, Medicare's inpatient hospital payments averaged a yearly jump of 18.5 percent.[17] But in 1984, thanks to prospective payment and a general inflation rate that is now under control, the rate was held to just 7 percent. We simply cannot afford to let a runaway medical technology wipe out that progress. If we can continue to control Medicare's inpatient hospital costs, we are on the way to ensuring Medicare's financial future.

This does not mean curtailing medical progress; it does mean ensuring that the kind of progress we do approve represents a real benefit to the patients involved. It also means making sure that the cost of any new technology does not undermine the future fiscal integrity of a program that 30 million Americans depend on for their access to medical care. Balancing these considerations will not be easy, and to succeed we will need straightforward and clear thinking.

NOTES

1. 42 U.S.C. §1395y(l)(A) (1982, supp. I, 1983).
2. 21 U.S.C. §360e *et seq.* (1982).
3. Health Promotion and Disease Prevention Amendment of 1984, Pub. L. 98-551, §5 (1984).
4. *Id.* at §5(g)(l).
5. Pub. L. 98-507 (1984).
6. *Id.* at §372.
7. Eggers, *Analyzing the Cost Effectiveness of Kidney Transplantation,* in PROCEEDINGS OF THE NINETEENTH NATIONAL MEETING OF THE PUBLIC HEALTH CONFERENCE ON RECORDS AND STATISTICS (National Center for Health Statistics, Hyattsville, Md.) (1983) at 216–19.
8. *Id.*
9. *Id.*
10. 42 C.F.R. §412 (1985).
11. *See* R. W. EVANS, *et al.,* THE NATIONAL HEART TRANSPLANTATION STUDY: FINAL REPORT (Battelle Human Affairs Research Centers, Seattle, Wash.) (1984).
12. *Id.* at ch. 9.
13. *See* New York Times (December 2, 1982) at A24.
14. EVANS, *supra* note 11.
15. PUBLIC HEALTH SERVICE ASSESSMENT OF THE PANCREAS (U.S. Government Printing Office, Washington, D.C.) (July 26, 1984).
16. *See* Jackson, ch. 12, of this volume.
17. 1985 Annual Report of the Board of Trustees of the Federal Hospital Insurance Trust Fund (Washington, D.C.) Table A.1, p. 62.

16

Blue Cross and Blue Shield Coverage for Major Organ Transplants

Barbara W. Mayers

BLUE CROSS AND BLUE SHIELD COVERAGE BACKGROUND

This chapter will begin with a description of some important background components against which the Blue Cross and Blue Shield system is responding to the major organ transplantation phenomenon. This background includes characteristics of both the system itself and the surrounding environment that shapes its response. Some basic understanding of what the overall health insurance picture looks like, while not answering or even necessarily pointing the way toward answers to the larger question of how, for example, to develop principles of limitation on expenditures for health care, does explain much about how coverage decisions are made today. Once the background has been established, it will be followed by a summary of the system's response and a comment on policymaking.

The Blue Cross and Blue Shield system comprises ninety Plans, each of which is a separate, nonprofit corporation and a member of the Blue Cross and Blue Shield Association. The Association does not insure health benefits, but instead provides its member Plans with coordinated research and development, centralized administration of inter-Plan programs and communications systems to serve a mobile and multistate population of subscribers, and various kinds of specialized information, analysis, and advice. One such Association program evaluates available data on the safety, efficacy—and, in some instances, the cost—of new medical technology.

While Blue Cross and Blue Shield Plans' combined enrollment is nearly eighty million Americans, the size of their individual membership varies dramatically, and their geographic service areas range from a few counties to entire states. Despite this diversity, all Plans are organized and operated for the common purpose of offering prepaid health care benefits on a nonprofit basis at a reasonable cost to as many people in their communities as possible. In order to do this, Blue Cross and Blue Shield Plans typically contract with local health care providers to furnish covered services to their subscribers. Although these provider agreements generally do not shift underwriting risk from Plans to providers, they do serve as a means whereby Plans can manage, and thus better predict, that risk. As an overabundance of providers has developed in many locales in this country and costs have escalated, Plans have become increasingly selective and demanding in their provider contracting requirements.

Most Blue Cross and Blue Shield Plans are licensed and regulated under special state health service corporation laws. The state insurance department typically is responsible for overseeing subscriber contracts and rates, provider contracts, payment arrangements, claims practices, solvency, and other operational aspects. Plans generally are in the middle of a continuum from highly regulated health maintenance organizations (HMOs) to less regulated commercial insurance companies.

As is true for all forms of private health insurance, the majority of Blue Cross and Blue Shield subscribers are enrolled through employer groups. Health benefits are a form of employee compensation and, as such, are a mandatory subject of collective bargaining. Thus, where employees are unionized, their contract may include detailed health benefit specifications as is true, for example, of the most recently executed General Motors-United Auto Workers contract, or the contract may cover the subject only in broad outline. For nonunionized employees, the level and scope of health benefits is left almost completely to labor market forces and employer discretion. The federal Employee Retirement Income Security Act (ERISA) has the effect of preempting nearly all state regulation of employee health benefit plans, while itself imposing only basic reporting and disclosure requirements and certain minimal fiduciary standards.

The various providers of health insurance—HMOs, service benefit plans such as Blue Cross and Blue Shield Plans, and commercial insurers—are, however, directly affected by a growing body of state-mandated benefits laws that require them to cover various health services rendered. To the extent that employee health benefits are insured through these regulated carriers, the state benefit mandates are indirectly imposed on the employee benefit plan itself. Only one state has moved in that direction with respect to coverage of organ transplantation. The Illinois Experimental Organ Transplantation Act prohibits insurers, HMOs, and the Blue Cross and Blue Shield Plan in Illinois from denying benefits for what are referred to as "otherwise covered transplants" on the ground that they are experimental procedures. It is not an absolute mandate of coverage for transplants. In 1985, a bill similar to the Illinois law was introduced, but not passed, in Pennsylvania. It would have affirmatively required health insurance coverage of major organ transplants. Thus, there really is no body of law that directly governs the substance of employee health benefits in general, and almost none that indirectly requires coverage of organ transplants by requiring them to be provided by health insurers.

Almost without exception, the questions of whether and to what extent health insurance covers new medical technology are matters of private decision making, but the quasi-public nature of Blue Cross and Blue Shield Plans affects the decision-making process. Blue Cross and Blue Shield Plans are aware of the economic and social welfare imperatives to apply limited health benefit dollars toward efficient delivery of services that actually benefit their subscribers' health status. For this reason, most benefit contracts expressly exclude coverage for procedures that are determined to be not medically necessary and those that are still experimental or investigational.

FACTORS AFFECTING BLUE CROSS AND BLUE SHIELD TRANSPLANT COVERAGE

Three developments of the past decade have had a significant effect in shaping the environment in which Blue Cross and Blue Shield Plans address questions regarding benefits for major organ transplants, and other new and emerging technologies which have unusual characteristics similar to those of human organ transplantation.

First, and perhaps most pervasive, is the strong and rising customer dissatisfaction with the escalating cost of health benefits. The perception of uncontrollability and the skepticism about whether there has been any commensurate increase in general well-being probably have been as important as the absolute dollar increases themselves. This dissatisfaction has reached the point where it has produced some very profound changes in employee health benefit plans. One is a significant shift to self-insurance—and even self-administered benefits—to the point where more than one-third of such plans are today self-insured, something that was extremely rare ten years ago. Another is the very active and direct employer involvement in efforts to manage costs, including redesign of benefits and the selection of providers and types of care.

Additionally, there has been a substantial reduction in benefit levels for employees through the increased use of deductibles and coinsurance arrangements that have served to shift more of the costs of care to the employees who receive that care.

The second environmental factor within the last decade that affects how Plans approach benefit design and administration consists of changes in the antitrust laws that have significantly increased health care providers' and insurers' exposure to litigation and liability. One result of this has been a group of cases in which provider plaintiffs sue other providers and insurers on a variety of restraint-of-trade and monopolization theories. One species of this kind of litigation comprises cases in which it has been alleged that benefit denials for experimental or investigative services or medically unnecessary services are really the result of and a means of effectuating agreements among competing providers to unreasonably restrain competition in providing a particular health service, thereby stifling medical innovation.

Although the law in this area is minimal and unsettled, the potential exposure to antitrust defense costs alone is threatening and may well chill efforts to determine the safety and efficacy of new medical procedures, drugs, and devices and to exclude from coverage those that are unproven. One particularly noteworthy case, *Vest* v. *Waring*,[1] was a large antitrust action filed by a group of ophthalmologists in the federal district court in Atlanta several years ago. They alleged that the thirty-five defendants—including physicians participating in a series of clinical trials funded by the National Institutes of Health to evaluate radial keratotomy, a number of National Eye Institute physicians, and several ophthalmology organizations—were engaged in a conspiracy to falsely designate radial keratotomy as an experimental procedure for the purpose of unreasonably restraining competition in the procedure and monopolizing its performance. After three years of litigation the case was settled.

What is both interesting and disturbing is that one of the terms of the settlement was an agreement by the principal clinical investigator to issue a statement to the effect that he no longer considers the procedure, still under study, to be experimental. Health insurers all over the country have been sent copies of the settlement statement, and a number of breach of contract suits have been filed by individuals who were denied insurance benefits for radial keratotomy on the ground that coverage for experimental procedures is excluded. All of this has taken place while the balance of the five-year clinical evaluation of the procedure and publication of final results is pending.

The third relevant environmental factor of the last decade also involves changing and unsettled law plus large amounts of money. This refers to the phenomenon of insurer exposure to extracontract damages for "bad faith" breach of contract; that is, compensatory and punitive court-awarded amounts in addition to the amount of insurance contract benefits involved. The allegations in such cases typically include benefit misrepresentation and various unfair and unreasonable claims administration policies and practices. In some instances this has been construed to mean failure to meet what is deemed to be the insured's "reasonable expectations" of coverage, even in the face of express contract exclusions.

Under the influence of an array of factors, Blue Cross and Blue Shield Plans address the questions of whether and how to cover major organ transplants. Emerging high-cost, low-frequency, life-saving technology presents Plans with problems of information, evaluation, and prediction. On one hand, attempts to limit health benefit cost escalation, the infrequency of these procedures, and uncertainty about their effectiveness have all limited demand. On the other hand, when a Plan subscriber—whose contract excludes experimental procedures, or even expressly excludes transplants—does need such a procedure, its life or death nature and very high cost exert nearly irresistible pressure to find the means necessary to provide such benefits.

RISK MANAGEMENT AND TRANSPLANT COVERAGE

High-cost, low-frequency, life-saving technology also presents risk-spreading problems. The Plans' enrolled populations vary dramatically in size, and are increasingly fragmented as insurable groups among various employee-choice health benefit options. This necessitates the development of new risk-pooling arrangements to protect small groups against unpredictable catastrophic costs.

Employee benefit plan customers are determined to limit their health benefit costs and are often highly prescriptive about benefit design. There is increased risk of liability for failure to give subscribers clear and complete information about their coverage and failure to administer benefits in a matter that meets shifting judicial standards of fairness and reasonableness. There is the phenomenon of providers using the antitrust laws to attempt to redress what they perceive as economically threatening decisions about health insurance coverage and group purchasing of health care services.

Within this context, the Blue Cross and Blue Shield system has created a national major organ transplant reinsurance pool that currently includes more than ten million Plan and Plan-affiliated HMO enrollees as a necessary risk-management strategy in addressing this question. The system has developed the capacity to provide uniform organ transplant benefits for multistate employee groups that want such coverage. It is actively engaged in gathering cost and outcome data from transplant providers to try to improve its understanding of these procedures. The Association is encouraging Plans, where they are able, to limit their coverage only to services provided through transplant programs that: (1) have demonstrated the ability to achieve consistently good outcomes; (2) gather and make available usable data to support sound benefit design and administration; and (3) demonstrate the willingness and ability to reduce the costliness of this very expensive care through negotiation of global prices and agreement to other appropriate contract incentives. Plans are also advised to exclude coverage of major organ transplantation where, in fact, that is the intent of the contract, rather than relying on a general exclusion for experimental or investigational services.

During the past several years, Blue Cross and Blue Shield Plans have provided benefits for more than two hundred heart and liver transplants. Today, more than half the Plans, whose enrollment constitutes well over half the total Blue Cross and Blue Shield Plan enrollment, offer benefits for at least heart and liver transplantation. The Association participated on the federal Task Force on Organ Transplantation and is hopeful that this group's collective wisdom can enhance its own.

Conclusion

This chapter has described the context in which one group of interrelated organizations that do not enjoy central authoritative control is addressing major organ transplantation. Nobody makes a decision about organ transplantation coverage for eighty million U.S. Blue Cross and Blue Shield subscribers. That is not necessarily a bad thing. There will continue to be diversity in approaches to this and other health care issues, because in the United States important competing value hierarchies challenge not only "health policy" decision making, but agreement on what the decision-making process itself should be. Experience suggests that we will develop all the new medical technologies we can imagine, and continue to struggle for consistent and fair means both to evaluate and to distribute their benefits.

Notes

1. Vest v. Warings, 565 F. Supp. 674 (N.D. GA. 1983).

17

Organ Transplantation:
Future Directions
for Federal Policy

Bernadine P. Healy

Medicine has dramatically changed in the past decade and a half, and high technology typifies the change.

Not long ago, the great physician was a master diagnostician who had few therapies but was skilled at recognizing the disease, defining its natural course, and helping the patient and family through that course. This was especially true for end-stage organ failure of the kidney, heart, liver, and lungs. Thanks to advances in medical science, we now have numerous technologies to change the course of illness. The maturing field of organ transplantation has already helped many patients and promises to help even more live longer and more fruitful lives.

In the broadest terms, organ transplantation is a phenomenal success. It has captured the public's imagination and provides hope for a whole class of people whose condition is otherwise hopeless. The public clamors to use new technology, regardless of its cost-effectiveness, and transplantation is no exception. Medical scientists and practitioners are ready to move the frontiers forward—that is their mission. Indeed, the golden era of medicine is symbolized by "high-tech" items. Industry plays a key role here; in the case of transplants, it has made the current era possible by developing new and better drugs. In high technology, the United States is the world leader.

However, all of this benefit comes with a price: the ubiquity of the federal government. There are three stages of federal involvement in transplantation that parallel the emergence of most new science and technology into widespread practice. For organ transplantation in particular, only at the brink of the third and final stage of emergence do we confront the major uncertainties of the future and the major controversies we are now witnessing.

Phase I—Basic Science Investment

The first stage, and possibly the most important, is the federal investment in basic science. For forty years, the federal government has been the major source of support for basic biomedical research. It has funded the broad efforts in basic biology, including the physiology and pathology of organs, the pathophysiology of the variety of diseases that lead to end-stage organ failure, and the long-growing field of transplant biology and immunology. The investment has been extensive, since much of the research is targeted at specific diseased organs, such as the cornea, bone, kidney, heart, liver, pancreas, and bone marrow, and at the host of disorders that affect them. Probably all of the institutes of the National Institutes of Health have contributed. There has been little controversy with federal involvement at this level or with a governmental role that is limited to financial investment. This is not likely to change, although there have been concerns about the future implications for new technology. This country has always been wise, however, about focusing on new technology and not tampering with or trying to control the scientific exploration or experimentation that leads to it.

Phase II—Clinical Testing

The second level of federal involvement is in the support for clinical investigation and clinical trials—again, research investment in a few centers that are pioneering development. The extent and duration of the "experimental" testing phase have been determined largely by the force of the data, that is, by the results, the effectiveness, and the benefit of new medical procedures. The clinical benefit and safety of a procedure are by no means proved before a new procedure or therapy is accepted for clinical use. For example, within three years of its introduction, coronary angioplasty moved into widespread clinical use. Now about six years old, this procedure will be performed about 70,000 times a year, with little information on long-term results. Even though a therapy is only moderately expensive, adopting it so quickly is not necessarily justifiable. Coronary angioplasty is only one new and moderately expensive technology in the medical arsenal that has emerged so quickly and effortlessly. In contrast, in the case of organ transplants, a longer "Phase II"—some sixteen years—has generally been the case.

For organ transplants, there have been restraints and limits to the experimental trials and to the transition from experimentation into accepted therapy. These restraints have occurred primarily because of: (1)

dismal failures that tended to scare off the casual investigator, particularly before the use of cyclosporin and better surgical techniques; (2) a limited organ supply; and (3) the high cost of clinical studies. Here again, the federal role has been limited mainly to providing funds to make the clinical trials and investigations possible. The government has also worked, primarily through peer review, to limit the clinical studies to the centers best suited for this purpose.

Phase III—From New Technology to Accepted Therapy

For most new advances, the transition from experimental to accepted therapy is smooth. For example, by the time most new drugs are put on the market, they are long awaited, readily introduced, and rather easily accepted. But for organ transplantation, particularly for the major organs—kidney, heart, pancreas, and liver—this debut has been difficult. We are now in the midst of this emergence, and it is the transition phase that poses the greatest challenge for the future of organ transplantation. Clearly, much, though by no means all, of that responsibility is in the federal government's hands.

Why does the acceptance of organ transplantation seem so difficult, especially when compared to other great medical advances? Aside from the problem of cost, several difficulties mirror the reasons that transplantation has had such a long gestation in clinical investigation:

1. Transplantation is drastic therapy—replacing a heart that is not yet dead, for example, especially with the threat of the body rejecting the transplanted heart.
2. The therapy replaces the end-stage disease with other transplant-related diseases that in some cases are almost as bad. Most of these are complications of immunosuppression:
    —Infection is a major killer.
    —Cancer in the form of lymphomas occurs among heart transplants.
    —Hypertension remains a problem, even more so with the use of cyclosporin.
    —Accelerated atherosclerosis and myocardial infarction pose major problems among some renal and heart transplant patients.
3. The supply of suitable donor organs is limited.

In 1968, in an editorial prepared shortly after the first human heart transplant in South Africa, Dr. Michael DeBakey cited three major critical problems: control of graft rejection, limited availability of organs, and complications of immunosuppression.[1] Eighteen years later, these same problems still plague transplantation. The major recent advance is cyclosporin. This drug has partially mitigated two of the three major problems cited by DeBakey: rejection can be controlled somewhat, and the complications of immunosuppression are less severe.[2] Cyclosporin has thus increased the benefit of the procedures to the patients and, secondarily, has brought down the cost. Therefore, after a long Phase II where most of the activity was clearly focused on experimental use, organ transplantation has shifted significantly into the final transitional phase, mainly because of the scientific breakthrough of a more selective immunosuppressive therapy.

On the brink of Phase III, we now face the widespread debut of organ transplantation into clinical practice. Suddenly we are forced to confront a range of legal, ethical, and economic issues that until now have been abstract concerns.

Again, why is there all this fuss about organ transplants? Why the broad debate? Why the stronger governmental role? The reasons, which have received much publicity, are simple: the limited organ supply and enormous cost. The future direction of federal policy in these areas merits discussion.

Cost is a problem for many medical advances, particularly in Phase III when widespread use is anticipated. Here the impact of an expensive therapy is realized—and here very difficult questions are asked, which never were posed during the purely experimental phases, nor should they have been. These questions arise more frequently today because many people want to limit health care spending and because so many new medical technologies are constantly emerging.

As an aside, it should be noted that medical science differs from the physical sciences in the following regard. In physical sciences the cost of the basic science is often so high that questions about costs and benefits are often asked during Phase I. For example, the superconducting supercollider (SSC) has a price of five billion dollars or more, and that is for only one large accelerator. That SSC is needed, however, for the most fundamental research in small-particle physics. If the technology is not funded, Phase I research is constrained. The wisdom of making this substantial basic research expenditure has been widely questioned and debated. But, for medical advances, these questions come late in Phase III—at the practice level. We are hearing these questions loud and clear about organ transplantation:

—Can the nation afford all of the costly innovations emerging from the laboratory?

—Will the new medical technologies undermine efforts to reduce health care costs?

—How much is society willing to pay for the big-ticket items to maintain our high-technology medical system?

—Will other, less costly health care programs possibly suffer because of these big-ticket items?

These are broad issues of setting priorities—a painful task when resources are limited.

These issues are not unique to organ transplantation, nor should they be settled based on this single high-technology issue. Ronald Bayer described this broader confrontation between exploding technological advance and increasing demand as "the confrontation of Prometheus with Malthus."[3] Prometheus, the conqueror of powerful fire, symbolizes technology; Malthus represents our increasingly limited resources as the population increases. These issues of cost are "macro issues" and affect each new medical technology.

The federal government and the public do not seem ready to answer these macro issues, whether arising from transplantation or from other technological advances. Rather, the approach has been micro—case by case—and for a while will continue to be so. Case-by-case policymaking occurs at two levels. One level is that of the individual patient who is the subject of personal appeals—on television, radio, and in the newspapers. Local communities, the general public, state governors, and even the president respond to these heartbreaking pleas for organs. Policymaking at the individual level can also be exemplified by the individual doctor at the bedside who cannot bear to see his or her patient die if there is anything at all that can be done—even if it is a long shot. We want these qualities of compassion and humanity in our doctors, in our communities, and in elected officials. Indeed, reverence for human life and human dignity, and tolerance and compassion for others, are essential to our way of life and to our goodness as a nation. Providing these humanitarian benefits on the basis of visibility and media access may not, however, be the best policy.

The second level of case-by-case policy setting is better. In it, the federal government plays a major role through its regulatory authority and its responsibility to determine reimbursement policy for Medicare and Medicaid. This approach involves generic case-by-case analysis. For example, when and for what illnesses should heart transplants be used?

What is the generic case for liver transplants? This most difficult task, which involves treatment for thousands, not just a few people, must be developed in a fashion that recognizes that the process is dynamic, and that the facts change. For transplants, at least two dynamic things are happening: (1) science is increasing the probability of successful transplants, and (2) with better immunosuppression and more transplants being performed, the price should come down.

The federal attitude toward transplantation is fairly clear.[4] The federal government decides to cover a specific kind of transplant when it deems that the transplant is no longer experimental. Although the federal government makes this decision only for its own Medicare population, it can affect the market price by setting rates for diagnosis-related groups (DRGs). The Health Care Financing Administration has the data base to set a reimbursement level that will allow for some market competition and yet be a reasonable figure.

These clear roles give the federal government considerable influence in national transplant policies. Yet it is unknown whether these roles will satisfy our future needs. For example, who should decide when a big-ticket technology emerges from experimental status into practice? Is it necessary to show only that it is scientifically valid? Another problem concerns uniting all the appropriate players to develop the more difficult cost-benefit analysis. Any cost-benefit analysis must be soundly based on scientific information and on a sufficient and unbiased data base; thus, medical investigation must be part of the decision. But should the other key groups such as the public—especially when they are paying—be part of the dialogue? Traditionally, those who pay have not been involved in the decision about other new technologies. An even more unsettling question concerns whether the courts should be involved, as in *Vest* v. *Waring*.[5]

The federal government could also begin to designate and fund specific transplant centers. These "centers of excellence" would be a break from our traditional approach to medical technology, and they would put restraints on medical practice and on patients—restraints that have never existed except in the research setting of Phase II. Such restraints may be feasible for research but are quite a different matter for accepted practice. The concept of the center of excellence raises legal issues of antitrust and the question of who decides. The full implications of the concept, both for transplants and medicine today, should be weighed carefully.

Another governmental route is to designate more diseases in Medicare and to broaden the scope of Medicare coverage, as has occurred for end-stage renal disease (ESRD). The federal government pays

80 percent of the cost of kidney dialysis and transplantation.[6] What was predicted to be thousands or millions of dollars rapidly became billions. The government now dominates the market, and private insurers do little. Moving further in the direction of ESRD programs for all organ transplants could put our health care system, which is a carefully balanced public-private partnership, in jeopardy. An example of such a move would be payment for cyclosporin. The government's avoidance of such disease-specific procedures preserves the blend of private and public in our overall medical care system.

A current major issue in Washington is whether the federal government needs to expand its role in organ procurement. State regional efforts, some claim, are adequate and possibly more efficient. Should the federal government act as a catalyst or as the central manager? The government has taken the former role and may not need to change, particularly in light of success stories in several parts of the country that have developed cooperative regional organ procurement efforts.

The answers to these questions will change, with the passage of time, as other factors modulate; forecasting future policy directions is thus extremely difficult. We can identify the factors that will shape the future. One factor is how fast science changes. For example, even better immunosuppressives and better organ preservation will increase the medical benefit of transplants and decrease the costs.

When most transplants cost approximately $20,000 per year or less, much of the dialogue on transplantation may not be so worrisome. In fact, if the costs fall into that range, then the costs of transplanting an organ in a patient and returning him or her to a more vigorous life may be no more expensive than maintaining a patient with end-stage disease to the end of life. These end-stage patients make many trips to the hospital, and utilize much of our medical resources, but without much hope. If costs lessen, then transplants may become just one element of the broader debate on strained resources and rising health care costs.

Finally, if other organ sources, such as primates, become available, or if mechanical organs can replace or augment the function of end-stage living organs and decrease the demand for transplants, the answers to many questions will change.

However, in the course of this debate about future policies and the roles of the various sectors of society, it is most important not to lose sight of the fact that medicine moves ahead and science brings change. Whatever policies develop must be flexible and consistent with the kind of health care establishment this country needs.

Abraham Lincoln once said that the dogmas of the quiet past are inadequate to the stormy present. We should take that maxim further: they may be even less suited for the uncertain future. In our flurry of concern about transplants, we must not forget that our wisdom today may not be right for our children tomorrow. Whatever we do must be reasonable and flexible so that our children can also have a say.

NOTES

1. DeBakey, *Human Cardiac Transplantation,* JOURNAL OF THORACIC AND CARDI-OVASCULAR SURGERY 55(3):447–54 (March 1968).
2. Oyer, *et al. Cyclosporin in Cardiac Transplantation: A 2½-Year Follow-Up,* TRANS-PLANTATION PROCEEDINGS 15(4):2546–52 (December 1983).
3. *See generally,* Bayer, *Prometheus Meets Malthus,* BUSINESS AND HEALTH 22–25 (July-August 1984).
4. *See* Davis, ch. 15, of this volume.
5. Vest v. Waring, 565 F.Supp. 674 (N.D. Ga. 1983).
6. 42 U.S.C.A. §1395(b)(2)(A) (West Supp. 1985).

Part II

Background on Issues

Regulating Heart and Liver Transplants in Massachusetts: An Overview of the Report of the Task Force on Organ Transplantation

George J. Annas, J.D., M.P.H.

Organ transplantation has been a favorite topic of health lawyers since its inception. Organ procurement was addressed with the adoption of the Uniform Anatomical Gift Act in all fifty states, and "brain death" has been recognized both judicially and legislatively across the country. Nonetheless, it is now apparent that the major problems in organ transplantation are not legal and thus neither are their solutions. Heart and liver transplants are extreme and expensive interventions that few individuals can afford and few hospitals can offer. In an era of economic scarcity, how (if at all) should organ transplant procedures and other extreme and expensive treatments be introduced into the health care delivery system?

Although it seems reasonable to expect federal leadership to establish a limited number of high-quality transplant centers, federal efforts to date have focused almost exclusively on trying to help the scattered organ procurement agencies become more efficient. By default, the individual states have had to develop their own policies. A number of them, like California and Connecticut, have concentrated on Medicaid reimbursement requirements. Ohio has worked to develop a statewide "consortium" approach. But until late 1984, only Massachusetts had established a statewide public task force to make recommendations concerning how heart and liver transplants should be introduced. The Massachusetts Task Force grew out of a recommendation, made by Dr. Harvey V. Fineberg's earlier Liver Transplantation Task Force, that a broadly based public group examine the social issues involved with transplantation technology. The Massachusetts experience is important not only because it is the first state to utilize the strategy of a public task force, but also because of the strong medical institutions in Massachusetts, the vigorous use of determination-of-need mechanisms to regulate the introduction of liver and heart transplants, and the almost overwhelming desire of at least four Boston hospitals to do liver transplantation and of four Boston hospitals to do heart transplantation. Indeed, at times the political aspects of whether one hospital or more than one hospital should do either of these procedures have eclipsed all of the other critical issues involved in using these extreme and expensive technologies.

The recommendations themselves went to public hearing on November 5, 1984, and on November 27, 1984, the policy-making body of the Massachusetts Department of Public Health, the Public Health Council, unanimously adopted the recommendations as official policy guidelines and used the Report itself as explanatory text for the Department in reviewing determination-of-need applications for organ transplantation.

MAJOR CONCLUSIONS

Although sometimes lost in bland prose, several significant conclusions were reached by the Task Force, which structured its set of recommendations. The basis of the Report can be stated in one long sentence. Because transplants are extreme and expensive procedures that nevertheless do not cure disease but replace the patient's underlying disease with a lifetime of immunosuppression, and because introducing transplantation into the current cost-constrained health care system threatens to displace other, higher priority health care services (including services to the Medicaid population and the poor), transplants should not be performed at all unless they are done on those who are likely to benefit from them, unless the total cost is controlled, and unless resources are not diverted from higher priority care. In fleshing out this basic principle, the Task Force concluded that public regulation would be ineffective if the burden of proving health care priorities was placed on the Department of Public Health. Accordingly, the Task Force recommended that the analysis of health care priorities begin with a presumption that all currently offered health care services have a higher priority than organ transplantation. Therefore, any hospital applying to perform transplants should have the burden of demonstrating that "transplantation has a higher priority than any other currently available health service from which organ transplantation diverts funds and/or support systems."

On the underlying value issues of fairness and equity, the Task Force concluded that access to a transplant must be "independent of the individual's ability to pay for it." Thus, if offered at all in the system, heart and liver transplants must be considered part of the "minimum benefit package" to which all are entitled. But how could the health care system, which arguably could not handle organ transplants at all, introduce them in a manner that would make them available to everyone? The key is to restrict the total number of transplants done. However, this must be accomplished in a manner that optimizes the quality of care and benefit of those procedures actually performed, eliminates arbitrary patient selection excluders (such as income, age, and personal habits), and provides an equitable manner of selecting among suitable candidates when not all can be served. The most crucial element is to define "clinical suitability" for transplantation in a manner that concentrates on benefit to the patient in terms of life-style and rehabilitation rather than simple survival. In the words of the Task Force, medical suitability should be an attempt to predict "those who can benefit the most from [transplants] in terms of probability of living for a significant period of time with a reasonable prospect for rehabilitation." Critical to maintaining a strict definition of "clinical suitability" is the restriction of total system capacity to perform transplants, as explained in the summary of the economics section later in this article.

APPLICATION OF THE REPORT

The utility of the Task Force Report, its recommendations, and the new policy guidelines of the Massachusetts Department of Public Health will face their first test when they are used to determine the public need for a four-hospital consortium to do heart transplants in Massachusetts in early 1985. A separate four-hospital consortium was approved to do liver transplants for a three-year period in January 1984. Conditions were placed on that determination of need, including requirements that the hospital not consider ability to pay or insurance status in patient selection, not reduce Medicaid services as a trade-off for liver transplantation, not reduce free care for nontransplant services below that provided in the most recent fiscal year, and have its liver transplantation protocols reviewed and approved by an institutional review board. The members of the Consortium objected to these conditions, and appealed them to the Health Facilities Appeals Board, which ordered a remand on procedural grounds. On remand, the Public Health Council explicitly adopted the conditions, with some modifications, over the objections of the Consortium. The Institutional Review Board (IRB) review requirement was modified most significantly to read:

> The hospital will have its liver transplant protocols, including consent and withdrawal of consent policies, organ procurement policies, recipient selection policies and confidentiality policies, reviewed and approved by an ethics committee of the Boston Center for Liver Transplantation, which will contain significant public representation, or by a special board set up for this purpose by the Department of Public Health.

It remains to be seen whether the Liver Consortium can live up to the policy guidelines. While the hospitals did not have to satisfy the guidelines originally, they will serve as minimum requirements for any renewal of their determination of needs (DONs) two years from now.

OTHER SECTIONS OF THE REPORT

Portions of the Report not included here are sections on economics, religious views, and the consortium approach. The latter two can be dealt with relatively quickly. The Task Force found no religious tradition that prohibited organ donation or transplantation, and the perspectives included in the Report from the Catholic, Protestant, and Jewish traditions were all supportive of organ transplants. As previously mentioned, the consortium approach is primarily a political issue. It was grafted onto the original draft of the Report at the request of the Commissioner of Public Health. In March 1984, Commissioner Bailus Walker asked the Task Force's opinion about the advisability of granting a temporary exemption from determination of need to the Brigham and Women's Hospital, a tertiary care hospital, to do heart transplants. Such a single-hospital exemption was seen as preferable to having multiple hospitals request "emergency waivers" for individual patients while they pursued an institutional DON (this procedure was used for liver transplants in the Commonwealth by the Deaconess Hospital for more than six months). The commissioner found it impossible to refuse such requests, and the use of emergency waivers in heart transplantation would have undercut any reasonable planning efforts.

The commissioner's request for advice quickly became politicized, and a loose "consortium" of hospitals was thrown together to provide an alternative to the single-hospital exemption. The Task Force met three times on this issue. At its final meeting on this subject, May 15, 1984, the Task Force appeared for the first time in its entirety. Following a two-hour discussion, which was highlighted by a comment from State Senator Ed Burke that the paper consortium looked more like a "fig leaf" to cover "naked rivalry" among the hospitals, rather than a serious effort at cooperation, the Task Force voted unanimously to recommend a DON exemption for heart transplants in Brigham and Women's Hospital until the end of 1984. In addition, the Task Force voted to attempt to develop guidelines for a "truly cooperative consortium." A summary of guidelines for a "worthwhile consortium" appears in the group's final recommendation.

Economics

Since it was the cost of these extreme and expensive procedures that initially led to the formation of the Task Force, the Report's economic section and its conclusions are critical to any understanding of the recommendations. The analysis describes the many different ways of determining "costs" of transplants, and uses the specific figures generated by various agencies as examples of how divergent figures are calculated.

In general, hospitals have used only direct costs in the figures they have relied on to support their applications for determinations of need. Figures from the Massachusetts Liver Transplantation Task Force and Massachusetts Blue Cross, on the other hand, utilized fully allocated average costs. While arguments can be made for both views, the Task Force decided to use "fully allocated average costs for one year of survival" as a benchmark for determining the cost of transplants and comparing it to the costs of other extreme and expensive medical procedures. In computing the costs of heart and liver transplants, the cost of the surgery itself is generally the smallest item, amounting to only about 5 percent of the cost, for example, of a liver transplant. About one-fourth of the cost is attributable to readmission to the hospital due to complications, and almost one-half of the total is attributable to ancillaries such as laboratory, blood, intravenous lines, radiology, social work, and physical therapy. The most important cost determiners are the number of ICU days that will be used by the patient and the cost of these days. Fully allocated average costs will be a function not only of this, but also of the probability of surviving for one year and thus using the ICU bed for a longer period of time (and for additional years, if we want to arrive at average total costs).

Using this model, the Task Force derived costs of $230,000 to $340,000 per liver transplant patient alive at the end of one year (using a 70 percent survival rate), and $170,000 to $200,000 per one-year survival for heart transplant patients (also using a 70 percent survival rate). Additional years of survival would add from $10,000 to $20,000 in costs per year to these figures. Compared to other extreme and expensive medical care examined by the Task Force (including neonatal ICU care, adult ICU care, end-stage renal disease care, hemophilia, bone marrow transplants, and variceal bleeding) on the basis of fully allocated average one-year costs, the cost of heart and liver transplantation is four to ten times more expensive than any of these. That's the bad news.

The good news is that these procedures can be performed for substantially less than this fully allocated cost to the health care system at least in a state like Massachusetts, which utilizes a prospective revenue cap on individual hospital budgets. Indeed, this cap on prospective total revenue may actually make innovation easier by limiting the costs to the system. A summary of the argument, which is the economic underpinning of the Report, runs like this. First, a significant portion of fully allocated costs goes toward amortization of the physical plant. Thus, if procedures can be "squeezed into" existing capacity without displacing other procedures, this cost will not have to be borne by the system. Second, and most important, since cost is primarily a function of ICU days, and since ICU days are a function of readmission and complications, the cost will be less if readmissions can be lowered. This is likely only if patient selection is kept very strict, that is, if transplants are given to only those patients with strong clinical suitability, in the sense of being able to survive the transplant for a significant period of time with reasonable prospects for rehabilitation. Thus, cost becomes a function of patient selection criteria.

Patient selection criteria, however, tend to expand to include almost everyone in the absence of restraints on the system. This was well demonstrated in the end-stage renal disease program in which universal entitlement has led to universal treatment, whether medically beneficial or not. No one wants to repeat this experience with heart and liver transplantation, and thus no national politician has even suggested that heart and liver transplants be covered by Medicare. Indeed, even though he has made nationwide appeals for livers for children, President Ronald Reagan threatened to veto an organ transplant bill that would have provided federal money to pay the $6,000 needed annually for cyclosporin to immunosuppress transplant recipients, unless this portion of the bill was deleted—which it was.

Clinical suitability is not an immutable scientific fact, but one that is highly influenced by the environment. It is the Task Force's view that clinical suitability criteria will depend to some significant degree on system capacity. Thus, if system capacity is restricted, the clinical suitability criteria would remain relatively stringent. This would help ensure that only good candidates received transplants, and thus that the health care system would not have to be expanded to accommodate large numbers of patients. This would, in turn, ensure a cost-effective transplant program. The conclusion is that in order to maintain a cost-effective program, one must limit volume. And this, of course, makes determination of need a logical regulatory mechanism, one in which demand is adjusted to system capacity, rather than system capacity being adjusted to demand. The chief architect of this model, and author of the economics section of the Final Report, is Professor Marc Roberts of the Harvard School of Public Health.

It should be noted that limitation is a fair policy so long as we make transplants available in an equitable manner to all who are clinically suitable. In this way, we can permit organ transplants to become part of the "minimum benefit package" for Medicare and Medicaid recipients and even for the uninsured, without "breaking the bank." A suggested way to achieve equity of access is outlined in the Report's section, "Patient Selection and Rationing Schemes."

CONCLUSIONS

Is all this merely an academic exercise? Won't the public demand expansion of the health care system to accommodate all who can obtain any conceivable benefit from transplants, no matter what the system costs? Possibly, but the experience with end-stage renal disease has been radicalizing. There are, for example, 80,000 individuals on dialysis in the United States today, yet only about 7,000, or fewer than 10 percent, are on waiting lists for kidney transplants. Because of the shortage of available organs, physicians have determined that more than 90 percent of all possible kidney transplant candidates are not "clinically suitable." Capacity of the system plays a critical role in this, and if we can directly limit the system's capacity, we not only can limit the system's costs, but also can provide the service to those who can benefit the most from it. A national system which limited heart and liver transplants to perhaps twenty high-quality centers is preferable. But in the absence of any national leadership on this subject, states will be forced to make their individual ways as best as they can. There will be tremendous pressures on the states from the hospitals, the media, and the public who cannot understand why such restrictions on capacity are being imposed. These pressures may be irresistible. But it may also be that these pressures can be resisted, at least during the three-year "Phase I" envisioned by the Task Force, and that after this period of limited transplantation and data gathering, we will have learned enough about this issue to be able to make sound public policy that can be persuasively articulated to the public so that the policy is acceptable. So long as the entire procedure is public and perceived as fair, the potential for regulatory success should not be discounted.

My physician friends are fond of quoting the following line from *Hamlet* in describing organ transplantation, "Diseases desperate grown by desperate appliances are relieved, or not at all." The more appropriate passage for the regulator appears seven lines earlier in the King's declaration: "How dangerous is it that this man goes loose! Yet must not we put the strong law on him. He's loved of the distracted multitude. . . ." (IV.iii) In this context, the man is organ transplantation. The challenge is to put "the strong law on him" long enough to persuade the public that a free-for-all in organ transplantation is reckless, while a controlled system has pay-offs in terms of quality of care, equity, and cost savings.

Excerpts from the Report of the Massachusetts Task Force on Organ Transplantation

SECTION I: INTRODUCTION AND RECOMMENDATIONS

The Task Force on Organ Transplantation was announced on September 26, 1983 by the secretary of Human Services and the commissioner of Public Health, and charged with "the development of standards and processes for evaluating the use of organ transplantation" in Massachusetts. It was asked to:

—Make recommendations concerning how organ transplantation should be introduced and financed, including mechanisms to assure equality of access
—Determine what priority should be placed by the state on extreme and expensive medical interventions
—Determine what criteria should be used in patient selection
—Determine how and by whom decisions concerning transplantation availability and patient selection criteria should be made.

The seventeen-member Task Force is composed of citizens with personal or professional interest and expertise in organ transplantation including public officials, health care providers, representatives of major religious groups, insurance company officials, business leaders, and fac-

The Report of the Massachusetts Task Force on Organ Transplantation was presented to the Commissioner of Public Health and to the Secretary of Human Services of the Commonwealth of Massachusetts on October 18, 1984. Sections 1, 2, 4, and 7 appear here. Complete copies of the *Report* may be obtained from the Department of Public Health, Commonwealth of Massachusetts, 150 Tremont Street, Boston, Massachusetts 02111.

ulty members of local schools of public health. The Task Force held its first meeting in September 1983 and has held fifteen meetings, including a public hearing, over a twelve-month period. All meetings were open to the public, and there were no executive sessions. This Report sets forth the final recommendations of the Task Force as well as a summary of the reasoning and facts on which these recommendations are based. Preliminary recommendations were announced by the Task Force in early January 1984, and these final recommendations clarify them, and add a section on the "consortium approach."

The Task Force has been well aware throughout its deliberations that its role in the public policy debate about organ transplantation is very circumscribed. The introduction of new medical technologies in the United States tends to take on a life of its own, and the impact of government policy on its diffusion has been very limited. Nevertheless, experience with kidney dialysis and transplantation has taught us that failure to plan can lead to tremendous unanticipated public expenditures and resource allocation problems. The Task Force has reviewed the kidney transplant history for the lessons it holds for the two procedures the Task Force decided to concentrate on: liver and heart transplantation. These are not only the ones currently clamoring for wider introduction into the system, but also provide useful policy models for decisions regarding other extreme and expensive procedures.

During the year the Task Force has worked, the transplant environment has continued to evolve. There was a series of congressional hearings concentrating on organ procurement, sales, and federal financing, and the National Organ Transplant Act made its way through Congress. The Surgeon General continued his initiative to involve the private sector in organ procurement. In Massachusetts, four hospitals were granted certificates of need to do liver transplants under a "consortium" arrangement and, based in part on the recommendation of this Task Force, a single hospital was given a temporary exemption from determination of need (DON) to do cardiac transplantation. Massachusetts Blue Cross/Blue Shield initiated a "Transplant Insurance Program" (TIP) for its group subscribers, and in early 1984 decided to include organ transplants as part of its basic coverage. Massachusetts Medicaid also pledged to cover necessary heart and liver transplants. A statute was enacted in Massachusetts in late December 1983 to set up a separate fund, financed by donations and contributions made from state income tax refunds, to help pay for organ transplants for those unable to finance them themselves. This "checkoff" system will begin in 1985.

Why all this interest in organ transplantation, and why a Task Force to examine "the difficult ethical and financial decisions" involved?

There is no single reason, but the following combination of factors together appears to account for the current focus on liver and heart transplantation:

—Those needing them are easily identified, need them quickly to survive, and have often been able to get their plight highly publicized.
—Transplants are viewed by the public as life-saving.
—The transplant procedure is extremely expensive, so that its general provision may have a significant impact on the health care system, and this is the first time rationing such a procedure has been seriously discussed by public officials.
—Denial of a transplant on the basis of inability to pay seems to unfairly restrict the procedure to the wealthy, and seems to place a specific price on life.

The issue has also taken on special importance in Massachusetts for at least four reasons: (1) Massachusetts has been blessed with some of the most outstanding hospitals and medical schools in the country and has always been seen as a major medical research center; (2) the first kidney transplant and the second series of liver transplants were done in Massachusetts; (3) the Trustees of the Massachusetts General Hospital explicitly decided not to engage in heart transplant surgery in 1980 because of the tremendous cost of a program which would benefit only a few patients (this unique step by a major hospital was not rescinded until 1984); and (4) Massachusetts is the home of Jamie Fiske, who received a liver transplant in Minnesota in October 1982, and whose father, Charles Fiske, has done more than any single person to publicize the inadequacies of the present system of financing and obtaining a liver transplant.

Nonetheless, although the Task Force was asked to prepare a set of recommendations in a four-month time period, the Task Force did not view this as a major policy emergency from the point of view of Massachusetts citizens as a whole. In 1983, for example, only five (four liver and one heart) Massachusetts citizens had to leave the state to seek nonkidney organ transplantation; and only eight procedures were done within the state. The individuals involved could, of course, have been better served if public policy had been in place. But in such a new, expensive, complicated, and rapidly evolving field about which little is known concerning the need, outcome, quality control requirements, or cost of procedures, these problems are inevitable. The Task Force decided it was prudent to examine them critically and carefully rather than rushing to conclusions that might, in the long run, cause more suffering and problems than they prevent.

On the federal level, the almost exclusive concern is increasing the supply of transplantable organs by making the organ procurement system more efficient. In Massachusetts and New England, organ procurement problems are real, but this has not been the primary factor limiting use of this technology, and witnesses before the Task Force indicated that it is not likely to be the major issue in the foreseeable future for our region. Accordingly, exclusive concentration on organ procurement is at least premature. The reason for this region's position in organ procurement is the success of the New England Organ Bank, and its work deserves wider public attention and support.

The major public policy issue in organ transplantation is how to move toward three goals simultaneously: quality of services, equality of access to services, and cost containment. Even assuming that we can maintain the high quality of care offered to Massachusetts citizens, will it be possible to simultaneously increase equity of access to services, and decrease or limit its cost? Assuming a limit on total health care and medical expenditures, some trade-offs must be made. In a country in which organs for transplant are routinely sought from other states, and in which citizens may freely travel to seek medical assistance, a national approach to organ transplants is both desirable and necessary. No individual state can develop an effective organ transplant program without utilizing a multistate organ procurement network. Nor can any state act as an organ transplant center without reasonable reimbursement policies in place in the states from which it draws its patients. Nonetheless, in the absence of any federal leadership in the area of organ transplantation, it would be equally irresponsible for the individual states to do nothing. Even though we cannot do as well as we would like, we should do as well as we can.

Ultimately, of course, one would like to eliminate the need for organ transplantation. It is a powerful and often life-saving technique, but while it may circumvent the patients' underlying illness by replacing a diseased organ with a nondiseased organ, it gives the patient a new lifelong problem: coping with immunosuppression to prevent organ rejection. The Task Force's mandate did not include making recommendations on basic science research or the comparative value of preventive programs (including public health programs to encourage exercise and reduce weight, smoking, and alcohol consumption). Nonetheless, the Task Force believes that efforts in both basic science research and preventive approaches should be vigorously encouraged as the long-term approach to major organ failure.

We are under no illusions that these recommendations are the "final word." Our hope is that this is a helpful report and that other states and those working toward a coherent national policy will find it constructive.

FINDINGS AND RECOMMENDATIONS

The Task Force finds that the primary values at stake in organ transplantation are human life, equity, and fairness. Organ transplants are extremely expensive; the fully allocated average one-year cost is $230–340,000 for liver transplants and $170–200,000 for heart transplants. This is in the range of four to ten times the cost of the other most expensive currently employed medical technologies. Nonetheless, the Task Force believes that these procedures should be performed on those who are likely to benefit from them, so long as the total cost is controlled and resources are not diverted from higher priority medical procedures to liver and heart transplantation. The question of what a "higher priority" procedure is will be based on the total number of individuals affected and the importance to their lives of the intervention. For example, it may be appropriate to shut down an underutilized maternity program to do organ transplants. The burden of demonstrating that such a trade-off is appropriate, however, should be on the hospital proposing it. Accordingly, in the determination of need process, all currently available health care services should be presumed to be higher priority than transplantation. The applicant should have the burden of demonstrating that transplantation has a higher priority than any other currently available health care service from which organ transplantation diverts funds and/or support systems.

On the issues of equity and fairness, we concur with the conclusions of the President's Commission for the Study of Ethical Problems in Medicine and Biomedical and Behavioral Research: society has an ethical obligation to ensure equitable access to health care for all; and the cost of achieving equitable access to health care ought to be shared fairly.[1] Transplantation of livers and hearts should therefore only be permitted if access to this technology can be made independent of the individual's ability to pay for it, and if transplantation itself does not adversely affect the provision of other, higher-priority health care services to the public. We believe it is possible to achieve this goal only by the gradual introduction of this technology in the Commonwealth, a close and careful monitoring of quality care, costs, outcomes, and patient selection, and provided that liver and heart transplantation can be done in the Commonwealth in a manner that does not necessitate additional capital expenditures for this purpose. The existence of Ch. 372, the DON procedure, and rate setting give us some confidence that this is possible.

Recommendation 1

Liver and heart transplantation should be introduced into the Commonwealth in a controlled, phased manner that provides the opportunity for effective evaluation and review of its clinical, social, and economic aspects by a publicly accountable body after an initial phase of two to three years of limited transplantation.

Discussion. The Task Force's basic conclusion is that heart and liver transplantation should be introduced into the Commonwealth of Massachusetts, but that the introduction should be done in a deliberate and cautious manner through a carefully monitored, phased approach. The findings and recommendations of the Task Force concentrate primarily on "Phase I," which may be termed the phase of "Initial Social Assessment." During this phase a limited number of heart and liver transplants should be performed in an atmosphere that maximizes the potential for clinical, economic and social data gathering. The anticipation is that sufficient data will be gathered during this two to three year phase to provide the basis for a decision by the Public Health Council and other publicly accountable bodies to determine the direction and scale of the next phase.

Recommendation 2

The decision of when extreme and expensive medical technologies, like heart and liver transplantation, should be generally available should be made only after the clinical, social, and economic consequences of introducing the procedure, including cost-effectiveness, ethical implications, and long-term effects on society, are studied and reviewed by a publicly accountable body.

Discussion. Tests currently used to determine when a new procedure should be generally available, like experimental versus therapeutic or pretherapeutic, or "safe and effective," tend to concentrate the discussion on the technical aspects of a new procedure without consideration of its impact on society in terms of values, financing, skewing the system, or allocating resources. Whatever the appropriateness of such tests in the past, these technical-assessment-based tests cannot serve as a reasonable or useful threshold test for the general introduction of extreme and expensive procedures in an era of resource constraint. Bodies like the Task Force can act as appropriate forums for examining the "social consequences" involved in introducing new medical technologies into the system, and making recommendations to publicly accountable agencies like the Public Health Council.

The decision of whether particular, extreme and expensive procedures should be generally reimbursed should be made in such a way that Medicaid does not become the de facto insurer for all such procedures. One possible mechanism would be a joint committee with representation from the state and the insurance companies, with input by external evaluation groups like the Task Force and federal agencies like the Office of Technology Assessment. Using this or some other analogous mechanism could help ensure fairness in the distribution of burdens regarding reimbursement.

Recommendation 3

In making a decision regarding an application for a determination of need for heart and liver transplantation, the Public Health Council should attempt to minimize and track the total incremental cost of adding these procedures to the health care system.

Discussion. Although the Task Force endorses the limited and controlled introduction of organ transplantation in Massachusetts, it does so only because it believes that it can be done without decreasing services in other medical sectors, and that the total demand can be met without additional capital expenditures. Whether or not this assumption is correct, of course, remains to be seen. Testing this view will require careful monitoring of the impact of organ transplantation performed at major university facilities on such things as ICU utilization in community hospitals, as well as on the general case mixes in the hospitals. While it might optimistically be hoped that both heart and liver transplantation can be introduced in Massachusetts without capital expansion by increased efficiency and "taking up the slack in the system," it is uncertain what the "spill over" effects will be and how many (if any) more similar technologies can be "painlessly" introduced in the future. As a principle, the Task Force believes that if it turns out that liver and heart transplantations take resources away from higher-priority health care services, and decrease their accessibility to the public, these transplantation procedures should not be performed.

To help evaluate the effects of organ transplantation on the system, as well as its cost and quality control mechanisms, and monitor Phase I, the Commonwealth of Massachusetts should contract with an independent evaluation group with medical and economic expertise to collect and analyze data on liver and heart transplantations during Phase I.

Current information about the need for, costs of, and outcomes of liver and heart transplantation is insufficient to justify any more than the very limited and controlled introduction of these technologies in Massachusetts. For example, the "additional evidence about the effectiveness and safety" of liver transplants anticipated by the Fineberg report has not yet materialized. An independent evaluation group could collect and analyze comprehensive data during Phase I, and present it to the Public Health Council in a credible manner, as an essential aid in their decision-making process.

Recommendation 4

Until such time as there are reasonably reliable data on the need for, costs of, and outcomes of liver and heart transplantation (end of Phase I) hospitals proposing to do these procedures in the Commonwealth should not be given a certificate of need unless they agree to (1) support the operating expenses for heart and liver transplantation within current reimbursement limits set by the hospital's maximum allowable cost under Chapter 372 of the Acts of 1982 (provided that an exception may be granted for expenditures that are unique to organ transplantation: the cost of the organ itself and the cost of the cyclosporin A); (2) collect evaluative data on the costs, outcomes, and displacements caused by transplant candidates who receive transplants as well as those who do not, in a manner approved by the Department of Public Health, and agree to make these data available to the Department and an independent evaluation group; and (3) have the protocols reviewed, approved, and monitored by the Institutional Review Board (IRB), or by a special review board set up for this purpose by the Department of Public Health.

Discussion. Implicit in this recommendation is the Task Force's view that the determination of need process is an appropriate one for required review and prior approval of this extreme and expensive technology because of the major impact it is likely to have on the health care system. The requirement of working under the "MAC" or maximum allowable costs echoes the Fineberg Task Force recommendation which it believed should hold until "the representative advisory body [this Task Force] has rendered a judgment about adding costs to the health care system for such extreme and expensive procedures."[2] As previously noted, the factual data upon which such a judgment can be rendered are not yet available.

Finally, subparts (2) and (3) of this recommendation recognize the need to collect data in a systematic and complete manner, and recognize that whether they are characterized as experimental, pretherapeutic, therapeutic, or by some other designation, both heart and liver transplants require and demand significant research and data collection activities that make IRB review or analogous protocol review by a similarly constituted body both warranted and useful. Special attention in this review should be focused on the consent procedure utilized by the institution, procedures used to withdraw consent and order the withholding of future treatment (if and when the patient determines he or she does not want further treatment, even if such a decision will result in death), organ procurement procedures, patient selection procedures, and issues of confidentiality.

Recommendation 5

Patient selection criteria should be public, fair, and equitable. Primary screening should be based on medical suitability criteria made available to the public which are designed to offer transplantation to those who can benefit the most from it in terms of probability of living for a significant period of time with a reasonable prospect for rehabilitation. If there are insufficient resources to transplant all who can so benefit, selection from the medically suitable group should be based primarily on a first come, first served basis. The selection criteria and process should be filed with a publicly accountable body.

  Discussion. Fairness and equity demand that no one be excluded from the pool of potential recipients because of social class, ability to pay, family situation, or place of residence in New England. Referral patterns need to be examined, but all candidates who are referred for transplant should undergo the same medical screening examination. In this screening examination, age can be taken into account as one factor (insofar as it may affect longevity and prospects for rehabilitation), but cannot be used alone as an arbitrary disqualification. Likewise, the policy should recognize that Massachusetts has a special, historical relationship to our neighboring states, and that residents of the New England states that have been involved with the New England Organ Bank's program should be eligible for transplants on the same basis as Massachusetts citizens. Their state of residence should adopt mechanisms to reimburse Massachusetts hospitals for their transplants.

  For liver transplants especially, active alcoholism may be taken into account insofar as it might affect the longevity and prospects for functional rehabilitation, but not as an absolute contraindication. As the President's Commission has properly noted: "In light of the special importance of health care, the largely undeserved character of differences in health status, and the uneven distribution and unpredictability of health care needs, society has a moral obligation to ensure adequate care for all."[3]

  Similarly, although family support networks may be extremely important in after-hospital care, the absence of a family or the existence of an unconventional substitute should not serve as a reason to exclude the patient from evaluation. Society should develop mechanisms, in cooperation with the transplanting hospitals, to provide sufficient support resources for such patients during their recuperation. The cost of aftercare, including visiting nurses or other needed medical support for a transplant candidate without a family or other social support, should be included in the analysis of the cost of the transplant procedure itself. Hospitals should develop plans for dealing with such patients, and these plans should be included in their DON applications.

If the pool of medically acceptable candidates is larger than available resources, patient selection should be made on a first come, first served basis with consideration of the donor organ "match." This is expected to be close to a random allocation, and is probably the fairest we can do at this time. Individual adjustments in the system may be called for in a medical emergency, or where some on the waiting list are from outside New England. New England residents can be given preference so long as this policy is made known to non-New England residents before they are medically evaluated for transplant; and during Phase I, non-New England residents should not be screened unless they have demonstrated the ability to finance their transplants.

In the event that an individual believes he or she has been discriminated against unfairly in the selection process, the hospital should have an appeals mechanism in place to enable the individual to present his or her case promptly and fairly to a neutral decision maker with authority to have the patient's case reviewed again by the selection team.

Recommendation 6

If more than one hospital is granted a certificate of need to do heart or liver transplantation, all hospitals so involved should be required to coordinate services in a way that comes as close as possible to a single, integrated medical service. Each hospital should be able independently to demonstrate either its ability to perform the procedure, or to act in concert with the other hospitals in a particular aspect of the procedure. All hospitals should establish and use a single set of patient selection and treatment protocols, agree to joint publication of research results, use a common patient recipient pool and a common organ procurement pool, formalize a program for the interchange and common use of staff and students, develop a common training program, share facilities and equipment, use a common format for data collection, and establish a formal organization, central staff, and records file.

Discussion. In general it seems best to inaugurate extreme and expensive medical technologies like heart and liver transplantation either at a single facility or at a "consortium" that meets the criteria set forth in this Report. This is consistent with recommendation 1, that liver and heart transplantation be introduced into the Commonwealth in a "controlled, phased manner." Looked at purely from an economic point of view, one cannot make out a case for initiating organ transplantation at more than one hospital. Nonetheless, truly cooperative efforts have some other potential advantages. In the case of liver transplantation, the Public Health Council has already granted certificates of need to four individual hospitals that have agreed in principle to work together. On the other hand, an exemption from DON for heart transplantation has been granted to a single hospital for a limited period of time.

As a result of the debate regarding the "consortium" approach to liver and heart transplantation, the Task Force has developed guidelines for a "worthwhile" consortium, consistent with our other basic recommendations. In order to prevent duplication, minimize the new capital expenditures, prevent the displacement of significant numbers of patients, and help assure high quality care, we believe a formal cooperative agreement among all the hospitals involved in a consortium should be required by the Public Health Council. This agreement should ensure that the multiple-hospital consortium arrangement is truly cooperative and is run like a single, integrated medical service.

Each applicant must, of course, independently demonstrate its clinical ability, and the necessity of its involvement in transplantation from the public's perspective. A single set of patient selection and treatment protocols must be agreed upon and used, as well as a single set of data collection criteria and an agreement to joint publication of all research, so that there will be a sound basis on which to make policy judgments after Phase I. To help formalize cooperation and maximize the utility of a group effort, written agreements regarding the interchange and common use of staff and students should be entered into, as well as agreement regarding the development of a common training program, and efficient joint use of facilities and equipment. To coordinate all of this, and maintain records on it, a formal organization with a central staff and record file will be required.

SECTION II: THE STATE OF THE ART

The first successful transplantation of a vascularized whole kidney under immunosuppressive chemotherapy was carried out in Boston in March

1962. This transplant was the culmination of studies and experience spanning a decade of intensive work in the field. Since that time remarkable progress has taken kidney transplantation from the realm of experimental surgery to a viable approach for the treatment of end-stage renal (kidney) failure. While scientific and technical problems were being overcome, many social and ethical issues were raised. The medical community could not as easily address the political, economic, and logistic questions created by this new technology.

This section contains a brief survey of the current status of organ transplantation as it pertains to the work of the Task Force. The emphasis is on experience with kidney transplantation; the development, current volume, and outcomes of liver and heart transplantation; and on the development of organ banking. Our intent is to present a broad overview of transplantation for the general reader. This precludes an exhaustive review of the most current literature which reflects changes reported each month.

Discussion of any type of transplant must address the goals of this treatment modality. It is often assumed that a transplant cures a patient of disease. This is simply not true. For instance, atherosclerosis (hardening of the arteries), the major cause of heart disease and death, is not eliminated when a new heart is transplanted. The disease process of narrowing of the blood vessels continues, even in the transplanted heart. With every transplant, the body also has the burden of a foreign tissue (the new organ) with which to contend, and immunosuppressive drugs must be taken for the remainder of the patient's life to prevent rejection. Transplantation can improve life both in quantity and quality, but it rarely returns a patient to fully normal health. The primary goal of modern medical research remains that of understanding the cause, and prevention, of diseases so that eventually the need for transplant, and many other temporizing measures, will be eliminated. Until such time many technically complex procedures offer an improved quality of life for many patients.

TRANSPLANTATION OF THE KIDNEY

Since the first transplant in 1962, it is estimated that more than 100,000 kidney transplants have been performed throughout the world. Publications in the medical literature concerning transplantation continue to grow rapidly, and today approximately 3,000 medical articles appear annually on the subject.

In 1982, more than 5,300 kidney transplants were performed in the United States. At present, nine hospitals in New England, seven of them in Massachusetts, each perform from ten to fifty-seven procedures each year. The total number of procedures performed in New England has steadily increased from 193 in 1978 and 257 in 1982, to an all time high of 313 in 1983 (including 19 pediatric patients),[4] with kidneys harvested from both cadavers and living related donors.

As increasing numbers of transplants have been performed, survival rates of both the patient and the kidney graft have improved. In a recent study,[5] 86 percent of recipients of kidneys from unrelated donors survived one year, and 78 percent survived to three years. Of those receiving kidneys from related donors, 95 percent survived to one year and 91 percent to three years. The reason that overall survival is better for people who have related donors is because there is less chance for kidney rejection. Kidney graft rejection exacts a huge toll on the patient with increased stress, higher likelihood of infection and a consequential higher mortality. Return to dialysis and the possibility of a second graft remain an option. Graft retention rates have been lower than patient survival rates, and removal of rejected kidneys in cases where the graft is not successful has resulted in greatly reduced patient mortality. Retention rates for transplants from unrelated donors are 56 percent for one year and 45 percent for three years, while 75 percent of organs from related donors have been retained for one year, and 67 percent for three years. Due to improved immunosuppression, graft retention rates have shown progressive and substantial increases. Patient survival rates improved drastically, and have recently remained stable.[6]

Kidney disease differs from other terminal, organ-specific diseases in two important ways. Since human beings possess two kidneys, and can live comfortably with one, it is possible to obtain a healthy, well-matched kidney from a donor (living or recently deceased). Secondly, and more importantly, dialysis is available as an alternative life-sustaining measure to assume the functions of the diseased kidney either on a long-term basis or while the patient awaits a transplant. In addition, patients from whom a rejected kidney is removed are able to return to dialysis. In 1983, of the 69,409 patients on dialysis in the United States, 2,399 were in the New England area. Fewer than half of these patients are considered potential candidates for a transplant, and in the entire United States only about 6,000 are on a formal waiting list. Being a candidate is a function of organ availability, patient selection criteria, and patient preference.

Treatment selection for patients with kidney failure is a choice between dialysis and transplantation. If a patient suffers severe concomitant disease (e.g., widespread cancer, emphysema, or liver failure) that will not be improved by receiving a transplanted kidney, the patient will be a dialysis candidate. If the patient has a disease, such as high blood pressure or diabetic retinopathy, which is likely to be improved by transplantation, then the patient will preferably be selected for transplantation. Another factor favoring transplantation is availability of a suitably matched, living related donor. The patient's own wishes are paramount in any decision to seek transplantation.

The transplant team itself is, of course, critical. There is an important skill and experience factor in successful performance of any complex medical team effort. Transplants seem to function best when supervised by a well-balanced professional group in a medical center. Ideally, transplantation should involve physicians and surgeons possessing a variety of skills and backgrounds and a hospital with services broad enough to carry the added burdens of blood banking, chemical treatments that are sometimes toxic, treatment of severe disease in other organ systems, and rejection. A well-balanced professional group in the field of kidney transplantation involves many skills including medical nephrology, cardiology, bacteriology, immunology, surgery, vascular surgery, urology, social services, psychiatry, and teams experienced in troubleshooting both dialysis and transplantation. Even though it seems intuitively correct that medical centers with a larger number of patients, hence more experience, would be more successful in transplantation, some small groups have done well on measures of mortality and morbidity. Unfortunately, other small groups have produced results which are not as encouraging. At present, factors such as experience and professional balance must be weighed in determining the likelihood of a favorable outcome.

Throughout this Report, kidney transplantation is discussed as a useful benchmark because it is established. Now the foundations for transplantation of heart, liver, and other organs must be established. The experiences with kidneys, and the lessons learned in the procurement of organs, patient selection, reimbursement, and broad social policy, are often applicable to other organ transplants. For example, kidney transplantation has brought into sharp focus questions concerning public financing of costly high technology procedures. Moreover, increasing acceptance of the procedure by clinicians has coincided with greater public awareness of the availability of these procedures and a willingness to participate in organ donor programs to utilize organs that would otherwise be lost in the unfortunate deaths of family members. The experience with kidney transplantation has demonstrated the importance of having social, financial, and ethical factors considered, debated, and, if possible, resolved, simultaneously with the development of medical techniques.

TRANSPLANTATION OF THE HEART

Since 1967, approximately 900 heart transplants have been performed worldwide, 635 of those in the United States.[7] World experience in heart transplantation has been dominated by the work of Dr. Norman Shumway at Stanford University Medical Center, Palo Alto, California. Heart transplants performed on dogs by Dr. Shumway in 1958 anticipated the first human heart transplant in 1967 by Dr. Christiaan Barnard in South Africa. Within a year, about 100 heart transplants were performed worldwide, but with dismal survival rates.[8]

Data for survival of heart transplant patients at Stanford University were collected in four distinct temporal phases. First came a period when potential transplant patients were identified. Shumway found candidates for the operation, but a transplant was not performed. Ninety percent died within two months, and all died within nine months. Second came the period between January 1968 and December 1973, in which there was an initial 45 percent survival rate. The remaining 55 percent of patients were lost in the operative or early hospital period. Survivorship subsequently declined to 25 percent at five years. In the third phase, January 1974 through December 1980, initial survival rates improved to 62 percent at one year, and 45 percent at five years. In the fourth and most recent phase, December 1980 through May 1983, survival rates improved to 82 percent at one year, and 78 percent at two years, with estimates of 65 percent at five years.[9]

The fairly dramatic improvement in survival rates appears to be the result of at least three medical factors: improved clinical and operative management, improved immunosuppression, including the introduction of a new and seemingly more effective drug, cyclosporin A, and improved patient selection. No one factor can be isolated as the most important reason for increased survival rates.

An enhanced outlook for both survival and a return to normal life appears to have added momentum to interest in transplantation: the 172 heart transplants performed in the United States in 1983 represent nearly one-third of the total heart transplant operations since 1967. These transplants were performed at eleven transplant centers throughout the nation. Worldwide, heart transplant operations are conducted in Canada, Great Britain, France, and South Africa. Of the 635 United States heart transplants, 295, or 46 percent, are still living. The current total one-year survival rate is 80 percent and a two-year survival rate of 75 percent is projected.[10] One-year survival has gone from 44 percent in 1973 to 88 percent in 1983. Presently the leading causes of deaths are infection, acute rejection, graft arteriosclerosis, and malignancy.[11]

Estimates of potential annual need are extremely variable and range from 1,000 to 75,000 nationwide, and from 20 to 1,800 in Massachusetts. Conditions which may necessitate heart transplantation include intractable heart failure of several causes, coronary obstructive disease, cardiomyopathy and, in young people, congenital heart disease and tumors. The larger national estimate assumes that one out of every four patients less than fifty years of age and dying of cardiac disease might be a candidate for cardiac transplantation.[12] The smaller national estimate is based on a series of selection criteria and contraindications to transplantation developed at Stanford University.[13] For Massachusetts, the larger estimate is simply a proportionate share of the national figure based on population. A more conservative figure of 109 operations annually was arrived at by applying more rigid criteria: limiting patient age to fifteen to forty-nine, eliminating those with kidney disease or diabetes, and subtracting the one-third who unfortunately might be expected to die while awaiting a transplant. The estimate of about twenty was put forth to the Task Force by the three hospitals in Massachusetts proposing to do heart transplantation in May 1984. The great variability in these estimates leads to a conclusion that we simply do not know what either the "demand" or "need" for heart transplants is likely to be with any degree of certainty.

TRANSPLANTATION OF THE HEART AND LUNGS

The transplantation of heart and lungs is still in its nascent stage. It remains in the realm of such experimental procedures as the artificial heart and pancreatic transplant. Initial exploration of the double transplant (heart and lungs) is encouraging, but the procedure has not yet been employed on a scale large enough to provide mortality parameters similar to the worldwide experience with kidneys, hearts, and livers.

Approximately twenty-three heart-lung transplants have been performed, including seventeen at Stanford University under the direction of Dr. Shumway. Other centers performing the procedure are the University of Pittsburgh and Johns Hopkins University. Of the seventeen transplants performed at Stanford, eleven patients are alive including the first patient transplanted in March 1981.[14]

Patients needing a heart-lung transplant suffer either from pulmonary hypertension or Eisenmenger's syndrome. These two conditions are unusual diseases of varied etiology which have in common concomitant disease of heart and lungs. No single replacement of either heart or lungs ameliorates these conditions and at present no other mode of treatment has met with success. Both pulmonary hypertension and Eisenmenger's syndrome are relatively rare but serious illnesses with a high mortality. Successful transplantation of the heart and lungs together involves identical determinants of success (immunosuppression, team experience and balance, specialized clinical knowledge) that characterize all other organs.

TRANSPLANTATION OF THE LIVER

Initial experimental whole organ transplantation of the liver by the method now used in patients was reported from Boston in 1959;[15] four clinical liver transplants were conducted in Boston in 1963–1965 without success. Since that time, the major work in this field has been conducted by Dr. Roy Calne at Cambridge University, England, and Dr. Thomas Starzl, formerly of Denver, Colorado, now in Pittsburgh, Pennsylvania.

Recently tabulated results by Calne[16] from four centers cover 466 liver transplants in 434 patients from 1963 to 1982. Of these, 163 are now alive, while 36 died within six months. A total of 123 (28 percent) are living three years or more after the transplant. Dr. Starzl has prepared actuarial curves contrasting the data from his Denver-Pittsburgh centers for 1963–79 with that from 1980–82. One-year survival has increased from approximately 30 percent prior to 1979[17] to approximately 60 percent in 1980–82.[18]

Projections of the need for liver transplants in Massachusetts are based on estimates of the prevalence of certain liver diseases. About 90 percent of all deaths from liver disease in Massachusetts are a result of cirrhosis (alcoholic and post-hepatitic) and hepatitis. Important minor causes are primary biliary cirrhosis and biliary atresia. Dr. Starzl estimates the potential need for liver transplantation to be approximately 20 per million population or 114 patients in Massachusetts and 246 in New England, although based on actual experience in Massachusetts, these estimates seem high.

A unique feature of liver transplantation is the presence of two distinct patient populations in need of transplants. Adults, who have several causes of liver failure (e.g., hepatitis and alcoholic cirrhosis) and various underlying diseases (e.g., coronary artery disease and emphysema), and children, of whom 90 percent of those suffering liver failure have a congenital disease called extrahepatic biliary atresia (a disease affecting the secretion of bile). The problems that face these groups are very different, and these distinct patient populations are often evaluated separately. A group may be prepared to do liver transplants in children based on their own experience or based on prognostic, ethical or technical considerations. The same group may not be prepared to do liver transplantation in adults. A second clinical center may decide just the opposite. Projections for liver transplantation in children are based on several data sets. Extrahepatic biliary atresia has an incidence of one in 8,000 to 10,000 live births. About 30 percent of these cases will be aided by other surgical procedures and will not require an early transplant. On the basis of existing data, seven Massachusetts children annually could be expected to have biliary atresia requiring a transplant.

ISSUES IN IMMUNOSUPPRESSION

One of the major problems inherent in organ transplantation is rejection of the grafted organ by the recipient's immune system. To control rejection, drugs which suppress the immune system are administered post-operatively. Since its introduction in Boston in 1961, Azathioprine (Imuran) has been the standard drug, often used with cortisone. Now, cyclosporin offers promise of improvement. Cyclosporin A is produced by the Sandoz Corporation, in Basel, Switzerland, and marketed under the name Sandimmune. Although many have attributed the increased survival of transplant patients to cyclosporin, it is premature to give it full credit. The drug has been in use in the United States for a limited period of time and the most current data[19] reveal more profound toxicity than previously appreciated. Considering the limited data, apparent toxicity, and a cost of $6000 per year, the drug should not be used as the sole or major impetus for encouraging expanded transplantation volume. More credit should be given to the growing experience, better surgical technique, better patient selection, and better postoperative management and immunosuppressive regimens. Further research and time is needed to evaluate more fully the role of cyclosporin in transplant immunosuppression. The potential benefits of using cyclosporin are exciting, but enthusiasm must be tempered until more information is available.

ORGAN PROCUREMENT AND BANKING: COORDINATION AND REGIONALIZATION

Organ transplantation is unique in that it involves two human beings in a technology-mediated exchange of live organs: one human (alive or dead) donates an organ to a diseased recipient. Living kidney donors (either related or unrelated) were initially used because kidneys are paired organs. Even at the very outset of the kidney program, however, it was clear that cadaver tissues would also be used and that timing, preservation, and transportation of organs would be central to success. For livers, hearts, and heart-lungs, all donors must be deceased persons who meet brain death criteria and whose respiration is mechanically maintained; in many instances postmortem survival of other organs is assured by temporary pump-oxygenation support of the circulation.

With the growing need for fresh and viable organs, it became apparent that kidney transplants could be managed best on a regional basis with a central clearing house of clinical information on donors and recipients. The New England Organ Bank was one of the first regional organ banks established, and today transplant patients in Boston receive organs from as far away as the Midwest and Southeast. Moreover, the various regional banks in the country trade organs extensively according to supply and demand: a recent study showed that transplantations conducted in Richmond, Virginia, used organs harvested as far away as Massachusetts and Texas. An expanded regional organ banking system would have to be an integral part of any initiatives taken in Massachusetts for the transplantation of livers, hearts, or hearts and lungs.

Successful organ banking requires cooperation at five levels of public and professional activity: public education, hospital preparedness, surgical training, organ preservation and transportation, and centralized coordinating and dispatching.

A *central coordinating* organization must possess a list of potential organ recipients and maintain communication with regional hospitals in the event an organ becomes available. In addition to data assembly and information dispersal a central organization has the responsibility of acting within the time restraints that perishable organs require.

The New England Organ Bank serves as a role model. It is rapidly expanding its tissue procurement programs, and continues to build public support that will benefit additional transplant programs. The New England Organ Bank, however, cannot function without adequate support from all agencies; fiscal support of its work must be considered an integral part of the cost of tissue transplantation.

Public Education. Media attention given to several recent transplant patients has heightened public awareness of the procedure, and a new level of awareness was reached in the spring of 1984 with the proclamation by President Ronald Reagan of National Organ Donation Awareness Week, April 22–28. With activities such as this, the possibility of donating or bequeathing organs is gaining public acceptance. Even though laws in all states permit individuals to sign donor cards, very few doctors and hospitals will use the organs of such a person without the added consent of the next of kin. A vigorous campaign to educate the public and health professionals including doctors, hospital personnel, medical examiners, and coroners would be extremely helpful. The media could educate by indicating to the public the need for their cooperation and the benefits to society of active participation. The airing of documentaries and public service announcements would probably best achieve these goals rather than the publicizing of dramatic isolated cases. In several instances the families of recently deceased teenage children have been the prime movers in making those precious organs available to others; they have found some solace, in their grief, in helping others. The public, through the media, is most receptive to such knowledge, and is educated thereby; but careful steps should be taken to guard the confidentiality of patient information and maintain the anonymity of donors.

Hospital Preparedness. Tissue destined for transplant must be obtained by an experienced physician. Respiration is generally maintained mechanically, and is continued after death to permit the organs to survive. As many as eight tissues or organs may be harvested: eyes, skin, bones, heart, kidneys, liver, and lungs. To maximize the value of these scarce resources, hospitals involved in the chain of donation require trained personnel, sophisticated equipment, communication systems, and cooling devices.

Surgeon Training. The surgical procedure for harvesting kidneys is fairly simple. In New England, surgeons cooperating with the Organ Bank have obtained expertise in removing kidneys. In the case of livers and hearts, a surgeon from the hospital where the recipient is being cared for will most likely be dispatched to remove the tissue from the donor and supervise its return. Such capability and preparedness require special training, communication networks, and transportation systems.

Preservation and Transportation. "The faster, the colder, the better," best describes the goal of teams that carry living organs from one hospital to another. Properly handled and attached to a special oxygenating device, a kidney can remain viable for seventy-two to ninety-six hours after harvest; presently, hearts and livers perish after twelve hours.

The excitement and urgency of the transportation of a liver or heart make for a dramatic newsworthy event. The media often cover these stories, which can help in public education as already mentioned.

CONSIDERATIONS OF BRAIN DEATH

In the area of death, the law has always been and remains that an individual is dead when a licensed physician pronounces him dead, so long as the physician makes the determination based on "accepted medical standards."[20] Brain death has been an "accepted medical standard" for more than a decade, and every court that has examined the question, including the Massachusetts Supreme Judicial Court, has agreed that brain death is a legally proper determination for a physician to make whether or not there is a state statute on the subject.[21] Where physicians are unclear about this, education is indicated.

Uniform legislation does not, however, overcome deeply held convictions or conventions. For example, although the Uniform Anatomical Gift Act, which is law in all fifty states, makes a person's donation of an organ by use of a donor card effective upon declaration of death, almost no physician or hospital will in fact use the person's organ without permission of the next of kin. This permission is not legally required, but appears to be sought for personal, psychological, and perhaps public relations reasons. The presence of the donor card, however, probably does make the relatives more likely to agree to the donation.

SALES

One of the most bizarre proposals to increase the supply of kidneys has been to develop a "kidney exchange" which would put willing sellers in touch with willing buyers. This proposal has occasioned an outcry from those who believe it will exploit the poor, bring commercialism into the transplantation field, and decrease the supply of donated organs. The Congress and a number of state legislatures are currently considering legislation to outlaw such sales, although there have as yet been no reports of actual sales having taken place in the United States, and the position of the transplant surgeons is that they will not transplant an organ which has been privately paid for. Since we do permit the poor to take all sorts of occupational risks with their bodies, it does seem somewhat paternalistic not to permit them to take this one. Nonetheless, this is a highly visible and symbolic exploitation, and one that has the potential to undermine society's belief in the integrity of the entire transplantation enterprise.[22] Therefore it seems reasonable to the Task Force to strongly oppose organ sales, and if a credible attempt to establish a sales network ever develops, state laws directly outlawing such sales would be appropriate.

SECTION IV: PATIENT SELECTION AND RATIONING SCHEMES

In an era of scarce resources, decisions concerning which patients will receive the resources must be made.[23] Unless we decide to make heart and liver transplantation available to no one, or available to everyone, some rationing scheme must be used to choose among potential transplant candidates. The debate has existed throughout the history of medical ethics. Traditionally it has been usually stated as a choice between saving one of two patients, both of whom require the immediate assistance of the only available physician to survive. More recently, national attention was focused on decisions regarding the rationing of kidney dialysis machines when they were first used on a limited basis in the late 1960s. As one commentator described the debate within the medical profession:

> Shall machines or organs go to the sickest, or to the ones with most promise of recovery; on a first-come, first-served basis; to the most "valuable" patient (based on wealth, education, position, what?); to the one with the most dependents; to women and children first; to those who can pay; to whom? Or should lots be cast, impersonally and uncritically?[24]

In Seattle, Washington, an anonymous screening committee was set up to pick who among competing candidates would receive the lifesaving technology. One lay member of the screening committee is quoted as saying:

> The choices were hard ... I remember voting against a young woman who was a known prostitute. I found I couldn't vote for her, rather than another candidate, a young wife and mother. I also voted against a young man who, until he learned he had renal failure, had been a ne'er-do-well, a real playboy. He promised he would reform his character, go back to school, and so on, if only he were selected for treatment. But I felt I'd lived long enough to know that a person like that won't really do what he was promising at the time.[25]

When the biases and "selection criteria" of the committee were made public, there was a general negative reaction against this type of arbitrary device. Two experts reacted to the "numbing accounts of how close to the surface lie the prejudices and mindless clichés that pollute the committee's deliberations," by concluding that the committee was "measuring persons in accordance with its own middle-class values." The committee process, they noted, ruled out "creative nonconformists" and made the Pacific Northwest "no place for a Henry David Thoreau with bad kidneys."[26]

To avoid having to make such explicit, arbitrary, "social worth" determinations, the Congress in 1972 enacted legislation that provided federal funds to cover virtually all kidney dialysis and kidney transplantation procedures in the United States.[27] This decision, however, simply served to postpone the time, which is fast arriving, when identical decisions will have to be made about candidates for heart and liver transplantation in a society that does not provide sufficient financial and medical resources to provide all "suitable" candidates with the operation.

There are four major approaches to rationing scarce medical resources: (1) the market approach; (2) the selection committee approach; (3) the lottery approach; and (4) the "customary" approach.[28]

THE MARKET APPROACH

The market approach would provide an organ to everyone who could pay for it out of his/her own funds or through private insurance. It puts a very high value on individual rights, and a very low value on equality and fairness. It has properly been criticized on a number of bases, including that the transplant technologies have been developed and are supported with public funds, that medical resources used for transplantation will not be available for other, perhaps higher priority, care, and that financial success alone is an insufficient justification for demanding a medical procedure. Most telling, however, is its complete lack of concern for fairness and equity. In the words of the President's Commission for the Study of Ethical Problems in Medicine and Biomedical and Behavioral Research: "In light of the special importance of health care, the largely undeserved character of differences in health status, and the uneven distribution and unpredictability of health care needs, society has a moral obligation to ensure adequate care for all."[29]

A "bake sale" or charity approach that requires the less financially fortunate to make public appeals for funding is demeaning to the individuals involved, and to our society as a whole. Rationing by financial ability says that we do not believe in equality and that we do believe that a price can and should be placed on human life and that it should be paid by the individual whose life is at stake. Neither belief is tolerable in a society in which income is inequitably distributed.

THE COMMITTEE SELECTION PROCESS

The Seattle Selection Committee represents a model of the committee process. "Ethics committees" set up in some hospitals to decide whether or not certain handicapped newborn infants should be given medical care may represent another. These committees have developed because it was seen as unworkable or unwise to explicitly set forth the criteria on which selection decisions would be made. But only two results are possible, as Professor Guido Calabresi has pointed out: either a pattern of decision making will develop or it will not. If a pattern does develop (e.g., in Seattle, the imposition of middle-class values), then it can be articulated and those decision "rules" codified and used directly, without resort to the committee; if, on the other hand, a pattern does not develop, the committee is vulnerable to the charge that it is acting arbitrarily, or dishonestly, and therefore cannot be permitted to continue to make such important decisions.[30]

In the end, public designation of a committee to make selection decisions on vague or nonspecific criteria will fail because it too closely involves the state and all members of society in explicitly preferring specific individuals over others, and in disregarding the interests those others have in living. It thus directly undermines, as surely as the market system does, society's view of equality and the value of human life.

THE LOTTERY APPROACH

The lottery approach is the ultimate equalizer which puts equality ahead of every other value. This makes it extremely attractive, since all comers have an equal chance at selection regardless of race, color, creed, financial status, etc. On the other hand, it offends our notions of efficiency and fairness since it makes no distinctions among the strength of the desires of the candidates, their potential survival, their quality of life, etc. In this sense it is a "mindless" method of trying to solve society's dilemma which is caused by its unwillingness or inability to spend enough resources to make a lottery unnecessary. By making this macro spending decision clear to all, it thereby also undermines society's view of the pricelessness of human life. A first come, first served system is a type of lottery since referral to a transplant program is generally done randomly in time. Nonetheless, higher income groups may have quicker access to referral networks and thus have an inherent advantage over the poor in a strict first come, first served system.[31]

THE CUSTOMARY APPROACH

Traditionally, society has attempted to avoid explicitly recognizing that we are making a choice not to save individual lives because it is too expensive to do so. As long as such decisions are not explicitly acknowledged, they can be tolerated by society. For example, until this year there was said to be a general understanding among general practitioners in Britain that individuals over fifty-five suffering from end-stage kidney disease not be referred for dialysis or transplant. In 1984, however, this unwritten practice has become highly publicized, with figures that show a rate of new cases of end-stage kidney disease treated in Britain at 40 per million (versus the United States figure of 80 per million) resulting in 1500–3000 "unnecessary deaths" annually.[32] This has, predictably, led to movements to enlarge the National Health Services budget to expand dialysis services to meet this need, a more socially acceptable solution than permitting the now publicly recognized situation to continue.

In the United States, the "customary" approach permits individual physicians to select their patients on the basis of "medical criteria" or "clinical suitability" which may, in fact, contain much that we would consider "social worth" criteria if they were explicitly spelled out. For example, one criterion, common in the transplant literature, requires an individual to have sufficient family support for successful after-care. This discriminates against individuals without families and those who have become alienated from their families.[33] The criterion may be relevant, but it is hardly medical.

Similar observations can be made about "medical" criteria that include I.Q., mental illness, criminal records, employment, indigency, alcoholism, drug addiction, or geographical location. Age is perhaps more difficult, since it may be at least impressionistically related to outcome. But it is not medically logical to assume that an individual who is forty-nine years old is necessarily a better medical candidate for a transplant than one who is fifty years old. Unless specific examination of the characteristics of older persons that make them less desirable candidates is undertaken, such a cut-off is arbitrary and thus devalues the lives of older citizens. The same can be said of blanket exclusions of alcoholics and drug addicts.[34]

In short, the customary approach has one great advantage for society and one great disadvantage: it gives us the illusion that we do not have to make choices; but the cost is mass deception, and when this deception is uncovered, we must deal with it either by universal entitlement or by choosing another method of patient selection.

A COMBINATION OF APPROACHES

Any approach selected, to be socially acceptable, must be fair, efficient, and reflective of important social values. The most important values at stake in organ transplantation are fairness itself, equity in the sense of equality, and the value of life. To promote efficiency, it is important that no one receive a transplant unless he or she is likely to obtain benefit from it in the sense of increased length of life at a reasonable level of functioning.

Accordingly, it is appropriate for there to be an initial screening process that is based exclusively on medical criteria designed to measure the probability of a "successful" transplant, that is, one in which the patient survives for a considerable length of time and is rehabilitated. Of course there is room in "medical criteria" for social worth judgments, and there is probably no way to avoid this completely. For example, it has been noted that "in many respects social and medical criteria are inextricably intertwined" and that therefore medical criteria might "exclude the poor and disadvantaged because health and socioeconomic status are highly interdependent."[35] Roger Evans notes an example. In the End-Stage Renal Disease Program, "those of lower socioeconomic status are likely to have multiple comorbid health conditions such as diabetes, hepatitis, and hypertension" making them both less desirable candidates and more expensive to treat.[36]

To prevent the gulf between the haves and have-nots from widening, we must make every reasonable attempt to develop medical criteria that are objective and independent of social worth categories. One minimal way to approach this is to require that medical screening criteria in the state be uniform and that the criteria adopted be reviewed and approved by an ethics committee with significant public representation, filed with a public agency, and made readily available to the public for comment. In the event that more than one hospital in the state is offering a particular transplant service, it would be most fair and efficient for the individual hospitals to perform the initial medical screening themselves (based on the uniform, objective criteria), but to have all subsequent nonmedical selection done by a method approved by a single selection committee composed of representatives of all hospitals engaged in the particular transplant procedure, as well as members of the Department of Public Health and significant representation of the public at large.

As this implies, after the medical screening is performed, there may be more acceptable candidates in the "pool" than there are organs or surgical teams to go around. If (and only if) this is so, some selection among waiting candidates will have to be made. This situation occurs in kidney transplantation now, but since the organ matching is much more sophisticated than in hearts and livers (permitting much more precise matching of organ and recipient), and since dialysis permits individuals to wait almost indefinitely for an organ without risking death, the situations are not close enough to permit use of the same selection criteria for hearts and livers.[37] On the other hand, to the extent that organs are specifically tissue- and size-matched and fairly distributed to the "best-matched" candidate, the organ distribution system itself will be a natural random allocation system.

At present in Massachusetts there is no shortage of hospital space or surgical teams to perform transplants. Nevertheless, it is possible that at some time in the future there will develop a "pool" of acceptable candidates and that choices will have to be made among members of this pool as to who gets the next available, suitable organ. It is here that we must make a choice between using conscious, value-laden, social worth selection criteria (including a committee to make the actual choice), or some type of random device. In view of the unacceptability and arbitrariness of social worth criteria being applied, implicitly or explicitly, by committee, the Task Force does not believe such a process is viable or proper. On the other hand, strict adherence to a lottery might create a situation where an individual who has only a one in four chance of living five years with a transplant (but who could survive another six months without one) would get an organ before an individual who could survive as long or longer, but who will die within days or hours if he or she does not immediately receive a transplant. Accordingly, we believe the most reasonable approach would be to generally allocate organs on a first come, first served basis to members of the pool, with individuals being able to "jump" the queue if the second level selection committee believes they are in immediate danger of death and the person who would otherwise get the organ can survive long enough to be reasonably assured that he or she will be able to get another organ.

We adopt the first come, first served method of basic selection (after a medical screen) because it most closely approximates the randomness of a straight lottery, without having the obviousness of promoting equity as the only value. Some unfairness is introduced by the fact that the more wealthy and medically astute will likely get into the pool first, and thus be ahead in line, but this advantage should decrease sharply as public awareness of the program grows. The possibility of unfairness is also inherent in permitting individuals to jump the queue, but the necessity for approval by a committee with significant public representation on it decreases the likelihood of medical favoritism, and such an exception seems reasonable to protect our view of the value of life (see Figure).

Society will have to face the reality that should the resources devoted to organ transplantation be limited (as they are now and are likely to be in the future), at some point it is likely that significant numbers of individuals will die in the "pool" waiting for a transplant. There are three things that can be done to avoid this: (1) medical criteria can be made stricter, perhaps by adding a more rigorous notion of "quality" of life to longevity and prospects for rehabilitation; (2) resources devoted to transplantation and organ procurement can be increased; or (3) individuals can be persuaded not to attempt to join the pool.

Figure: Screening Procedure

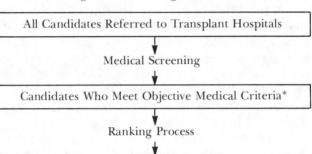

*As determined by physicians at the transplant hospitals.

†Ranked on first-come, first-served basis so that highest ranking candidate who "matches" first available donor organ gets it, unless lower ranking candidate is in immediate danger of death and first candidate has a reasonable chance of surviving to receive the next available donor organ (jumping the queue must be approved by a system-wide selection committe with public representation).

Of these three options, only number 3 has the promise of both conserving resources and promoting individual autonomy. While we assume that most persons medically eligible for a transplant would want one, we also assume that at least some would not—at least if they understood all that was involved, including the need for a lifetime commitment to daily immunosuppression medications and periodic medical monitoring for rejection symptoms. Accordingly, it makes public policy sense to publicize the risks and side effects of transplantation, and to require that careful explanations of the procedure be given to prospective patients before they undergo medical screening. It may be that by the time patients come to the transplant center they have their minds made up and would do anything to get the transplant. Nonetheless, if there are patients who, when confronted with all the facts, would voluntarily elect not to proceed, we enhance both their own freedom and the efficiency and cost-effectiveness of the transplantation system by screening them out as early as possible.

SECTION VII: REIMBURSEMENT POLICIES FOR ORGAN TRANSPLANTATION

Faced with rapid advances in technology and increasing costs, health planners, regulators, and third-party payers are being challenged to develop new policies and programs for payment of organ transplantation. This section describes the policies of the federal government, Medicare, state Medicaid programs, Blue Cross/Blue Shield, commercial insurers, and policies in some other countries.

FEDERAL POLICY

With the exception of kidney transplants funded by the End-Stage Renal Disease (ESRD) program of Medicare, there is no federal policy on organ transplantation. The Medicare program is administered by the Health Care Financing Administration (HCFA), a division of the Department of Health and Human Services (HHS), which determines procedures covered and appropriate levels of reimbursement. Medicare has labeled heart and liver transplants as experimental and has thus not authorized payment for these procedures. However, transplantation is moving rapidly from the realm of human experimentation to therapy, and new criteria for reimbursement are emerging. In 1980, Patricia Roberts Harris, secretary of HHS, announced that new technologies must be evaluated not only on the traditional bases of safety and efficacy, but also on cost-effectiveness and long-range social, economic, and ethical considerations. At a press conference on June 12, 1980, Secretary Harris stated:

> A final decision on coverage of heart transplants under Medicare, whatever that decision shall be, must be fully justified by a clear and careful analysis of all pertinent facts about which the public is fully informed. Heart transplantation illustrates the complex policy issues presented by rapidly advancing medical technologies and procedures. It is incumbent on all of us—the government, the medical profession, and the public—to assess carefully the safety, efficacy and the social consequences of new procedures before financing their wide dissemination. I fully expect that studies of the sort we propose for heart transplantation will become increasingly necessary in the years ahead.

In November 1979, HCFA authorized Medicare payment for heart transplants at Stanford University Medical Center. Payment, which was authorized temporarily pending development of final criteria for coverage, was discontinued effective June 13, 1980 due to lack of sufficient information concerning a patient selection process, long-term social, economic, and ethical consequences of the procedure, and the potential for national expansion of the transplant procedure. Several months later the Medicare program solicited hospitals and medical centers to participate in a study of heart transplants. The study was to include all aspects of heart transplants including scientific, social, economic, and ethical issues. This $1.5 million study was submitted to HCFA by the Battelle Center in Seattle in September 1984, scheduled for public release in early 1985. The hospitals which performed transplants in the study were Stanford University, Medical College of Virginia and Richmond Veterans Administration Hospital, in Richmond, Virginia, Columbia-Presbyterian in New York, and the Universities of Minnesota, Pittsburgh, and Arizona.

The Office of Health Technology Assessment, a division of the National Center for Health Services Research, has been asked by HCFA to evaluate the safety and effectiveness of heart, pancreas, and liver transplantation. The assessment of liver transplantation, requested by HCFA in August 1982, was finished in 1983. The report concluded that liver transplantation was technically feasible, extremely expensive, and a very complicated operation capable of extending the lives of carefully selected patients with end-stage liver disease. The report went on, however, to raise questions about selection mechanisms, organ availability, costs, institutional capabilities, and equality of access.

Based on this report, HHS announced that at this time the Administration supports federal recognition of liver transplantation as nonexperimental for children with biliary atresia and other rare congenital abnormalities. It has been reported that the Department of Defense will issue regulations for its CHAMPUS program permitting reimbursement for liver transplantation. Some transplants are financed by federal health research funds through the National Institutes of Health (NIH). NIH is financing heart transplants at Stanford and will continue until 1987. Other federal agencies funding heart transplants include the Veterans Administration's program at Richmond, Virginia.

MEDICARE

The Medicare program is one of a number of programs administered by HCFA. Medicare benefits are available to those sixty-five or over, those who are disabled, and those who are suffering from ESRD. HCFA determines the procedures covered and the appropriate level of reimbursement.

Presently the only major organ transplants covered by Medicare are kidney transplants. Renal transplants and dialysis were included in the Medicare program under section 229 of Public Law 92-603, effective October 30, 1972. This program has been successful from the point of view of improving access and providing health care to those suffering from ESRD, and has grown rapidly since 1972. The number of beneficiaries has risen from 10,000 in 1974 to more than 65,000 in 1982, while the annual cost rose from $242 million in 1974 to almost $2 billion in 1982, and a projected $5.5 billion for 90,000 patients in 1995.

A number of commentators have noted the disproportionate share of Medicare funds spent for ESRD recipients. For example, in 1980, ESRD beneficiaries were less than one-half of 1 percent of total beneficiaries for Supplementary Medical Insurance (professional and ancillary services); but ESRD costs represented 5 percent of the total Medicare budget for these services. Another high figure for the kidney program is the dialysis rate. The United States provides dialysis for patients at a rate which far exceeds that of Europe and Israel. The United States dialysis rate is 204.7 per million. Of the countries studied, Israel has the next highest rate (144 per million) and France (123 per million) has the highest rate in Western Europe. The dialysis rate in the United Kingdom is 52 per million. Among the states in the United States, the highest is the District of Columbia (983 per million) and the lowest is Wyoming (20 per million).

MEDICAID

Medicare policy on acceptable procedures strongly affects policies of many states in the establishment and implementation of Medicaid standards. The Medicaid program is a federal-state program. While states are required to pay for a basic set of acute, outpatient and skilled nursing home services, other optional services can be added to the state program under the same federal-state cost sharing arrangements. Several groups of clients are covered by Medicaid, including the elderly, dependent children and their families, and the disabled. Also covered by many states are those who have spent a portion of their income on medical care or have "spent-down" and have become "medically indigent."

The federal government will not fund heart and liver transplants through Medicare, but will pay the federal portion of Medicaid transplant coverage in states which choose to fund them. To learn more about Medicaid-funded transplants, the Task Force carried out an informal survey of eleven states, including the contiguous New England states (Connecticut, Rhode Island, Vermont, New Hampshire), and states in other regions (Arizona, California, Maryland, Michigan, New Jersey, New York, and Pennsylvania). Medicaid central offices in these states were asked if they had received any requests for liver, heart, or heart-lung transplants, if requests had been approved, and if a prior authorization mechanism or case management technique was used for these requests. If the respondent mentioned the Medicare criteria as part of the explanation or rationale for state policy, this was also noted.

Nine of the eleven states had at least one request, and eight had approved at least one transplant. All three states receiving requests but not granting approvals cited the Medicare criteria in explaining their decision. Seven states had approved at least one liver transplant, five states had approved at least one heart transplant, and four states had approved at least one heart-lung transplant. All states but one which had approved at least one transplant had a prior authorization mechanism. This is not unusual because for many Medicaid-eligible patients, organ transplantation will be an out-of-state service which automatically requires prior authorization. Several states emphasized that recent transplants were exceptions and were not established state policy. Other states reported that transplants were the subject of ongoing discussion or that reimbursement arrangements for transplants limited the hospitals to the standard per diem rate for the stay. In another state, liver transplants were being approved for biliary atresia only. Finally, Medicaid may not be the only state program capable of covering transplantation. One state reported that two residents turned down by Medicaid received a transplant through the vocational rehabilitation agency in the state. The Department of Welfare in this state paid for the hospitalization and related costs.

New England States. Of five other New England states, only Vermont at present has received no transplant requests. Two states, Maine and Connecticut, have authorized transplants. Maine has authorized a heart transplant; Connecticut has authorized a heart-lung transplant and three heart transplants. All New England states contacted have staff working on transplant issues.

Massachusetts. The Medicaid program in Massachusetts will pay for heart, heart-lung, and liver transplants for eligible patients. Potential recipients must meet both federally established Medicaid financial eligibility criteria, and medical criteria developed by the Massachusetts Medicaid Review Committee to determine medical necessity. Financial eligibility criteria include provision for those who have spent-down by spending their income on medical expenses. Medicaid is the payer of last resort on these procedures. All available resources are applied to the cost of the procedure before Medicaid contributes.

Medical criteria for each type of transplant define the medical conditions and circumstances for which the procedure is appropriate. Examples of these standards are age criteria, clinical diagnosis, and the presence of specific clinical signs. Based on the criteria, the Medical Review Committee, a physician advisory group representing a number of medical specialties, makes case-by-case determinations of appropriateness. To allow time for the prior authorization procedures, requests for approval should be made fourteen days prior to the need for surgery. In a medical emergency, review of the material can be completed by central office staff within two days.

The Massachusetts Medicaid program has paid for several out-of-state transplants in the past, and following the implementation of organ transplant in-state, has approved payment for several in-state recipients.

NATIONAL BLUE CROSS/BLUE SHIELD POLICY

Currently, the policies of "the Blues" vary by state. The plans closest to the major transplant centers have been compelled to address the issue to a greater extent than the outlying plans. Although a few plans have tried to provide coverage through innovative methods, several have taken the position of addressing each transplant request on an individual consideration basis. In a number of plans, no requests have been made to cover such services and, therefore, the need for a specific policy statement has not been forced.

Twenty plans have formal policies to pay for one or more of the types of transplants. All twenty plans cover liver transplants. Nineteen cover heart transplants as well. At least one of the twenty covers all organ transplants. Ten additional plans have paid one or more cases based on an administrative decision, and ten plans have specifically denied claims. Many plans have exclusions in their contracts for experimental-investigational procedures.

Among the New England states, the policy varies widely:

1. *Blue Cross/Blue Shield of Rhode Island* is offering a rider to its current contracts which would cover all investigational transplant procedures. They recognize heart, liver, heart-lung, pancreas, and small intestine transplants as coverable.

2. *Blue Cross of Vermont, Blue Cross/Blue Shield of New Hampshire and Blue Cross/Blue Shield of Maine* have had a limited number of requests for coverage. The number of subscribers in these plans has been too small to underwrite such expensive surgery and the plans are looking for ways to put coverage in place without excessive cost. A suggestion under discussion in Vermont is a statewide insurance pool to share the risks. Blue Cross/Blue Shield of New Hampshire will cover liver, heart, heart-lung, and pancreas transplants as of June 1, 1984. Blue Cross/Blue Shield of Maine has obtained reinsurance for transplant and expects to offer coverage as of January 1985.

3. *Blue Cross/Blue Shield of Connecticut* provides coverage for heart, liver, and heart-lung transplants and has paid for several transplants. They are presently completing a study which will assist them in developing a more complete transplant policy.

Most plans, whether or not they have developed a policy, are experiencing frustration in attempting to address the issue on a local level. Issues such as clinical indications for the various types of transplants, viable funding mechanisms, the optimal number of transplant centers, and the criteria for their certification, remain unanswered.

BLUE CROSS/BLUE SHIELD IN MASSACHUSETTS

Blue Cross/Blue Shield of Massachusetts provide coverage for medical procedures which are considered "generally accepted." The corporations rely on the advice of the Interspecialty Medical Advisory Committee (IMAC) for a determination of which procedures meet the established criteria for general acceptability.

Established in 1941 to advise the Board of Directors on medical issues, IMAC is comprised of thirty-eight professional physician and paramedical members, representing over twenty-six medical and surgical specialties. Subcommittees for each specialty provide IMAC with an advisory resource of over 300 medical and paramedical professionals throughout the state.

Decisions of IMAC do not in and of themselves constitute Blue Cross/Blue Shield policy changes. The Central Professional Service Committee (CPSC), a bylaw committee of the Blue Shield Board of Directors, must approve IMAC recommendations for conformity to "generally accepted guidelines" established for surgical and medical procedures. A generally accepted surgical or medical procedure is defined as a procedure which:

1. Has completed the research or experimental stage of development
2. Does not involve, as an integral part of the procedure, the use of any drug, substance, or device which has not been released by the Food and Drug Administration or other governmental licensing agencies for general use by qualified physicians
3. Is in general use for patient care by physicians qualified to perform the procedure
4. Is of demonstrated value for the diagnosis or treatment of an illness, injury, or bodily function.

Using these review procedures, the corporations approved corneal transplants in the 1950s, kidney transplants in the 1960s, and, in 1980, certain bone marrow transplants. Heart transplants were first reviewed by IMAC in 1977 and liver transplants were considered in 1978. At that time IMAC recommended, and CPSC concurred, that neither procedure met the criteria for "generally accepted." Liver transplants had another review in September and November 1982, but IMAC voted in November that it was not a generally accepted procedure. This recommendation was upheld by CPSC in February 1983. Then, in July 1983, IMAC reviewed heart transplantation and the following vote to defer final approval of heart transplants was taken:

> Motion was made and seconded that the procedure, heart transplantation, *appears* to be a generally accepted procedure. However, because the procedure requires the use of a *non-FDA approved drug,* cyclosporin A, the Committee recommends *deferral* of *final approval at the present time.* (20 yeas, 4 nays, 1 abstention.)

Cyclosporin A received FDA approval on November 14, 1983. Liver, heart, and heart-lung transplants were considered again by IMAC in January 1984, and by CPSC in February 1984. Both groups voted that these three transplants were now generally accepted.

In response to public pressure, in August of 1983, Blue Cross/ Blue Shield of Massachusetts announced a program for insuring the costs of liver, heart, and heart-lung transplants, called the Transplant Insurance Program (TIP). It was a stand-alone program that provided its own level of benefits, rather than adding to existing basic Blue Cross/ Blue Shield coverage.

Current Policy. Massachusetts Blue Cross/Blue Shield, as of February 1, 1984, will pay for heart, liver, and heart-lung transplants as part of the regular benefit package rather than under the Transplant Insurance Plan. The coverage will cost $24 a year for a family, about $10 million total. This is about 1 percent of the average statewide family premium. In 1986 the cost will increase to $35.4 million. The Transplant Insurance Plan will continue to be offered by Blue Cross/Blue Shield and may be attractive to small employee groups since it is "community-rated" rather than "experience-rated" and thus more favorably priced.

COMMERCIAL INSURANCE

Over three-fourths of the thirty major commercial health insurers will pay for heart or liver transplants under their group major medical health plans. An informal survey prepared by the Health Insurance Association of America in June of 1983 showed that 82 percent of the companies were willing to pay for liver transplants and 85 percent were willing to pay for heart transplants. In covering these procedures, reimbursement by many insurance companies will depend on compliance with certain criteria. Examples of conditions and questions asked by many carriers include:

—Is the procedure medically necessary?
—Have all other conventional methods of treatment been tried?
—Is the patient's condition life-threatening?
—Is the procedure safe and effective?
—Has the policy holder requested coverage for this procedure?

In addition, some policy holders have contracts which specifically exclude certain procedures.

New medical procedures are reimbursed by commercial insurers after a study of safety and effectiveness. Sources of information used by insurance companies include the medical profession, specialty medical associations, state or national medical societies, new research studies, articles in medical journals, and government reports. If the procedure is controversial or has not been proven safe and effective, a company may decide against reimbursement. Officials of the Health Insurance Association of America say an industry-wide decision to cover transplants could come within one year.

REPRESENTATIVE POLICIES FROM OTHER COUNTRIES

Sweden. Heart and liver transplants are not done in Sweden, but Swedish citizens have received transplants in England. The procedures are approved individually, and are paid for by the Swedish County councils.

England. Heart, liver, and a limited number of heart-lung transplants are performed in England. One center for liver transplant and two for heart transplant are funded by the National Health Service. The Health Service recently announced plans to provide a further year's support for the two heart transplant centers. This decision was based on the interim report of a research study group sponsored by the Department of Health and Social Security. The final report is due at the end of 1984.

Netherlands. Liver, but not heart transplants, are performed in Holland. Permission for establishment of the liver transplant center in Gronigen was granted by the government and financed with funds from private insurance companies.

Canada. Organ transplants in Canada are financed by the individual provincial health plans and vary according to the comprehensive nature of each plan. Kidney transplants are routinely covered. Heart, liver, and heart-lung transplants are considered more experimental and can be covered through prior authorization and special application to the Ministry of Health. Patients are referred at the recommendation of the attending physician and referrals may include out-of-province and United States locations. Heart and liver transplants are performed in London, Ontario, and Montreal, Quebec.

Notes

1. President's Commission for the Study of Ethical Problems in Medicine and Biomedical and Behavioral Research, Securing Access to Health Care: The Ethical Implications of Differences in the Availability of Health Services (U.S. Government Printing Office, Washington, D.C.) (vol. 1 1983) [hereinafter referred to as Securing Access].
2. Final Report of the Task Force on Liver Transplantation in Massachusetts (Fineberg Report) (May 1983) at 40.
3. Securing Access, *supra* note 1, at 25.
4. Coordinating Council, End-Stage Renal Disease Network #28, *Annual Report to the Secretary of Health and Human Services for Calendar Year 1982* (July 1, 1983).
5. Krakauer, H., *et al.*, *The Recent U.S. Experience in the Treatment of End-Stage Renal Disease by Dialysis and Transplantation*, New England Journal of Medicine 308(26):1558–63 (1983).
6. Personal communication with N. L. Tilney.
7. Griepp, R. N., *A Decade of Human Heart Transplantation*, Transplantation Proceedings 9:265–91 (1979).
8. Shumway, N. E., *Cardiac Replacement in Perspective*, Heart Transplantation 3:3–5 (1983).
9. Shumway, N. E., *Recent Advances in Cardiac Transplantation*, Transplantation Proceedings 15:1221–24 (1983).
10. Thompson, M. E., *Selection of Candidates for Cardiac Transplantation*, Heart Transplantation 3:65–69 (1983).
11. Pennock, *et al.*, *Cardiac Transplantation in Perspective for the Future: Survival, Complications, Rehabilitation and Cost*, Journal of Thoracic and Cardiovascular Surgery 83:168–77 (1982).
12. Reitz, B. A., Stinson, E. B., *Cardiac Transplantation 1982*, Journal of the American Medical Association 248(10):1225–27 (September 10, 1982).
13. *Cardiac Homotransplantation*, Current Problems in Surgery 16:3 (1979).
14. Reitz, B. A., *Heart-Lung Transplantation: A Review*, Heart Transplantation 1:8 (1982).
15. Moore, F. D., *et al.*, *Experimental Whole Organ Transplantation of the Liver and Spleen*, Annals of Surgery 152:374–87 (1960).
16. R. Calne, Liver Transplantation (Grune & Stratton, New York, N.Y.) (1983).
17. Public Health Service, Assessment of Liver Transplantation (U.S. Government Printing Office, Washington, D.C.) (1983).

18. Starzl, T., *et al.*, *Evolution of Liver Transplantation*, HEPATOLOGY 2:614–36 (1982).

19. Myers, B. D., *et al.*, *Cyclosporin-Associated Chronic Nephropathy*, NEW ENGLAND JOURNAL OF MEDICINE 311(11):699–705 (September 13, 1984).

20. G. J. ANNAS, L. H. GLANTZ, B. KATZ, THE RIGHTS OF DOCTORS, NURSES, AND ALLIED HEALTH PROFESSIONALS (Ballinger Books, Cambridge, Mass.) (1981) at 224–25.

21. Commonwealth v. Golston, 366 N.E.2d 744 (Mass. 1977), *cert. denied*, 434 U.S. 1039 (1978). *See* PRESIDENT'S COMMISSION FOR THE STUDY OF ETHICAL PROBLEMS IN MEDICINE AND BIOMEDICAL AND BEHAVIORAL RESEARCH, DEFINING DEATH (U.S. Government Printing Office, Washington, D.C.) (1981) at 136–38.

22. Annas, G. J., *Life, Liberty, and the Pursuit of Organ Sales*, HASTINGS CENTER REPORT 14(1):22–23 (February 1984).

23. Much of this section relies on ideas in or derived from the work of Professor Guido Calabresi of Yale Law School, especially from G. CALABRESI, P. BOBBITT, TRAGIC CHOICES (Norton, New York, N.Y.) (1978).

24. Fletcher, J., *Our Shameful Waste of Human Tissue*, in THE RELIGIOUS SITUATION (D. R. Cutler, ed.) (Beacon Press, Boston, Mass.) (1969) at 223–52.

25. R. FOX, J. SWAZEY, THE COURAGE TO FAIL (University of Chicago Press, Chicago, Ill.) (1974) at 232.

26. Sanders, D., Dukeminier, J., *Medical Advance and Legal Lag: Hemodialysis and Kidney Transplantation*, UCLA LAW REVIEW 15(1):357 (1968).

27. Rettig, R. A., *The Policy Debate on Patient Care Financing for Victims of End-Stage Renal Disease*, LAW AND CONTEMPORARY PROBLEMS 40(4):196 (Autumn 1976).

28. TRAGIC CHOICES, *supra* note 23.

29. SECURING ACCESS, *supra* note 1, at 25.

30. TRAGIC CHOICES, *supra* note 23.

31. Bayer, R., *Justice and Health Care in an Era of Cost Containment: Allocating Scarce Medical Resources*, SOCIAL RESPONSIBILITY 9:37–52 (1984). *See* Annas, G. J., *Allocation of Artificial Hearts in the Year 2002:* Minerva v. National Health Agency, AMERICAN JOURNAL OF LAW AND MEDICINE 3(1):59–76 (Spring 1977).

32. *Commentary: UK's Poor Record in Treatment of Renal Failure*, LANCET, p. 53 (July 7, 1984).

33. A 1969 study of the criteria employed by kidney dialysis centers in the United States found that the eight most frequently employed criteria were: (1) willingness to cooperate in treatment regimen (86 percent); (2) medical suitability (79 percent); (3) absence of other disabling disease (69 percent); (4) intelligence to understand treatment (34 percent); (5) likelihood of vocational rehabilitation (32 percent); (6) age (20 percent); (7) primacy of application for available vacancy (26 percent); and (8) psychiatric evaluation (25 percent). FOX AND SWAZEY, *supra* note 25, at 230. The family question, as put to candidates at Stanford's heart transplantation center has been, "Does the patient have a strong supportive family willing and able to withstand the apprehension, anxiety, fear, waiting, fatigue, separation, euphoria, disappointment, and grief that the different phases of cardiac transplan-

tation entail? Does the family have enough strength to provide continuous support to the patient as well as to manage the stresses of cardiac transplantation themselves? *Id.* at 310–11.

34. Most, but not all, liver transplant programs exclude active alcoholics from consideration for liver transplantation. The Boston Center for Liver Transplantation, for example, excludes alcoholics who have not abstained for [more] than two years, and more generally excludes "active drug or alcohol" users. The Brigham and Women's Hospital's Guidelines for Cardiac Transplantation are somewhat less explicit, asking referring physicians to consider "a history of alcohol or drug abuse, or mental illness that would complicate post-transplantation followup" as a "contraindication to cardiac transplantation." The Task Force concluded that blanket exclusions, like that of the Boston Liver Center, are arbitrary and tend to reinforce negative and destructive societal stereotypes. Accordingly, such individuals should not be *per se* excluded from screening if they want a transplant. On the other hand, it is reasonable and proper to consider the impact of the patient's substance abuse or mental illness on the probability of successfully following an immunosuppression regimen and being physically rehabilitated following transplant. Although such a judgment will also have large subjective elements, it is here, rather than on the disease of substance abuse itself, that the decision should focus.

35. Evans, R. W., *Health Care Technology and the Inevitability of Resource Allocation and Rationing Decisions, Part II,* JOURNAL OF THE AMERICAN MEDICAL ASSOCIATION 249(16):2208–17 (April 22/29, 1983).

36. *Id.*

37. The New England Organ Bank is in the process of changing its policy, but the following summarizes what it was. One of the two kidneys goes to the regional center that covers the hospital that procured it and the kidney is used at the hospital's discretion. The other is distributed on the basis of matching. Kidney matching is generally done on the basis of tissue compatibility to minimize the probability of rejection. Most importantly, the recipient must be crossmatch-negative; i.e., there must not be a reaction when the recipient's blood is mixed with the white blood cells of the donor. If there is, there is likely to be a severe and early rejection of the kidney. If there is not, a patient in immediate need of a kidney may obtain one on this basis alone.

　　More sophisticated immunological tests are usually performed, however, so that the kidney can go to the matching individual with the lowest probability of ever obtaining a kidney. The quest is to determine the recipient's allergic status to foreign substances, like blood and kidneys. The more highly allergic a patient is, the more difficult it will be to find the patient a suitable kidney. Past blood transfusions increase the patient's allergic reaction status, as, of course, do prior transplants. The patient's allergic status is "panel reactivity" and is expressed as a percentage, with 100 percent being the most allergic. The panel reactivity is determined by the presence of antibodies to 160 antigens, common in North American man. The more blood used, the higher percentage of antibodies to the 160 antigens. One hundred percent reactivity means that the patient has antibodies to all antigens.

Patients with high percentages get preference; if percentages are equal, the bank goes to the next two tissue matching tests: HLA-DR matching and no incompatibility for HLA-A,B antigens. The patient scoring the highest match on these tests should receive the kidney. In the unlikely event that two or more patients still score the same, hospitals with the better record of organ procurement are given priority. And if no patient in the region scores well enough to justify transplantation, the organ is referred to a national pool. These general criteria were supplied by the New England Organ Bank, whose priorities for kidney distribution of the second kidney are (1) medically urgent; (2) sensitized patient, negative cross-matches; 50–100 percent panel reactivity for greater than three months; (3) full house HLA-DR match; (4) no incompatability for HLA-A,B antigens; (5) NEOB institutional net credit rating; and (6) export of kidney to National Network.

Distribution systems for livers and hearts are much less sophisticated. Patient blood type and age/weight factors are first priorities. Hearts are generally cross-matched, while livers are not. After these criteria are met, medical urgency is usually the primary priority. Because hearts and livers survive less than twelve hours (versus seventy-two hours for kidneys) after removal from the donor, there are much stricter geographic and temporal constraints on distribution. *See generally,* ORGAN TRANSPLANTS: HEARINGS BEFORE THE SUBCOMMITTEE ON INVESTIGATION AND OVERSIGHT, HOUSE COMMITTEE ON SCIENCE AND TECHNOLOGY, 97TH CONGRESS, 1ST SESSION (U.S. Government Printing Office, Washington, D.C.) (1983).

With artificial organs, cross-matching will no longer be an issue, and we will have to directly confront distribution of replacement organs on more exclusively nonmedical terms. *See, e.g.,* Annas, *supra* note 31.

Equity and Costs

Mark V. Pauly, Ph.D.

The task of determining who should or should not have access to a life-prolonging procedure would not be easy even if cost were no consideration. In an era in which the health industry has largely converted to the cost-cutting religion, or at least the religion of budget limitation—a conversion for which health economics is partly responsible—the task becomes doubly difficult.

At one level, the Massachusetts Task Force on Organ Transplantation has dealt with this task simply by recommending that the final decision be postponed, and that a limited program of organ transplantation be introduced in an "Initial Social Assessment" phase. There is a faith that somehow this period will permit the gathering of data which, although unidentified, will "provide the basis for a decision." What sort of decision might that be? If the final version is anything like the recommended initial phase—a real possibility, given the general discussion in the Task Force Report—I would argue that a serious error would be made.

The Task Force obviously accepted most of the cost-cutting dogma, and the rituals—such as rate limitation and determination of need—which often accompany it. Indeed, the Task Force recommends that organ transplantation in Massachusetts, despite its already proven efficacy for patients with severe disease, take place only within a fixed total budget (for inpatient hospital care) and only to the extent that activities which have to be eliminated in order to free hospital resources for transplants can somehow be shown to have "lower priority." The implicit model is very much one in the spirit of a fully publicly controlled system with a fixed budget, in which individual choices and values have almost no role to play.

Reprinted with permission from *Law, Medicine & Health Care* 13(1). Copyright 1985, American Society of Law & Medicine, Boston, Massachusetts.

Economists are among the least likely to object to being concerned about resource costs in health care. Nevertheless, I am concerned that the Task Force, in accepting only the "cost" part of cost-benefit analysis (and its larger welfare economics framework), has been led to make recommendations which have some serious problems. These problems may well make the recommendations unacceptable, especially if viewed as the precursors of a more permanent solution. To put it bluntly, acceptance of the recommendations, even as an interim measure, would cause some people to die unnecessarily.

The major defect in the Task Force's analysis is its elevation of a political expedient—limitations on hospital spending—to the role of a moral postulate. Why are hospital costs limited in Massachusetts and in some other states? Given conventional forms of insurance and conventional ways in which information is transmitted to patients, it is believed that the current system would render care which is worth less than its cost. Although some politicians (and some budget directors) talk as if there were something intrinsically evil about having the health share of the gross national product exceed a certain percentage, this is only shorthand for the notion that we are not getting value for money. Even worse, it may be shorthand for the sentiment that publicly financed medical care costs cause problems for the public budget. Yet, if there should occur a medical innovation that is worth what it costs, the amount of resources available for this sector ought to be expanded by cutting inefficiency if that is possible; if it is not, we should reduce the amount we spend on other things—television, chocolate, books, bombs, and computers. That is, one ought require only that the resources used for the transplant have a lower priority in the economy as a whole, not that those resources be drawn necessarily (or even presumptively) from other health care services.

Suppose we then assume that there is no intrinsic merit to a fixed medical or hospital care budget. Suppose we also assume, as the Report itself suggests, that with feasible arrangements the supply of organs for transplantation will be adequate for all who desire transplants. Suppose that heart and liver transplants have passed the research stage, and are known to be effective, if expensive, ways of extending life, and that accurate information concerning the transplants is transmitted to patients and insurers. Finally, suppose that a financing method is developed in which someone who receives a transplant is charged the full resource costs of "producing" that transplant. The purchaser, in effect, causes no additional costs to be imposed on anyone except his household if he obtains a transplant. There could be insurance coverage of such expenses, but the premiums would apply only to those who had specifically elected transplant coverage; there would be no general spillover onto other insureds, either for the transplant surgery, or for the follow-up care. My understanding of the Task Force's recommendations is that they would prohibit a person who lives in Massachusetts from buying a transplant under such circumstances. In effect, the Task Force finds objectionable a family's decision that it is willing to sacrifice other things it might consume in order to prolong the life of one of its members.

Why would this be objectionable, even in the assessment phase? Ought it to be objectionable, so objectionable in principle that someone should die unnecessarily—that human life should be sacrificed? The consumption of this procedure in no way reduces the resources available to others, since the family is spending its own property, property which it would not make available to others in any case. Who gains from having such people die?

Another area where I have difficulty with the Task Force Report is the part that deals with the terrain most familiar to me: Section III's discussion of, and rationale for rejecting, cost-benefit analysis (not published in the preceding excerpts from the *Report of the Task Force*). The Task Force interprets cost-benefit analysis as based on this premise: "If, and only if, consumers are willing to pay more than the cost of producing what they consume, is it efficient to provide that output." The Task Force objects to the use of this method because "the views of the rich are given greater weight in the analysis"; such a procedure is inappropriate because "we do not believe that the only objective in allocating resources should be the satisfaction of current individual tastes and preferences. Instead, we are persuaded that most citizens want to serve a variety of objectives, including fairness and freedom."

Technically speaking, the interpretation that cost-benefit analysis applies to "consumers" is incorrect; instead, it refers to the valuations that people (or citizens) place on activities for whatever reason, whether they are direct consumers or not. For example, if people place positive values on additional consumption of primary education by others, or negative values on the consumption of cigarettes, these valuations ought in principle to be incorporated into any cost-benefit analysis. In this sense, if "citizens" value additional consumption by an individual as a way of improving "fairness" in the distribution of a service, these valuations ought to be added to the individual's valuations as a consumer of that service.

In regard to transplants, the economic notion that seems most plausible to me is that a taste for "fairness" on the part of the citizenry could be represented as a psychic benefit that higher-income persons achieve from lower-income persons' receipt of medical care. I would regard a situation in which all poor people were unable to afford transplants as unfair and unlovely; I would be willing to pay, via taxation, to subsidize their use of this undoubtedly life-saving measure. The number of such transplants for which I and others are willing to pay may unfortunately be smaller than the number at which there is no additional positive benefit, but it will surely be above the level which the poor—and the not-so-poor—could finance on their own.

In contrast, what does the Task Force mean by equity? Here we come to the critical part of the argument, in which the Task Force is vague. The report is replete with appeals to "equity" and "fairness," but there is no clear statement (except tautologically) of what fairness means, or how one determines how much of it one wants. The closest the Report comes to a definition is in the executive summary, where the conclusions of the President's Commission for the Study of Ethical Problems in Medicine and Biomedical and Behavioral Research are quoted with favor, and are alleged to support the Task Force's view. But how, in fact, does the President's Commission define "equitable access?" The Commission specifically rejects the notion that equity means a right either to "all care that others are receiving" or to unlimited care. In their place, the Commission proposes a standard of "an adequate level of care, which should be thought of as a floor below which no one ought to fall, not a ceiling above which no one may rise."[1] In contrast, as noted above, it is clear that the Task Force's recommendation, in prohibiting people from purchasing transplants they are willing to buy, does set a ceiling as well as (in fact, at the same level as) a floor.

I find myself more in agreement with the President's Commission than with the Task Force. Improving equity or equality of access to care in this country has always meant "bringing up the bottom" of the distribution of use or health. Under the guise of an artificial budget constraint, the Task Force proposes a radical departure from this tradition—achieving equity by "cutting off the top" of the distribution.

What can be said in favor of this sort of distribution? In a society shot through with envy, such a view might make sense, but the Task Force offered no empirical evidence for such envy (or for that matter, for its assertion about citizens' beliefs about fairness). In the absence of such evidence, I have serious difficulties about raising envy as a moral principle equal to altruism. In any case, envy would call for at most an excise (sumptuary) tax on purchased transplants, not a total prohibition.

I would like to offer some brief comments on some other aspects of the Task Force Report. First, it is clear that it would not be feasible to achieve the Task Force's idea of equity, given the low cost of domestic travel; "the rich" would still travel to other states (or countries) for transplants. The net impact of the proposal could be to widen the gap between the rich and the nonrich.

Second, the Task Force seems to have the idea that it can pressure hospitals to squeeze out alleged inefficiency through the mechanism of allowing them to obtain resources for transplants only by limiting these hospitals' budgets. However, I would suggest that having people die is not the best way to get hospitals to run their laundries more efficiently; there must be incentives that are not as lethal.

Finally, I believe that the Task Force probably overstates the current marginal resource cost of transplants, and surely overstates the cost that could be achieved after additional research and after an increase in the volume of transplants. Most of the current "costs" are taken from teaching-research situations; if the costs (or the benefits) of such activities are as large as I think they are, the costs attributable to patient care as such are likely to be well below the minimum costs of $60,000 and $30,000 per life year for livers and hearts respectively.

As to what one might expect to happen to patient care costs with the passage of time and an increase in volume, the renal dialysis program is instructive. The payment level for outpatient dialysis for that program was not changed at all between 1972 (when the program began) and 1983, with no apparent reduction in supply. This occurred in a period when the general medical care input price index rose by 250 percent, implying a 72 percent fall in the real price.[2] In 1983 the price for dialysis was reduced in nominal terms, with still no evidence of reduction in supply. This evidence is consistent with massive declines in the real cost of dialysis. (I might add that the Task Force Report greatly overestimates the saving from home dialysis; recent calculations put the saving at less than $5000 without adjusting for the better health of the home dialysis patient.[3]) In any case, "society" is today clearly willing to pay (or is at least unwilling to stop paying) $25,000 per life year for in-facility dialysis patients, which is about the same as what I suspect heart transplants would cost.

CONCLUSION

The Task Force wrote a report that was appropriately if not excessively cautious in its discussion of the phasing in of a new potentially life-saving technology. But its elevation of budget limitation to the level of a moral principle, and its full-scale transfer of the entire hospital budget to the public sector, with political directives replacing choice, are inappropriate.

NOTES

1. PRESIDENT'S COMMISSION FOR THE STUDY OF ETHICAL PROBLEMS IN MEDICINE AND BIOMEDICAL AND BEHAVIORAL RESEARCH, SECURING ACCESS TO HEALTH CARE (U.S. Government Printing Office, Washington, D.C.) (vol. 1 1983) at 4.
2. These data are derived from Gibson, R., Waldo, D., Levit, K., *National Health Expenditures, 1982,* HEALTH CARE FINANCING REVIEW 5(1):1–31 (Fall 1983).
3. Eggers, P., *Trends in Medicare Reimbursement for End-Stage Renal Disease, 1974–79,* HEALTH CARE FINANCING REVIEW 6(1):31–38 (Fall 1984).

If There's a Will,
Is There a Way?

Arthur L. Caplan, Ph.D.

The recent Report of the Massachusetts Task Force on Organ Transplantation represents a watershed in public policy formulation in the
health care field. The Report reflects the views of a diverse group drawn
from fields which include public health, religion, surgery, law, private
industry, and consumer affairs. As such, it is, happily, unlike nearly
every other advisory study of health care technology that has been commissioned by federal or state bodies during the past twenty-five years.

EXPERTISE AND TECHNOLOGY ASSESSMENT

All too often, assessments of medical technology commissioned by government or publicly funded scientific agencies, such as the National
Institutes of Health, the Office of Technology Assessment, or the Public
Health Service, have been confined to the views of "experts" in the area
of technology being assessed. A policy of relying primarily on medical
or scientific experts to evaluate new technologies frequently produces
a situation wherein physicians or scientists with a vested interest in a
particular technology are called upon to make an "objective" assessment
of the pros and cons of proceeding with the development of the technology. Not surprisingly, "expert-dependent" technology assessments
often result in reports or recommendations favoring generous funding
and unfettered development for new technologies in health care.[1]

The medical community has generally looked with disfavor upon
attempts by nonphysicians to become involved in decisions concerning

Reprinted with permission from *Law, Medicine & Health Care* 13(1). Copyright 1985,
American Society of Law & Medicine, Boston, Massachusetts.

the use and development of medical technology.[2] This resistance has been bolstered by the lack of standardized information concerning the safety and efficacy of many medical technologies, particularly those that do not depend upon new drugs or devices. As the Task Force Report correctly observes, it is particularly difficult to formulate sound public policy for such technologies as organ transplantation, when basic information regarding costs, protocols, and efficacy is not collected in any routine, systematic, and centralized manner.

Resolution of the issues raised by such new technologies as organ transplantation requires expertise that is not limited to that available from physicians or scientists. The policy issues of financing, allocation, patient selection, and pace of dissemination of new and expensive forms of medical technology raise questions of ethics, law, and policy that demand input from many segments of society.

The Massachusetts Task Force is thus to be commended for their efforts in drawing upon a diverse cross-section of public opinion. While there are many substantive political and philosophical issues that ought to be thoroughly debated concerning the composition of advisory bodies charged with conducting technology assessments in health care, perhaps the most important lesson to be drawn from the Task Force Report is that, in the future, local, state, and federal agencies must make serious efforts to involve broad segments of the public in assessments of new and expensive forms of medical technology.

IMPLEMENTING THE REPORT'S RECOMMENDATIONS

The Task Force Report concludes that the dissemination of new forms of organ transplantation technology, such as heart and liver transplantation, should proceed in a carefully controlled and phased manner that allows for periodic evaluation and review. It also recommends that patient selection criteria be public, fair, and equitable, and that organ transplant techniques not be allowed to skew the availability of other proven medical services that are available to the citizens of Massachusetts.

If these recommendations are sound, as I believe they are,[3] then their implementation will require the restructuring of existing regulatory mechanisms in the area of health care technology. The existing institutional and regulatory provisions for new technologies in health care are inadequate for implementing the policies and procedures that the Task Force recommends.

First, no hospital, whether public or private, should be allowed to proceed with the development of any form of extreme and expensive medical technology without both public input and publicly accountable monitoring. The recent involvement of for-profit hospital corporations in the funding of basic research on such devices as the artificial heart raises questions about the adequacy of the current system of using institutional review boards to ensure that the goals of thorough data collection and vigorous monitoring will be met. The absence of statutory authority for state and federal agencies in examining and monitoring research activities, such as xenografting or the artificial heart, which are currently being undertaken with private funds, highlights a serious regulatory lacuna in current federal and state mechanisms.[4]

Second, no single federal agency is at present mandated by law to require well-designed random clinical trials for any new medical technology or procedure. The recommendations of the Massachusetts Task Force regarding patient selection and data collection will be impossible to implement at either a state or a national level unless steps are taken to create an agency which can discharge these functions.

Third, the reluctance of public and private payers to address issues of reimbursement openly with respect to such technologies as heart and liver transplantation has resulted in an inchoate mass of conflicting state, federal and private reimbursement policies which are both unfair and confusing to those who must avail themselves of new and evolving forms of transplantation. A system that depends upon the ability-to-pay through bake sales, carwashes, and public pleas is blatantly unfair both to those who dislike begging and publicity, and to taxpayers whose monies have, over the years, supported the basic research that has permitted the development of techniques for transplanting solid and replenishable tissues. Congress and state legislatures should act quickly to create forums and agencies where reimbursement policies can be publicly discussed. These bodies must take seriously their moral responsibility to formulate consistent policies which do not leave desperately ill persons at the mercy of geography, charity, and the fancy of the media.

The Report of the Massachusetts Task Force on Organ Transplantation is a vast improvement over previous efforts at the state and federal level to conduct assessments of new technologies in health care. Steps must now be taken to institute standardized procedures for commissioning similar reviews of other new and evolving technologies at both the state and the federal levels. If this is not done, then, despite the quality of the Report, there is a danger that its insights will not be an effective antidote to the technological enthusiasm which currently pervades our health care system.

NOTES

1. *See, e.g.,* Kolata, G. B., *Liver Transplants Endorsed,* SCIENCE 221(4606):139 (July 8, 1983) (example of the usual consensus panel process at the National Institutes of Health).
2. *See* Wehr, E., *National Health Policy Sought for Organ Transplant Surgery,* CONGRESSIONAL QUARTERLY 42(8):453, 453–58 (February 25, 1984) (discussion of the resistance of the American Medical Association and the American Hospital Association to establishing federal standards for undertaking organ transplants).
3. Caplan, A. L., *Organ Transplants: The Costs of Success,* HASTINGS CENTER REPORT 13(6):23–32 (December 1983).
4. In a story about the Baby Fae xenograft, it is reported that Charles McCarthy, Director of the Office for Protection from Research Risks at the National Institutes of Health, declined to review the informed consent and research protocol used at Loma Linda Medical Center. McCarthy stated: "It is not NIH policy to investigate research work performed without federal funds. . . ." *See* Breo, D. L., *Interview with Baby Fae's Surgeon,* American Medical News, November 16, 1984, at 16. Unless NIH policy is changed, or unless an individual institution's institutional review board chooses to engage in review, research conducted with private funds will not be subject to review by IRBs or, if it does not involve new drugs or devices, by the Food and Drug Administration or any other federal agency.

Practical Issues
in Obtaining Organs
for Transplantation

Luke Skelley, R.N., M.S.N.

The medical and social fascination with organ transplantation, beginning with Dr. Barnard's pioneering work with heart transplantation in
the 1960s, has most recently resulted in the highly publicized and experimental baboon heart transplantation and artificial heart replacements. Transplants of proven efficacy, such as of corneas, kidneys, bone
marrow, heart-lungs, hearts, and livers, are a reality of modern medicine
and embrace the most fundamental ideals of medicine by alleviating
suffering and saving lives. Nevertheless, many question the increasing
allocation of such a large proportion of our scarce medical and financial
resources for such a relatively small population of recipients. The debate
over how much of our limited health care resources we are willing to
commit to transplantation has encouraged development of the federal
Task Force on Organ Procurement and Transplantation and of statewide committees, such as the Massachusetts Task Force on Organ
Transplantation.

The discussion of how much transplantation to perform and at
what cost is incomplete without a consideration of how many cadaveric
organs are available. The Massachusetts Task Force on Organ Transplantation recognizes the problem of organ procurement but chooses
to focus its Report on issues of quality, distribution, and cost of transplant services. However, the efficient utilization of transplantable organs
must be addressed. The United States' three-part system of identification and referral of potential donors, organ retrieval, and organ distri-

Reprinted with permission from *Law, Medicine & Health Care* 13(1). Copyright 1985,
American Society of Law & Medicine, Boston, Massachusetts.

bution is the best in the world, but could be improved. The step most in need of help is one involving health care professionals throughout the country—the recognition and referral of potential organ donors to the organ procurement network.

Available cadaveric organs in the United States are limited. According to a few estimates, we are currently using only 10–15 percent of the total number of vascular organs available from brain-dead donors.[1] Efforts to increase the pool of available organs include such legislative and organizational efforts as the passage of the National Organ Transplant Act and the establishment of such organizations as the United Network for Organ Sharing and the American Council of Transplantation.

Despite these endeavors, the most crucial effort to increase the supply of available transplantable organs lies in the increased participation of health care professionals in identifying and referring potential donors. The current method by which donors are identified and referred to the system presents obstacles to participation by the nurses and physicians who work in clinical settings.

The major barriers to participation by physicians, nurses, and other health care providers who have contact with potential donors cannot be dismissed as an unwillingness to obtain organs. Even in their professional education, physicians and nurses receive no information regarding their future role in organ donation. In the practice setting, the obstacles are practical. Organ donation is not an everyday priority to most physicians and nurses, especially in a nontransplant hospital setting. Unless the institution provides some type of transplantation services to its patients, it generally has no vested interest in organ donation. Because the staff lacks institutional support and direct contact with either waiting or successfully transplanted recipients, the staff is not externally reinforced for its efforts and must be intrinsically motivated by more humanitarian ideals.

One practical obstacle is the relative infrequency of potential organ donors. For the most part, potential donors constitute a small number of the total patient population and can easily be overlooked in the daily routine of patient care. Staff find it difficult to be constantly aware of the need to identify the potential donor and may not be convinced that one or two donors a year is worth the effort or that the identification of such individuals does not conflict with the provision of medical and nursing care. In smaller critical care units, practicality dictates that an infrequent procedure such as organ donation is not a priority, for it fails to yield direct, tangible results to the hospital staff.

Another problem is the perceived conflict between the medical and nursing care of the patient and the measures that must be instituted to evaluate and maintain the status of the transplantable organs. In short, the conflict is between saving the patient's life and salvaging the patient's organs. This conflict arises largely because most organ donor candidates are obviously terminal at the time of admission to the hospital. Often the decision is made to let nature run its course. In order to maintain the organs for transplantation, more intensive medical and nursing intervention is required. This more aggressive intervention may not be welcomed by the staff. The physician may resent the additional time and effort required and may be concerned that more aggressive treatment will prolong the patient's demise. Similarly, the nurses may question the additional care given to the potential donor patient over a patient with a similar condition who is not a potential donor. Steps to evaluate and maintain donor organs are consistent with patient care, although some staff may consider it to be overaggressive or nonproductive.

Once the nurse or physician has identified a potential donor, the candidate must be referred to an organ procurement or transplant program. The problem here is that a clear delineation of responsibility for referring the patient is generally lacking. Because the physician has ultimate responsibility for the patient's care, it would seem that the physician should be responsible for the referral process as well. Again, unfortunately, the failure to emphasize organ donation in the hospital inhibits most physicians' initiative. The critical care or emergency room nurse has greater contact with more patients, which enhances the possibility of the nurse's recognizing the potential for organ donation. Nurses, however, may be unsuccessful in convincing the physicians to make these referrals. Physicians may be wary of brain death declarations, even in states that explicitly allow it, may resent the implication that the patient is unsalvageable, may be concerned about supposed legal liabilities, may wish to avoid extraordinary involvement with the family, or may feel that investing more time in managing a terminal patient is impractical. Nurses who repeatedly fail to elicit the cooperation of physicians may minimize their efforts, thus worsening the situation.

Some hospital personnel may not be aware of how to initiate the donor process, and may be unfamiliar with the local organ procurement agency. The establishment of a 24-hour donor information and referral hotline (1-412-24-DONOR) by the North American Transplant Coordinators Organization is designed to facilitate participation by providing information about donor criteria and referring the call to the nearest transplant program or organ procurement agency.

The actual organ donation process can itself be an obstacle to health care professionals' involvement because they must invest uncompensated time and effort. The staff must aggressively treat a dead patient solely for the benefit of an anonymous recipient. The potential donor not only signifies more work but also prolongs the staff's exposure to death. In the operating room, where the staff's contact with patients is usually in the context of heroic measures to save life, the transfer of a dead patient for removal of organs and its subsequent transfer to the morgue can be unsettling. Afterwards, the staff's only reward is a letter from the transplant program or organ procurement agency giving sketchy details of the recipient and thanking the staff for their help. Again, there is a lack of concrete evidence that the staff's efforts were productive.

There are additional complications which involve obtaining consent to use the organs. Often the staff may be concerned about the impact of the donation request on the acutely grieving family and may preclude the family's opportunity to donate. To the contrary, organ donation may provide comfort to the bereaved family. In an unpublished survey by the Nashville Regional Procurement Agency, 66 percent of the families that donated their loved ones' organs felt that it provided a comfort during their time of grief, and 87 percent said that they would donate again.

Health care professionals may encounter ethical, although not legal, problems in the use of organs from a victim of child abuse. Here, the staff must often obtain consent from the parent who has been accused of the child abuse, and this brings to the fore many ethical uncertainties. Another problem is that even if the deceased had shown a verbal or written intent to donate his or her organs, the staff feels obligated to ask the family, who may then refuse to give permission. This perceived obligation is difficult and time-consuming to perform. In general, the process of obtaining consent and maintaining a donor is an added burden on an already overworked and understaffed critical care unit. In some situations, failure to refer a potential donor is the path of least resistance.

In order to minimize the effort expended by the hospital staff, an organ procurement or transplant program may employ a transplant coordinator who is a nurse, physician's assistant, or a specially trained person. This individual coordinates the donation process. He or she evaluates the donor, obtains consent, coordinates the removal of the organs, and places the organs with the best recipient.

Although the role of the coordinator is to facilitate the process, his presence may be an additional stress on the staff. Since the coordinator's presence is associated with death and the possibility of additional work, he may be viewed as an outsider because his goal of obtaining viable organs for unidentified recipients may be interpreted as conflicting with the staff's goal of providing quality patient care. Unless the role is performed with utmost respect for the donor and family, and with an intense desire to work collaboratively with the staff while recognizing the additional work involved, the transplant coordinator may hinder participation by the health professionals.

A solution to these problems is neither easy nor likely to be forthcoming. However, one practical issue fundamental to the future of organ transplantation will, if unsolved, effectively prevent any progress in increasing the number of cadaveric organs. That issue is the simple lack of commitment by the overwhelming majority of people in our country to decide to donate their own organs. One public opinion poll indicates that only 10 to 20 percent of the population have signed donor cards despite a willingness on the part of 70 to 80 percent to donate.[2] The refusal to make a personal decision is not only a failure to recognize the increasing possibility that we all are potential donors or recipients of transplantable organs or tissues, but also places an unfortunate and easily avoidable burden on our next of kin to decide for us at a time that they are least able to do so. Prior discussion with the family assumes that the individual's desires for or against organ donation are respected with a minimum of debate by the family.

A personal decision about organ donation by health care professionals is also important in facilitating their involvement with potential donors. Physicians' and nurses' resolution of their feelings about donating their own organs is fundamental to discussing the option with families of potential donors. It is important to be cognizant of one's own personal bias concerning organ donation when presenting the opportunity to a grieving family. If we are to continue our commitment to offering transplantation as an alternative to suffering from end-stage organ disease, then we must also improve the system for identifying and referring potential organs, and, more important, resolve our own feelings about donating our own organs.

Notes

1. Iglehart, J. K., *Transplantation: The Problem of Limited Resources,* New England Journal of Medicine 309(2):123, 125 (July 14, 1983); S. Rep. No. 382, 98th Congress, 2nd Session (March 26, 1984) at 2.
2. *See* The Gallup Organization, *Attitudes and Opinions of the American Public Toward Kidney Donation* (Prepared for the National Kidney Foundation, Washington, D.C.) (February 1983) (G08305).

Organ Transplants and the Principle of Fairness

Albert R. Jonsen, Ph.D.

The Report of the Massachusetts Task Force on Organ Transplantation can be described as an incunabulum. This strange word, properly referring to a book produced in the first decades of printing with movable type, literally means "in the cradle." The Task Force document appears in the infancy of a discussion that is certain to grow: the public policy debate over the allocation of scarce resources. The debate was born several years ago, but until now has either been argued in general terms or by way of administrative devices. The Task Force addresses a quite particular issue: how to or whether to make available to the citizens of the Commonwealth and their neighbors the medical technology of organ transplantation. It approaches the problem with a vivid awareness of the expense of this technology as well as the constraints on health care resources and financing. Previous policy determinations, such as the congressional decision to establish the End-Stage Renal Disease Program, have, in contrast, an almost dreamlike quality. The shining ideal of saving lives with marvelous machines inspired legislators and the public, who were undisturbed by the specters of rationing and cost containment. Only afterward did those specters appear.

The members of the Task Force did not enjoy the felicity of such a dream. Working ten years after the enactment of the end-stage renal program, their waking hours were filled with data about the excessive costs of care, the inefficiency of the health care system, the repeated fiscal assaults on federal and state health budgets, and the clinical anomalies created by that strange apparition, the diagnosis-related group. The Task Force clearly perceived that the technology of organ transplantation was not a "miracle" that, by some astonishing suspension of the laws of financial, fiscal, organizational, and political reality, would now save lives. Organ transplantation is one technology among many other techniques and activities that also contribute in some sense to saving lives. It is my perception, in reading the Report, that the members of the Task Force did not slip into the dream world in which the solution of one problem does not create some other problem. They seem not to have left the real world where the advent of a solution is the prelude to more problems. Effecting access to organ transplantation means that access to something else is likely to be restricted; seeing that its costs are met means that money for something else will disappear or not be found.

Recognizing this, the Task Force turned to another incunabulum, *Securing Access to Health Care,* a report by the President's Commission for the Study of Ethical Problems in Medicine and Biomedical and Behavioral Research.[1] That report was commissioned by Congress and the president to report on the ethical implications of differences in the availability of health services due to differences in individuals' income or residence. *Securing Access* has not received much attention from policy makers in the federal government. The current administration seems to have ignored it, even though, in its final form, it bore the approval of a commission largely appointed by President Reagan. The book is the first extended analysis of the problem of justice in health care. Many scholars in philosophy, economics, social policy and sciences, and health sciences contributed to its formulation. A considerable amount of data was amassed to provide an empirical basis for discussion. The commissioners struggled seriously and honestly with the implications of the philosophical arguments and the factual data. The central conclusion is expressed in these words: Society has an ethical obligation to ensure equitable access to an adequate level of health care for all.[2]

This simple formulation may appear vacuous. The appearance of such words as "obligation," "adequate level," "equitable access" will strike some as empty. Yet the principle is, in fact, substantial and is supported by sound arguments. I urge that this book be read. The generality of the terms is dictated by the nature of the document; it purports to look at the broader question of social justice in health care and therefore must remain at a level of abstraction.

The Massachusetts Task Force, on the other hand, is forced to be concrete and particular. It is required by its mandate to deal with a particular technology in the setting of a determined population, financial situation, and political reality. The Task Force uses *Securing Access* precisely as it should be used: as a statement of principle that can be applied to the Task Force's problem. This is shown by the recommendation that transplantation of livers and hearts should therefore only be permitted "if access to this technology can be made independent of the individual's ability to pay for it and if transplantation itself does not adversely affect the provision of other higher priority health care services to the public."

The Task Force expands on the ideal of the "higher priority" procedure, basing the definition on the "total number of individuals affected and the importance to their lives of the intervention." The Task Force illustrates this through the concrete example of the shutting down of an underutilized maternity ward in order to perform organ transplants, noting that the burden of showing underutilization lies with the hospital. Again, the Task Force states: "As a principle, the Task Force believes that if it turns out that liver and heart transplantations take resources away from higher priority health care services, and decrease their accessibility to the public, these transplantation procedures should not be performed."

Note the words, "as a principle." This principle was enunciated by the President's Commission in a statement which I believe to be the first formulation of the principle in these terms, although philosophers who had been writing about justice in health care had approached it and hinted at it. The principle proposes that there is a moral obligation to provide adequate care; from this, it can be inferred that the forms of health care that, in some fashion, endanger equitable access to an adequate level of care would not be morally obligatory. Indeed, they might be morally prohibited.

The most striking feature of this principle and our inference is that it moves away from the life-saving nature of health care technologies. It allows life saving to be put onto a scale for cost-benefit analysis. Other items can be placed on this scale. In the President's Commission's words, "assessment of costs must take two factors into account: the cost of a proposed option in relation to alternative forms of care that would achieve the same goal of enhancing the welfare and opportunities of the patient, and the cost of each proposed option in terms of foregone opportunities to apply the same resources to social goals other than that of ensuring equitable access."[3]

Immediate problems arise, however, from an attempt to draw inferences from the principle regarding any actual health care technology. The Task Force seems to recognize these problems. The first problem is the descriptive specification of the words "an adequate level of health care." Everyone familiar with health policy acknowledges the difficulty of giving concrete meaning to this phrase. The Commission offers the usual list of methods whereby specificity might be achieved.[4] The Task Force employs none of these methods in a specific way, giving only an oblique glance at the problem. In one place, the Task Force offers a negative example: "it may be appropriate to shut down an underutilized maternity program to do organ transplants." It thereby hints that maternity programs might be among the things belonging in the adequate level. The Task Force also avails itself of the refuge from ethical problems open to policy makers, an administrative approach. It calls for a "controlled, phased" introduction of transplantation technology, so that the "cost effectiveness, ethical implications, and long-term effect on society are studied and reviewed by a publicly accountable body." Studies must be done and administrative controls exercised. We must watch carefully and we may see over time how the introduction of the technology relates to the ethical principle.

This is a prudent but questionable course. First, the watchful wait will proceed, although the criteria of equitability and adequacy are still undefined. It depends to a great extent on intuition: we will know inequitable inadequacy when we see it. Second, and this is the more serious problem, this course of action presupposes that "a controlled, phased" introduction is possible in our health care system. Health policy experts have long mused about the health "nonsystem." Health care in the United States is provided in a diversity of ways by a multiplicity of providers working in different sorts of institutions and financed in various ways. The controls available to the government are relatively few and weak. The authority of the Food and Drug Administration (FDA) to regulate drugs and devices is limited to an evaluation of their safety and efficacy; state agencies are, I imagine, limited similarly. We have licensure and certification, but these too are quite restricted in scope. Our principal technique for regulating the provision of health care has become control of the tax money that finances the system.

Tax money, of course, flows in many channels, but at present, the widest health care channels are the Medicare and Medicaid programs. The Medicaid programs become the states' major indirect regulatory handle on forms of medical practice. The ways in which states define such restrictions as eligibility and reimbursement levels can dictate forms of practice. However, it is clear that this sort of regulation affects only those who are beneficiaries of these programs: those unable to pay or without insurance sufficient to cover their health care needs. These persons are not, of course, only the traditional welfare recipients. Many of them are persons of middle or even higher income who have dropped into poverty precisely because of enormous medical costs incurred by an illness in the family. Thus, the ethical principle governing the introduction of a new expensive technology is applied, not to the population as a whole, but to the segment that depends for its medical care upon tax-supported programs. If not funded by the government, transplantation will be available only to a person who can afford to purchase it out of pocket or from insurance or by charitable gifts stimulated by dramatic appeal of one's plight.

When applied to organ transplantation, the President's Commission's principle leads us to something of a paradox. On the one hand, organ transplants are potentially life-saving. Persons are threatened with death regardless of race, social class, or economic status. It seems radically unfair that, in the face of this great equalizer, only those who can afford this technology should benefit from it. Thus, to rectify this unfairness, we seem obliged to make the life saver available to all. In so doing we add a charge to the publicly supported medical budget that may have the effect of pushing other services—services that deserve to be among those judged adequate—to the fringes or out of existence entirely. We may find this itself an unfair solution to a problem of unfairness.

The paradox now appears fully. We rightly demand that a new technology not jeopardize access of all to an adequate level of care. We intuitively believe that prenatal care, availability to physicians for early diagnosis or reassurance, treatment of the many reversible disorders that would otherwise be lethal or crippling, palliation of ravages of chronic disease—all must fall within the definition of an adequate level of medical care. We envision that an expensive new technology made available to all, that is, supported by public funds, may jeopardize or restrict many of these useful and necessary services. But the only place that it will do so with any obviousness and probability—one might say certainty—is within the segment of health care supported by public funds. Medicare has a budget, although probably a very complex and messy one. It has a dollar limit. In contrast, the so-called "health care budget" of the United States is a fictitious or metaphorical one: it does not have fund balances. It is a bottom line added up from a diversity of sources over which no budget officer has any control, unless it be the one with the famed "invisible hand" of classical economics.

In the final analysis, the President's Commission's principle is noble. It is probably the best statement of the principle of justice in health care that our present wisdom can generate. Its invocation by the Task Force is valiant. The Task Force has seen that the principle is the right one and that new technologies must meet the test of fairness. But the ability to carry the principle into practice probably eludes us, given our current system: an expensive technology will not be financed by those tax dollars that now finance currently available health care if it appears that the new technology will derogate from those currently available services. Yet, the same technology will be on the market (at least until we find the will and the way to prohibit it and then until we succeed in prohibiting it in neighboring states and nations and in banning people from traveling). Thus, some individuals will acquire the embargoed device; others will not, although their need may be the same. Is this unfair or merely unfortunate? For reflections on that question, I refer you to H. Tristam Engelhardt's Shattuck lecture,[5] delivered before an audience of those same Massachusetts citizens that will read the Task Force Report (and some, I am sure, who wrote it).

NOTES

1. PRESIDENT'S COMMISSION FOR THE STUDY OF ETHICAL PROBLEMS IN MEDICINE AND BIOMEDICAL AND BEHAVIORAL RESEARCH, SECURING ACCESS TO HEALTH CARE (U.S. Government Printing Office, Washington, D.C.) (vol. 1 1983).
2. *Id.* at 4.
3. *Id.* at 37.
4. *Id.* at 37–43.
5. Engelhardt, H. T., *Shattuck Lecture—Allocating Scarce Medical Resources and the Availability of Organ Transplantation: Some Moral Presuppositions,* NEW ENGLAND JOURNAL OF MEDICINE 311(1):66–71 (July 5, 1984). Reprinted in Part II of this volume.

Sounding Board:
Ethical and Policy Issues
in the Procurement
of Cadaver Organs
for Transplantation

Arthur L. Caplan, Ph.D.

In the past few years there has been a dramatic rise in the demand for organs for transplantation. Advances in surgical techniques, tissue typing, and the development of powerful immunosuppressive drugs, such as cyclosporin, have made it possible to transplant both a larger number and an increasing variety of organs. Among organs and tissues currently being transplanted from cadavers are kidneys, hearts, lungs, livers, bone marrow, skin, corneas, and pancreases.

Although some of these procedures are still experimental, graft and recipient survival rates for transplantations have shown steady improvement during the past decade.[1,2] Many centers report five-year graft survival rates of 60 percent among patients who have received kidneys from cadavers. More than 95 percent of those who receive corneas from cadavers have their sight restored. Moreover, recent survival rates for heart transplantation are approaching 50 percent at five years.

This remarkable progress in the field of organ transplantation raises numerous moral and policy problems for the medical profession and the general public. Who ought to pay the high costs associated with these procedures? What rate of survival justifies the labeling of a procedure as therapeutic, and who should be responsible for making such determinations? When the number of organs is insufficient to meet the

Reprinted with permission from the *New England Journal of Medicine* (October 11, 1984). Copyright 1984, the Massachusetts Medical Society.

demand, what policies should be instituted to help increase the availability of these precious tissues?

It is the last question that, in many ways, is the most disturbing of all. The large gap that exists between the available supply and the demand for organs for transplantation has been well documented. The Centers for Disease Control has estimated that no more than 15 percent of the 20,000 persons who might serve as organ donors actually do so.[3]

The gap between supply and demand with respect to organ transplantation is not only large but growing in proportion to the rapid advances being made in this area. Nationwide, between 6,000 and 10,000 people are being maintained on either hemodialysis or peritoneal dialysis while awaiting a kidney transplant[3]; nearly 4000 are estimated to be in need of corneal transplants. Indeed, the public has grown all too familiar with televised pleas for a liver, heart, or other tissue to save the life of a relative or friend.

The potential demand for organs is much greater than present levels may indicate. For example, the majority of liver transplantations are performed in children with congenital defects. However, if liver transplantation should prove to be an effective therapeutic option for adults with cirrhosis of the liver, then tens of thousands of persons might be potential recipients. Similar projections can be made for transplantations involving the heart, lungs, and pancreas.[2,4]

Given the current and potential future demand for cadaver organs, there may be no way to avoid the problem of rationing for many forms of transplantation. Nonetheless, it would appear to be both ethically and medically sensible to examine current public policy with respect to the procurement of organs for transplantation, to determine whether legal or regulatory changes might be effected that would help maximize the supply of tissues available to those in need.

For the past fifteen years this country has been committed to a policy of what might best be termed "voluntarism" in the procurement of tissues for transplantation.[5] As transplantation of certain tissues between genetically related family members became possible during the early 1960s, it soon became evident that physicians required both legal and moral guidance in developing procedures to procure tissue for this purpose.

Since many of the organs used for transplantation during this period were procured from living donors, legal authorities and the courts tended to stress the importance of voluntary consent in the procurement process. There was an understandable concern that family members, particularly those who were minors or had diminished mental capacities, were at some risk of being coerced to make donations against their will. Various court cases recognized the legal right of a person to give consent to the transplantation of tissue as long as he or she was both free from coercion and well informed about the risks and benefits of the procedure. Courts even gave children and the retarded the right to donate, in the belief that they might suffer greatly from the loss of a sibling or other family member.

When the prospects for the transplantation of tissues from cadaver donors improved during the late 1960s, public policy was modified in order to encourage this form of donation. In 1968 the Uniform Anatomical Gift Act was enacted, which recognized the legal status of donor cards and "living wills," as well as the authority of the next of kin to make a donation in a situation in which the deceased had not indicated any opposition to donation.

Free choice and voluntarism played key parts in the moral and legal arguments that surrounded the passage of this legislation. Proponents of donor cards, donor statements on driver's licenses, and other forms of living wills argued that a system of cadaver organ procurement built on voluntarism would promote socially desirable virtues, such as altruism, and at the same time, protect the rights of persons who might, for various reasons, oppose the procurement of tissues from cadavers.

As noted above, this system has been only partially successful in securing organs for transplantation. In light of the fact that the demand for cadaver organs is likely to increase, the time has come for a reexamination of current public policy regarding the procurement of such organs.

Although many of those involved in organ procurement are making heroic efforts to increase the supply of organs from cadaver donors, there are a number of factors that severely inhibit the ability of the present system to take advantage of the supply of tissues potentially available from cadavers. Both economic and legal fears impede the present system of voluntary donation.[5,7] Moreover, there is a real danger that unless something is done to improve the efficacy of the voluntary system, advocates of a free-market solution will attempt to create a for-profit system to meet the large demand for organs.[6]

Among the factors that diminish the effectiveness of the current voluntaristic approach to cadaver donation are the lack of trust on the part of physicians and hospital administrators in the legal authority of donor cards, the failure of the public to sign and carry donor cards, the failure of hospital personnel to locate donor cards, and most important, the failure of physicians and nurses to inquire about the possibility of organ donation in the absence of a written directive on the part of the deceased.[7]

There would appear to be a number of incentives that work against the efficacy of the current voluntaristic policy in obtaining cadaver organs. First of all, many people simply find the subject of death and organ donation upsetting and distasteful. Although surveys show that the public is willing to support organ donation,[8] it is difficult to transform willingness into concrete realization on a donor card or driver's license.

Second, most physicians and nurses do not want to inquire about organ donation. The highly emotional circumstances under which such requests are made make it uncomfortable for both families and medical personnel to communicate about the subject of donation. Moreover, at least some health professionals doubt that family members are able to give informed, voluntary consent in the context of the sudden death of a loved one.[5]

Finally, many hospitals fear adverse legal and financial consequences from their involvement with organ procurement. Many hospital administrators refuse to allow their staff to become involved with a procedure that carries some risk of legal complications and no promise of financial return.

Current federal policy is aimed at improving the present system by centralizing the collection of information concerning donors and recipients and by encouraging further efforts at public and professional education.[2,9] However, these efforts are not likely to prove useful in improving the supply of organs available from cadaver sources, since they do not address the major factors hindering the efficacy of the current system.

There is a public-policy option available at both the federal and state levels, however, that might increase the supply of organs available from cadavers. Legislation could be enacted that would require a routine inquiry of available family members as part of the existing procedures in each state for discontinuing life-support measures in hopeless situations. Such a law would mandate that no one on a respirator who might serve as an organ donor could be declared legally dead (assuming that the medical requirements for such a declaration had been met) until a request for donation had been made of any available next of kin or legal proxy. The request would have to be made by a physician, nurse, or physician's assistant with no connection to the determination of the actual occurrence of death, in order to assure the public that declarations of death would be made without regard to the need to obtain organs for transplantation. If family members or guardians were not available, organs could be removed only if a donor card or other similar legal document existed.

A policy of "required request" directly addresses the major obstacles in procuring cadaver organs for transplantation. Such a policy requires that hospital personnel routinely consider the need for transplantable tissues. It ensures that the burden of decisions concerning donation is equitably allocated among all families whose relatives might serve as organ donors. A policy of routine required request standardizes the process of routine inquiring about organ donation in such a way that it lessens the psychological burden on both health professionals and family members at a time of great stress and emotional upheaval. Moreover, it removes the option not to inquire, which is often chosen under the present system because of fears concerning legal and financial consequences. Finally, a policy of required request preserves the right of individuals to refuse consent, since voluntary choice remains the ethical foundation on which organ donation rests.

The benefits to society in terms of an increase in the supply of cadaver organs for transplantation would appear to outweigh the loss of clinical freedom inherent in a required-request policy for cadaver organ donation. In view of the desperate needs of those who are now awaiting organs and the large number of persons who will be able to benefit from transplantation in the years to come, the loss of this freedom would seem to be a small price to pay.

NOTES

1. Van Thiel, D. H., Schade, R. R., Starzl, T. E., *After 20 Years, Liver Transplantation Comes of Age*, ANNALS OF INTERNAL MEDICINE 99:854–56 (1983).
2. Iglehart, J. K., *Transplantation: The Problem of Limited Resources*, NEW ENGLAND JOURNAL OF MEDICINE 309:123–28 (1983).
3. Kolata, G., *Organ Shortage Clouds New Transplant Era*, SCIENCE 221:32–33 (1983).
4. FINAL REPORT OF THE TASK FORCE ON LIVER TRANSPLANTATION IN MASSACHUSETTS. Prepared for the Department of Public Health, State of Massachusetts (1983).
5. Caplan, A. L., *Organ Transplants: The Costs of Success*, HASTINGS CENTER REPORT 13(6):23–32 (1983).
6. Chapman, D. E., *Retailing Human Organs Under the Uniform Commercial Code*, JOHN MARSHALL LAW REVIEW 16:393–417 (1983).
7. Overcast, T. D., *et al.*, *Problems in the Identification of Potential Organ Donors*, JOURNAL OF THE AMERICAN MEDICAL ASSOCIATION 251:1559–62 (1984).
8. The Gallup Organization, *Attitudes and Opinions of the American Public Toward Kidney Donations*. Prepared for the National Kidney Foundation, Washington, D.C. (1983) (GO 8305).
9. Koop, C. E., *Increasing the Supply of Solid Organs for Transplantation*, PUBLIC HEALTH REPORT 98:566–72 (1983).

Health Care Technology and the Inevitability of Resource Allocation and Rationing Decisions, Part I

Roger W. Evans, Ph.D.

Increasingly, it is recognized that resources available to meet health care needs are limited. Recently, this has been evidenced by reductions in federally funded health care programs and the leveling off of research funds made available to the National Institutes of Health. The problem of severely constrained resources is likely to become more acute, given new medical technology and the high cost of medical care. It is now apparent that both resource allocation and resource-rationing decisions will become inevitable, since not all persons with catastrophic or complicated medical conditions will be able to benefit from medical technology. While the careful assessment of health care technology can conceivably increase the efficiency of the health care delivery system, the methods by which allocation and rationing decisions are made must be improved. In doing so, it will ultimately be essential for this society to come to grips with life and death issues in a manner to which it is not accustomed. (*JAMA* 1983:249:2047–2053)

Discussions regarding the high cost of medical care in increasing numbers now include commentaries on the possibility that the resources available for medical care must be allocated across medical care pro-

---

Preparation of this article was made possible by grant 95-P-97887/0-01 and contract 500-81-0051, provided by the Health Care Financing Administration.

grams. While in the past, resources available for the medical needs of the nation have at least been perceived as unlimited, the appearance of numerous large and small medical technologies and their indiscriminate use among some physicians has thrust resource allocation decisions into the forefront.[1] It is questionable whether it will be possible, in the future, to redistribute to medical programs resources available for other purposes. For example, resources earmarked for defense could be reallocated to meet health care needs. Meanwhile, it is now obvious that the health care of the nation is being jeopardized in at least two ways, both of which have implications for resource allocation. First, resources available to health care programs for the needy and disadvantaged have been threatened by budget cuts or have already been reduced substantially. Second, funds available for health-related research are being subjected to budgetary reductions.

These cuts also may affect both public and private insurance programs. These actions have heralded a renewed concern over which groups of beneficiaries are likely to be adversely affected.[2] For example, it is possible that resource limitations and ad hoc rationing systems could threaten the benefits currently derived through Medicare for patients with end-stage renal disease (ESRD) and various categories of Medicaid beneficiaries.[3] Accompanying these developments have been decisions by private insurers to revise coverage policies. Recently, some major insurers have begun to consider the possibility of limiting coverage to only those situations in which a physician providing treatment has performed a given procedure, such as coronary artery bypass surgery, a specified number of times. Policy initiatives such as this certainly raise questions about how persons with catastrophic illnesses will be treated in the future. Will medical care be regionalized or will the current, relatively fragmented delivery system remain in place?[4-6]

In past months there has also been a substantial reduction in funds made available for health-related research. Iglehart,[7] in a review of the status of the National Institutes of Health (NIH), concluded that "the NIH seems destined to face bleaker real budgets in fiscal 1983 and beyond." Thus, biomedical research is being given a lower priority, and, consequently, it is reasonable to expect that in the long run, the health of the population will be adversely affected. For example, it is becoming increasingly difficult to earmark sufficient resources for clinical trials, one of the major methods by which the efficacy and safety of new technological innovations are assessed.[8-12]

A picture is now beginning to emerge in which, in the future, resource constraints are likely to make allocation decisions inevitable.[13] Consequently, the tasks of both the clinician and policymaker are likely to become more difficult. For example, in the absence of formal resource allocation rules and the failure to test new health technology adequately and to assess its broader social implications completely, clinicians to an increasing degree find themselves being forced to confront problems that traditionally have been reserved for biomedical ethicists.[14-19] Unfortunately, clinicians are often ill prepared to deal with complex bioethical issues. Few clinicians have previously been asked to participate proactively in the allocation, let alone the rationing, of health care resources. Many would argue that, in principle, this activity represents a conflict of interest and is contrary to the Hippocratic oath.

Policymakers, perhaps surprisingly, seem to be equally inept at resolving ethical dilemmas. As described by myself and co-workers,[20] this was particularly true of the End-Stage Renal Disease Program, in which it was decided that in a country where resources appeared almost limitless, the ethical and moral dilemma of selecting patients for treatment, based on a perceived need to limit treatment, was resolved rather easily by making additional resources available to treat people with ESRD. In describing the process by which Medicare benefits were extended to ESRD patients, my co-workers and I concluded the following:

> The federal government appears to have been more concerned with ridding itself of the moral dilemma of indirectly deciding who could live and who would die in a country of almost unlimited resources. The easiest way to eradicate this problem was to treat everyone equally by making everyone eligible for the same benefits.

Today, it is now apparent that this decision has only staved off the inevitable—deciding which patients should be treated under public and private insurance programs. The prospect that such decisions may become inevitable raises a number of important medical, social, ethical, legal, and economic questions. To the surprise and chagrin of many, such decisions are not completely foreign to the medical profession.[21,22] Problems of medical triage and the treatment of patients in intensive care units (including neonatal intensive care) and other "high-cost" users of medical care raise similar questions.[23-33]

LIFE EXPECTANCY, CHRONICITY, DISABILITY, MEDICAL TECHNOLOGY, AND MEDICAL CARE COSTS

The reason that bioethical issues have emerged among the more predominant issues in medicine today becomes clear when one considers the increased prevalence of chronic disease, the changing age distribution of the population, notable increases in life expectancy, the increased prevalence of disability, the introduction and widespread availability of new medical technology, and the high cost of medical care. The interrelationships among these are obvious. For example, the longer people live, the greater the likelihood that they will exhibit chronic disease, have subsequent disability, make use of new and expensive medical technology, and, ultimately, fall into the category of high-cost users of medical care.[34-38]

LIFE EXPECTANCY

The percentage of persons older than sixty-five years has steadily risen in all industrialized countries during the past century.[39] While the proportion of elderly persons in the United States has doubled since 1900, their numbers have increased sevenfold. Today, the life expectancy of males, regardless of race, is approximately seventy years and for females is seventy-seven years.[40] The average life expectancy for both groups is about seventy-one years. Overall, males are expected to outlive their earlier (1900) counterparts by twenty-two years, and females, their counterparts by twenty-nine years (Table 1). While the longevity of nonwhites lags behind whites, the gains achieved by nonwhites have been even more dramatic as minority life expectancy in this country has doubled.

The composition of the population is also changing. In 1950, 12.3 million persons in the United States, or 8.1 percent of the total population, were older than sixty-five years. By 1960, this group had grown to 16.6 million persons, or 9.2 percent. The number reached 23.5 million in 1977, an increase of 91.1 percent from 1950, and this figure represented 10.9 percent of the total population. It is now projected that the number of persons older than sixty-five years will be 31.8 million by the year 2000—12.2 percent of the total population and a 157 percent increase in fifty years.[40] As the population ages, chronic disease and disability are becoming increasingly visible problems. Chronic rather than acute diseases are now the most prevalent causes of death in industrial societies.[22,41]

CHRONIC DISEASE AND DISABILITY

Since the early 1900s, there has been a substantial decline in those infectious diseases that have proved to be so intractable in past years.[42] Heart attack, stroke, cancer, and leukemia are but a few of those retrogressive chronic diseases, often of slow insidious onset, that have replaced infections, viruses, and tubercular fatalities in the United States.

Table 1: Life Expectancy at Birth According to Race and Sex, United States, Selected Years from 1900 Through 1978*

	Total, Year			White, Year			All Other, Year†		
	Both Sexes	M	F	Both Sexes	M	F	Both Sexes	M	F
1900‡	47.3	46.3	48.3	47.6	46.6	48.7	33.0	32.5	33.5
1950	68.2	65.6	71.1	69.1	66.5	72.2	60.8	59.1	62.9
1960	69.7	66.6	73.1	70.6	67.4	74.1	63.6	61.1	66.3
1970§	70.8	67.1	74.7	71.7	68.0	75.6	65.3	61.3	69.4
1975§	72.5	68.7	76.5	73.2	69.4	77.2	67.9	63.6	72.3
1976§	72.8	69.0	76.7	73.5	69.7	77.3	68.3	64.1	72.6
1977§	73.2	69.3	77.1	73.8	70.0	77.7	68.8	64.6	73.1
1978§	73.3	69.5	77.2	74.0	70.2	77.8	69.2	65.0	73.6

*Data from Department of Health and Human Services.
†For 1900 through 1902, data for the "all other" category were for blacks only.
‡Death registration areas only. The death registration area increased from ten states and the District of Columbia in 1900 to the coterminous United States in 1933.
§Excludes deaths of nonresidents in the United States.

Given current available data sources, it is difficult to estimate the *true* prevalence of chronic disease. Few population-based epidemiologic studies have been undertaken to estimate explicitly the prevalence of all chronic diseases.[43] The Framingham Heart Study represents but one exemplary population-based epidemiologic study of cardiovascular disease. Results of this study have shown the now apparent decline in the prevalence of cardiovascular disease.[39,44,45]

Other statistics on chronic disease that have been published by the National Center for Health Statistics are based on self-reported illness and disability in the Health Interview Study. These reports indicate that in the early years of life, only about six of 1,000 persons endure chronic conditions. During young adulthood (age 25 or so), the rate increases to 35, and by the fourth decade that figure has almost tripled to 100 persons of every 1,000. By age 65, this number has again doubled and then doubled yet another time after age 75, until almost 90 percent of all persons older than 90 years live with a chronic illness.[46] Again ignoring the age factor, it has at times been estimated that approximately 50 percent of the civilian population, excluding residents in institutions, have one chronic condition or more.[47] As for the number of chronic conditions per person, one study has shown this to be 2.2.[47]

It is currently estimated that 80 percent of health care resources in the United States, including facilities, services, and biomedical research, are now devoted to chronic disease.[34] During 1978, an estimated 10.3 million persons, or 45 percent, of the civilian population aged 65 years and older not residing in institutions were reported in health interviews to have some degree of activity limitation caused by chronic disease or impairment (Table 2).[48] Of these 10.3 million persons, fully 85.2 percent indicated that they were limited in or unable to carry on major activities, affecting their ability to work or manage a household.[48] The remainder were limited but not in major activity.

Ignoring the age factor, 30 million Americans (14 percent of the total population) were reported to have dysfunction caused by chronic diseases, and, of these, 23 million, or 74.6 percent, were limited in or unable to carry on major life activities, affecting their ability to work, manage a household, or attend school.[48]

MEDICAL TECHNOLOGY

Over the years, medical technology has been most successful in dealing with infectious diseases. Thomas,[49,50] in his analysis of technology, notes that much of the technology germane to the treatment of infectious diseases "comes from a genuine understanding of disease mechanisms,

Table 2: Distribution of Persons With Limitation of Activity Because of Chronic Conditions, According to Age and Degree of Limitation, United States, 1978*

Age of Both Sexes, Year	Number of Persons, in Thousands			Percent			
	Total Population	With Activity Limitation (in Major Activity)	With no Activity Limitation	Total Population	With Activity Limitation	Limitation in Major Activity	With no Activity Limitation
All ages	213,828	30,306 (22,598)	183,523	100.0	14.2	10.6	85.8
<17	59,012	2,309 (1,178)	56,703	100.0	3.9	2.0	96.1
17–44	88,627	7,501 (4,621)	81,126	100.0	8.5	5.2	91.5
45–64	43,403	10,244 (8,063)	39,159	100.0	23.6	18.6	76.4
≥65	22,788	10,252 (8,736)	12,535	100.0	45.0	38.3	55.0

*Data from Givens.[46]

and when it becomes available, it is relatively inexpensive, relatively simple, and relatively easy to deliver." This technology is exemplified by modern methods for immunization against diphtheria, pertussis, and the childhood virus diseases and the contemporary use of antibiotics and chemotherapy for bacterial infections.[51] Other examples cited by Thomas[50] include the treatment of endocrinologic disorders with appropriate hormones, the prevention of hemolytic disease of the newborn, and the treatment and prevention of various nutritional disorders.

Major technological advances, however, have been made specifically for treating incurable chronic diseases, many of which have varying implications for the level of functional ability patients are able to regain. Since many of these interventions do not cure disease, they are frequently referred to as "halfway technologies,"[50,51] and the extent to which a patient is able to cope and regain maximum function becomes all important. As described by Crane,[22] technological changes have affected the very character of illness, permitting the physician to have greater control over the process of dying and the timing of death. She also notes that in less obvious ways, improvements in medical technology have produced increasing levels of disability in western society.[52] Moreover, technology has permitted the survival of more or less severely disabled persons such as diabetics and infants with myelomeningocele who would otherwise have died.

It is now estimated that each year, hundreds—perhaps thousands—of new technologies enter the medical care system. These include drugs, procedures, devices, and instrumentation, all constituting preventative, diagnostic, and therapeutic tools.[53] Many of these technologies have undoubtedly contributed to the substantial improvement in the health status of the American people. Also, relief of pain, amelioration of symptoms, and rehabilitation now have become possible for many patients with diseases that cannot be successfully prevented or treated.[53] The benefits of medical technology, in some instances, have been found to be more apparent than real.[54] For example, various inefficacious procedures have been practiced and then abandoned in this country. These include gastric freezing for peptic ulcer, colectomy for epilepsy, hypogastric artery ligation for pelvic hemorrhage, sympathectomy for asthma, internal mammary artery ligation for coronary artery disease, adrenalectomy for essential hypertension, and wiring for aortic aneurysm.[51,54-57]

While efficacy and safety (that is, medical technology's medical benefits and risks) have traditionally been the primary focus of health technology assessment,[51,53,58-62] attention has begun to focus on other aspects of health care technology.[63,64] For example, on June 12, 1980, Patricia

Roberts Harris, then secretary of the Department of Health and Human Services, announced that new health technologies must be evaluated not only on the basis of their medical efficacy and safety but also on the basis of their "social consequences" before "financing their wide distribution."[65] As noted by Knox,[65] the approach being suggested by Harris was even more comprehensive than that used by, for example, the Environmental Protection Agency in dealing with pesticides, the Food and Drug Administration in its treatment of pharmaceuticals, and the Occupational Safety and Health Administration's approach to carcinogens in the work place.[66-69] New health technology was to be evaluated concerning its cost-effectiveness, cost-benefit ratios, ethical implications, and "long-term effects on society." The all-encompassing intent of technology assessment has been characterized by Banta and Behney[59] as follows:

> Technology assessment is seen as a comprehensive form of policy research that examines short- and long-term social consequences (e.g., societal, economic, ethical, legal) of the application of technology. Technology assessment is an analysis of primarily social rather than technical issues, and is especially concerned with unintended, indirect, or delayed social impacts.

It is now becoming more evident that the assessment of any emerging or existing technology must, at least, include consideration of the following parameters: (1) the potential need for the procedure, device, instrument, or drug; (2) the relevant constraints on the availability of the technology (e.g., absence of donor organs for transplantation, location of treatment facilities, shortage of trained personnel); (3) the cost-effectiveness–cost-benefits of the technology assessed in terms of both economic and social costs, including lives saved; (4) the legal issues pertaining to the adoption and availability of the technology, including risks associated with its use (e.g., Where will the technology be made available? Who is eligible to receive the technology? What risks does the recipient incur in the use of the technology?); and (5) the ethical issues concerning the selection of recipients of the technology, the allocation of resources to health care programs, and individual patient rights to health care regardless of cost and availability. Failure to consider these issues will make it extraordinarily difficult to anticipate the long-term implications of any emerging or existing technology.[70-73]

COST OF MEDICAL CARE

In 1980, expenditures for medical care consumed 9.4 percent of the gross national product (GNP).[74] In this same year, health care spending increased by 15.2 percent, representing a moderate acceleration over the 12.5 percent increase during 1979. This figure is substantially higher than the 13.4 percent growth rate between 1978 and 1979 and is certainly much higher than the average of 12.2 percent annually over the period of 1965 to 1979.[74] Gross national product increases have averaged 9.2 percent per year for the same period. This substantially greater growth rate in the health care sector compared with the rest of the economy resulted in the health care share of the GNP rising from 6.1 percent in 1965 to the 9.4 percent level seen today. Between 1950 and 1978 alone, in the United States, total annual expenditures for health care and other forms of health-related activities increased 1,500 percent.[75] In 1950, medical care expenditures constituted 4.5 percent of the U.S. GNP.

In analyzing these increased health expenditures, it is obvious that third-party payers have, in many respects, contributed to the rise in health care costs, primarily because they have traditionally placed few constraints on expenditures. In 1979, personal health care funds supplied by third parties amounted to $147.0 billion of the $217.9 billion in personal health expenditures, or 68 percent.[74] Federal, state, and local governments financed the largest portion of that amount—about 40 percent of the total. Private health insurance payments covered an additional 27 percent of personal health care. In 1980, private insurers, including Blue Cross and Blue Shield plans, commercial insurance companies, and independent plans, paid benefits amounting to $58.1 billion, or 27 percent of personal health care expenditures. In 1980, approximately 76 percent of the U.S. population was covered by private hospital insurance.[74]

Often the cost of disability is ignored as a health-related factor. This is somewhat misleading, since every chronic disease requires a certain level of expenditure for medical care, but, at the same time, the person may be disabled and, consequently, draws on disability programs for various cash benefits. The total cost of illness should reflect not only actual medical treatment costs but the cost of services and other benefits the person receives because of his illness.[76-83]

Table 3 gives a complete breakdown of government expenditures for illness-tested welfare programs for fiscal year 1975.[84,85] As shown here, in 1975, cash payments to disabled persons under these public programs amounted to more than $23 billion. The growth of the disability program is also interesting. As noted by Stone,[84] disability benefits administered through the Social Security program, although smaller than retirement benefits in total dollar amount, are increasing at a much higher rate, and the number of disability beneficiaries is also growing faster than the number of retirement beneficiaries (Table 4). A close

Table 3: Government Expenditures for Illness-Tested Welfare
Programs for Fiscal Year 1975*

	Amount, in Billion Dollars		
Program	Federal	State-Local	Total
Disability insurance			
(Social Security Administration)	7.6	—	7.6
Civil service disability	1.4	—	1.4
Railroad disability	0.2	—	0.2
Black lung benefits	0.6	—	0.6
Uniform services			
Veterans Administration and military			
disability	4.7	—	4.7
Other (income-tested)	0.5	—	0.5
Temporary disability insurance	—	0.9	0.9
Workman's compensation	1.3	3.2	4.5
Public assistance			
Supplemental Security Income—disabled	2.3	—	2.3
Aid to families with dependent children			
(Disabled male head of household)	0.6	—	0.6
Total			$23.3†

*Data from Stone[84] and Skolnik and Dales.[85]
†Total does not include payments made through various private insurance arrangements or payments made for medical services.

Table 4: Growth of Disability and Retirement Programs Under
Old Age, Survivors, Disability, and Health Insurance, 1965
Through 1979*

	Number of Beneficiaries, in Millions		Percent of Increase	Amount of Benefits, in Billion Dollars		Percent of Increase
Program	1965	1979		1965	1979	
Retirement	13.9	22.4	61	12.5	59.3	374
Disability	1.7	4.8	182	1.6	12.5	681

*Data from the Department of Commerce, Bureau of the Census.[105]

examination of the Supplemental Security Income program presents a similar picture—federal payments to disabled persons grew by 13.6 percent between 1977 and 1980, as compared with an increase of only 8.0 percent in payments to the aged (Table 5).

The rapidly rising costs of health care have served to spur interest in health care technology assessment.[51,55,86-90] Recently, much blame has been placed on health care technology as the "culprit" behind high health care costs.[10,11,91-101] Although the total contribution of new technology to rising costs is controversial, estimates of the effect of technology on increased per diem hospital costs range from 33 percent to 75 percent, with 50 being an average figure.[51,54,99,101-103] Detailed case studies have been undertaken that illustrate the variable effect of technology on the treatment of chronic disease.[54] Scitovsky and McCall,[104] for example, looked at the changing cost of treating eleven different conditions at the Palo Alto Medical Clinic in California during a period of several years.[104] They found the real cost of treating five conditions fell, while the cost of treating six actually increased. Closer examination of these six conditions showed that there had been a notable increase in the use of diagnostic tests and therapeutic procedures per diagnosis. Laboratory tests per case of perforated appendicitis rose from 5.3 in 1951, to 14.5 in 1964, to 31.0 in 1971. Inhalation-therapy procedures for myocardial infarction rose from 12.8 per case in 1964 to 37.5 in 1971.[51,54,104]

Fineberg and Hiatt[89] have noted that, for several reasons, rising medical costs can be attributed to technology. First, although the trend is toward shorter hospital stays, this is accompanied by an increased consumption of resources during hospitalization. Second, more advanced equipment design may improve efficiency, but, with increased use of the equipment and other "induced costs," potential savings are never realized. Third, many new technologies do more than simply perform old services more efficiently—they provide new and expensive services. The intensive care unit, for example, is but a single innovation that in 1974 was found to account for 10 percent of all hospital costs.[87]

It is often argued that big, expensive technologies contribute disproportionately to the high cost of medical care, although the costs and benefits of a new technology largely depend on how and to which patients it is applied.[89,105,106] Moloney and Rogers,[92] however, have argued that the big and highly visible technologies such as the computed tomographic scanner "actually account for far less of the annual growth in medical expenditures than do the collective expense of thousands of small tests and procedures that are more frequently used by physicians and that individually cost little."

Table 5: Growth of Expenditures Under
Supplemental Security Income, 1979 and
1980*

| | *Federal Payments, in Billion Dollars* | | *Percent of Increase* |
	1979	*1980*	
Aged	2.5	2.7	8.0
Disabled	4.4	5.0	13.6

*Data from the Department of Commerce, Bu-
reau of the Census.[105]

The use of a technology is directly related to reimbursement for
its use.[10,51,107-109] Moloney and Rogers[92] suggest that one approach, although problematic, to slowing the use of a technology is to develop
protocols that instruct physicians to use technologies only when less
expensive methods cannot provide adequate information on patient
care; limit reimbursement to use according to these standards. At present, policies with regard to the reimbursement of new technologies, if
they exist, are often inconsistent. Under the Medicare program, the
major reason for excluding a technology for reimbursement occurs when
it has not been demonstrated to be safe and effective.[110,111] As described
by Bunker and associates,[10] "the government's reimbursement policy
has been left largely to the commercial and nonprofit carriers to whom
the government, by contract, has delegated the responsibility for processing claims." To accomplish this objective, some carriers, such as California and Massachusetts Blue Shield, have organized their own
technology assessment committees and procedures. California Blue Shield
has only recently placed limitations on procedures that are considered
experimental. Previously, the carrier was committed to reimbursing for
services that were "reasonable and necessary."[10] At present, there seems
to be no satisfactory uniformly applied approach to limiting the growth
of technology through alternative reimbursement policies.

Controlling the growth and distribution of technology is complicated by the fact that the medical technology industry is large and mul-
tinational.[51,68,112] To slow its growth through regulation surely would
have a multitude of political ramifications. Since World War II, the medical technology industry has experienced dramatic growth in sales, firms,
and establishments (Table 6).[113] Wenchel[113] attributes much of the growth
to the increased demand for health services supported by private, vol-

untary health insurance and government programs such as Medicare and Medicaid, Hill-Burton, and Regional Medical Programs. The roentgenography and electromedical industries have seen the greatest increase in sales, showing an increase of $1.8 billion between 1958 and 1977.[113] Consequently, it is difficult to imagine that the medical technology industry is willing to sit idle as new regulations are introduced to slow the growth of technology. Perhaps this is most true in those situations in which existing rather than emerging technologies are being scrutinized.

SUMMARY

The foregoing discussion points to several problems and developments that indicate the inevitability of resource allocations to health care programs. The U.S. population is aging; chronic disease is becoming more prevalent, disability a common occurrence. To meet the needs of an aging, chronically ill, and disabled population, a complex array of expensive and sophisticated medical technologies has emerged. The cost of these technologies will make it necessary to develop elaborate plans not only to enable them to be used but to ensure that people receiving them derive the maximum expected benefits. Thus, it is apparent that resource allocation decisions are likely not only to become a necessity but to become routine.[114,115]

In short, in the future, the demand for health care will doubtlessly outstrip available resources.[116,117] The problem then becomes one of determining how best to allocate the available resources to optimize the health of the population. To accomplish this objective, it will be necessary to study carefully new and existing technology to determine the magnitude of potential benefits.[10,11,51,58] At the same time, it will be necessary to increase the efficiency of the existing health care delivery system in an attempt to ensure that maximum benefits are being derived.[118] During this process, it is probable that some types of medical care can

Table 6: Growth in the Medical Technology Industry*

	1958	1977
Sales, billion dollars	1.0	8.1
Number of companies	1,366	1,442
Number of establishments	2,802	3,203

*Data from Wenchel.[111]

no longer be provided, or, if provided, they will be done so on a limited basis, since the derived benefits are too costly for all to benefit. The question then becomes one of determining the best method of implementing allocation decisions.[119,120] In doing this, it subsequently will become necessary to ration care within health care programs that have been spared from complete extinction. Although advanced technology will provide many persons with a new lease on life, not all are expected to benefit equally, if at all. As these allocation and rationing exercises are undertaken, a new appreciation of medical ethics will come about, accompanied by a more careful assessment of the nature of death and dying within this society.[121,122] These issues as they apply to this analysis are more completely delineated in part II.

REFERENCES

1. Russell, L., *How Much Does Medical Technology Cost?* BULLETIN OF THE NEW YORK ACADEMY OF MEDICINE 54:124–32 (1978).
2. Caper, P., *Competition and Health Care: A New Trojan Horse*, NEW ENGLAND JOURNAL OF MEDICINE 306:928–29 (1982).
3. Iglehart, J. K., *Medicare's Uncertain Future*, NEW ENGLAND JOURNAL OF MEDICINE 306:1308–12 (1982).
4. McGregor, M., Polletier, G., *Planning of Specialized Health Facilities: Size vs. Cost and Effectiveness in Heart Surgery*, NEW ENGLAND JOURNAL OF MEDICINE 299:179–81 (1978).
5. Luft, H. S., Bunker, J. P., Enthoven, A. C., *Should Operations Be Regionalized? The Empirical Relation Between Surgical Volume and Mortality*, NEW ENGLAND JOURNAL OF MEDICINE 301:1364–69 (1979).
6. Finkler, S. A., *Cost-Effectiveness of Regionalization: The Heart Surgery Example*, INQUIRY 16:264–70 (1979).
7. Iglehart, J. K., *Health Policy Report: Prospects for the National Institutes of Health*, NEW ENGLAND JOURNAL OF MEDICINE 306:879–84 (1982).
8. Chalmers, T. C., *The Clinical Trial*, MILBANK MEMORIAL FUND QUARTERLY 59:324–39 (1981).
9. Chalmers, T. C., *Who Will Fund Clinical Trials?* SCIENCE 22:6–8 (1982).
10. Bunker, J. P., Fowles, J., Schaffarzick, R., *Evaluation of Medical-Technology Strategies: I. Effects of Coverage and Reimbursement*, NEW ENGLAND JOURNAL OF MEDICINE 306:620–24 (1982).
11. Bunker, J. P., Fowles, J., Schaffarzick, R., *Evaluation of Medical-Technology Strategies: II. Proposal for an Institute for Health-Care Evaluation*, NEW ENGLAND JOURNAL OF MEDICINE 306:687–92 (1982).
12. Frederickson, D. S., *Biomedical Research in the 1980s*, NEW ENGLAND JOURNAL OF MEDICINE 304:509–17 (1981).
13. Office of Health Economics, *Scarce Resources in Health Care*, MILBANK MEMORIAL FUND QUARTERLY 57:265–87 (1979).

14. P. RAMSEY, THE PATIENT AS A PERSON: EXPLORATIONS IN MEDICAL ETHICS (Yale University Press, New Haven, Conn.) (1970).

15. READINGS ON ETHICAL AND SOCIAL ISSUES IN BIOMEDICINE (R. W. Wertz, ed.) (Prentice-Hall, Inc., Englewood Cliffs, N.J.) (1973).

16. T. L. BEAUCHAMP, J. CHILDRESS, PRINCIPLES OF BIOMEDICAL ETHICS (Oxford University Press, New York, N.Y.) (1979).

17. J. STEIN, MAKING MEDICAL CHOICES: WHO IS RESPONSIBLE? (Houghton Mifflin Co., Boston, Mass.) (1978).

18. Callahan, D., *Shattuck Lecture: Contemporary Biomedical Ethics*, NEW ENGLAND JOURNAL OF MEDICINE 302:1228–33 (1980).

19. Tancredi, L. R., *Social and Ethical Implications in Technology Assessment*, in CRITICAL ISSUES IN MEDICAL TECHNOLOGY (B. J. McNeil, E. G. Cravalho, eds.) (Auburn House, Boston, Mass.) (1982) at 93–112.

20. Evans, R. W., Blagg, C. R., Bryan, F. A., Jr., *Implications for Health Care Policy: A Social and Demographic Profile of Hemodialysis Patients in the United States*, JOURNAL OF THE AMERICAN MEDICAL ASSOCIATION 245:487–91 (1981).

21. Crane, D., *Decisions to Treat Critically Ill Patients*, MILBANK MEMORIAL FUND QUARTERLY 53:1–33 (1975).

22. D. CRANE, THE SANCTITY OF SOCIAL LIFE: PHYSICIAN'S TREATMENT OF CRITICALLY ILL PATIENTS (Russell Sage Foundation, New York, N.Y.) (1975).

23. Becker, E. L., *Finite Resources and Medical Triage*, AMERICAN JOURNAL OF MEDICINE 66:549–50 (1979).

24. Civetta, J. M., *The Inverse Relationship Between Cost and Survival*, JOURNAL OF SURGICAL RESEARCH 14:265–69 (1973).

25. Cullen, D. J., *et al.*, *Survival, Hospitalization Charges and Follow-Up Results in Critically Ill Patients*, NEW ENGLAND JOURNAL OF MEDICINE 294:982–87 (1976).

26. Turnbull, A. D., *et al.*, *The Inverse Relationship Between Cost and Survival in the Critically Ill Cancer Patient*, CRITICAL CARE MEDICINE 7:20–23 (1979).

27. Thibault, G. E., *et al.*, *Medical Intensive Care: Indications, Interventions, and Outcomes*, NEW ENGLAND JOURNAL OF MEDICINE 302:938–42 (1980).

28. Detsky, A. S., *et al.*, *Prognosis, Survival, and the Expenditure of Hospital Resources for Patients in an Intensive Care Unit*, NEW ENGLAND JOURNAL OF MEDICINE 305:667–72 (1981).

29. Martin, S. W., *Inputs into Coronary Care During 30 Years: A Cost-Effectiveness Study*, ANNALS OF INTERNAL MEDICINE 81:289–93 (1974).

30. Zook, C. J., Moore, F. D., *High-Cost Users of Medical Care*, NEW ENGLAND JOURNAL OF MEDICINE 302:996–1002 (1980).

31. Schroeder, S. A., Showstack, J. A., Schwartz, J., *Survival of Adult High-Cost Patients: Report of a Follow-Up Study from Nine Acute-Care Hospitals*, JOURNAL OF THE AMERICAN MEDICAL ASSOCIATION 245:1446–49 (1981).

32. Silverman. W. A., *Mismatched Attitudes about Neonatal Death*, HASTINGS CENTER REPORT 11:12–16 (1981).

33. Bridge, P., Bridge, M., *The Brief Life and Death of Christopher Bridge*, HASTINGS CENTER REPORT 11:17–19 (1981).

34. Cluff, L. F., *Chronic Disease, Function and Quality of Care*, JOURNAL OF CHRONIC DISEASES 34:299–304 (1981).

35. S. J. REISER, MEDICINE AND THE REIGN OF TECHNOLOGY (Cambridge University Press, New York, N.Y.) (1978).

36. L. B. RUSSELL, TECHNOLOGY IN HOSPITALS: MEDICAL ADVANCES AND THEIR DIFFUSION (The Brookings Institution, Washington, D.C.) (1979).

37. J. H. V. BROWN, THE HEALTH CARE DILEMMA: PROBLEMS OF TECHNOLOGY IN HEALTH CARE DELIVERY (Human Sciences Press, New York, N.Y.) (1978).

38. D. L. ELLISON, THE BIO-MEDICAL FIX (Greenwood Press, Inc., Westport, Conn.) (1978).

39. McGinnis, J. M., *Recent Health Gains for Adults,* NEW ENGLAND JOURNAL OF MEDICINE 306:671–73 (1982).

40. DEPARTMENT OF HEALTH AND HUMAN SERVICES, HEALTH: UNITED STATES, 1981 (DHHS Publication (PHS) 82-1232) (National Center for Health Statistics, Hyattsville, Md.) (1981).

41. Lerner, M., *When, Why, and Where People Die,* in THE DYING PATIENT (O. G. Brim, Jr., *et al.,* eds.) (Russell Sage Foundation, New York, N.Y.) (1970) at 5–29.

42. R. DUBOS, MAN ADAPTING (Yale University Press, New Haven, Conn.) (1965).

43. COMMISSION ON CHRONIC ILLNESS, CARE OF THE LONG-TERM PATIENT (Harvard University Press, Cambridge, Mass.) (vol. 2 1956).

44. PROCEEDINGS OF THE CONFERENCE ON THE DECLINE IN CORONARY HEART DISEASE MORTALITY, BETHESDA, MD., OCTOBER 24-25, 1978 (R. J. Havlik, M. Feinleib, eds.) (National Institutes of Health, Bethesda, Md.) (1979).

45. T. R. DAWBER, THE FRAMINGHAM STUDY (Harvard University, Cambridge, Mass.) (1980).

46. J. HENDRICKS, C. D. HENDRICKS, AGING IN MASS SOCIETY: MYTHS AND REALITIES (Winthrop Publishers, Inc., Cambridge, Mass.) (1977).

47. A. STRAUSS, CHRONIC ILLNESS AND THE QUALITY OF LIFE (C.V. Mosby Co., St. Louis, Mo.) (1975).

48. J. D. GIVENS, CURRENT ESTIMATES FROM THE HEALTH INTERVIEW SURVEY, UNITED STATES, 1978 (Vital and Health Statistics Series 10, No. 130, Dept. of Health, Education, and Welfare Publication (PHS) 80-1551) (National Center for Health Statistics, Hyattsville, Md.) (1979).

49. L. THOMAS, THE LIVES OF A CELL: NOTES OF A BIOLOGY WATCHER (The Viking Press, Inc., New York, N.Y.) (1974).

50. Thomas, L., *Notes of a Biology-Watcher: The Technology of Medicine,* NEW ENGLAND JOURNAL OF MEDICINE 285:1366–68 (1977).

51. H. D. BANTA, C. J. BEHNEY, J. S. WILLEMS, TOWARD RATIONAL TECHNOLOGY IN MEDICINE (Springer Publishing Co., Inc., New York, N.Y.) (1981).

52. Ford, A. B., *Casualties of our Time,* SCIENCE 167:256–63 (1970).

53. OFFICE OF TECHNOLOGY ASSESSMENT, ASSESSING THE EFFICACY AND SAFETY OF MEDICAL TECHNOLOGY, Stock 052-003-00593-0 (U.S. Government Printing Office, Washington, D.C.) (1978).

54. Larson, E. B., *Consequences of Medical Technology: Controversies and Dilemmas,* UNIVERSITY OF WASHINGTON MEDICINE 8:2–5 (1981).

55. Hiatt, H. H., *Protecting the Medical Commons: Who Is Responsible?* NEW ENGLAND JOURNAL OF MEDICINE 293:235–41 (1975).

56. T. PRESTON, CORONARY ARTERY SURGERY: A CRITICAL REVIEW (Raven Press, New York, N.Y.) (1977).

57. Fineberg, H., *Gastric Freezing: A Study of Diffusion of a Medical Innovation,* in MEDICAL TECHNOLOGY AND THE HEALTH CARE SYSTEM (Committee on Technology and Health Care) (National Academy of Sciences, Washington, D.C.) (1979) at 173–200.

58. Bunker, J. P., Hinkley, D., McDermott, W., *Surgical Innovation and its Evaluation,* SCIENCE 200:937–41 (1978).

59. Banta, H. D., Behney, C. J., *Policy Formulation and Technology Assessment,* MILBANK MEMORIAL FUND QUARTERLY 59:445–79 (1981).

60. Banta, D., Sanes, J., *Assessing the Social Impacts of Medical Technology,* JOURNAL OF COMMUNITY HEALTH 3:245–58 (1978).

61. Schwartz, W. B., Joskow, P. L., *Medical Efficacy Versus Economic Efficiency: A Conflict in Values,* NEW ENGLAND JOURNAL OF MEDICINE 299:1462–64 (1978).

62. S. ARNSTEIN, A. CHRISTAKIS, PERSPECTIVES ON TECHNOLOGY ASSESSMENT (Science and Technology Publishers, Jerusalem, Israel) (1975).

63. MEDICAL TECHNOLOGY (J. Wagner, ed.) (Dept. of Health, Education, and Welfare Publication (PHS) 79-3254) (National Center for Health Services Research, Hyattsville, Md.) (1979).

64. MEDICAL TECHNOLOGY RESEARCH PRIORITIES (J. L. Wagner, ed.) (Urban Institute, Washington, D.C.) (1979).

65. Knox, R. A., *Heart Transplants: To Pay or Not to Pay,* SCIENCE 209:570–75 (1980).

66. Brooks, H., Bowers, R., *The Assessment of Technology,* SCIENTIFIC AMERICAN 22:13–21 (1970).

67. Coates, J. F., *Technology Assessment,* in TECHNOLOGY AND MAN'S FUTURE (A. H. Tiech, ed.) (St. Martin's Press, Inc., New York, N.Y.) (3rd ed. 1981) at 229–50.

68. G. GORDON, G. FISHER, THE DIFFUSION OF MEDICAL TECHNOLOGY (Ballinger Publishing Co., Cambridge, Mass.) (1975).

69. Morrison, R. S., *Visions,* in TECHNOLOGY AND MAN'S FUTURE (A. H. Teich, ed.) (St. Martin's Press, Inc., New York, N.Y.) (3rd ed. 1981) at 7–22.

70. B. STOCKING, S. L. MORRISON, THE IMAGE AND THE REALITY: A CASE STUDY OF THE IMPACTS OF MEDICAL TECHNOLOGY (Nuffield Provincial Hospitals Trust, London, U.K.) (1978).

71. COMMITTEE ON TECHNOLOGY AND HEALTH CARE, MEDICAL TECHNOLOGY AND THE HEALTH CARE SYSTEM (National Academy of Sciences, Washington, D.C.) (1979).

72. HEALTH CARE TECHNOLOGY EVALUATION, Vol. 6 of LECTURE NOTES IN MEDICAL INFORMATION (J. Goldman, ed.) (Springer-Verlag, New York, N.Y.) (1979).

73. Frazier, H., Hiatt, H., *Evaluation of Medical Practices,* SCIENCE 200:875–78 (1978).

74. Gibson, R., Waldo, D. R., *National Health Expenditures, 1980,* HEALTH CARE FINANCING REVIEW 1–54 (September 1981).

75. Herrell, J. H., *Health Care Expenditures: The Approaching Crisis*, MAYO CLINIC PROCEDURES 55:705–10 (1980).
76. Evans, R. W., *Economic and Social Costs of Heart Transplantation*, HEART TRANSPLANTATION 1:253–51 (1982).
77. D. P. RICE, ESTIMATING THE COST OF ILLNESS (Public Health Service Publication 947-6) (U.S. Government Printing Office, Washington, D.C.) (1966).
78. Rice, D. P., *The Economic Value of Human Life*, AMERICAN JOURNAL OF PUBLIC HEALTH 57:1954–66 (1967).
79. Rice, D. P., *Estimating the Cost of Illness*, AMERICAN JOURNAL OF PUBLIC HEALTH 57:424–40 (1967).
80. D. P. RICE, T. A. HODGSON, SOCIAL AND ECONOMIC IMPLICATIONS OF CANCER IN THE UNITED STATES (Vital and Health Statistics Series 3, No. 20, Dept. of Health, Education, and Welfare Publication (PHS) 81-1404) (National Center for Health Statistics, Hyattsville, Md.) (1981).
81. Rice, D. P., Hodgson, T. A., *The Value of Life Revisited*, AMERICAN JOURNAL OF PUBLIC HEALTH 72:536–38 (1982).
82. Cooper, B. S., Rice, D. P., *The Economic Cost of Illness Revisited*, SOCIAL SECURITY BULLETIN 39:21–36 (1976).
83. Landefeld, J. S., Seskin, E. P., *The Economic Value of Life: Linking Theory to Practice*, AMERICAN JOURNAL OF PUBLIC HEALTH 72:555–66 (1982).
84. Stone, D. A., *Diagnosis and the Dole: The Function of Illness in American Distributive Politics*, JOURNAL OF HEALTH POLITICS, POLICY AND LAW 4:507–21 (1979).
85. Skolnik, A., Dales, S. *Social Welfare Expenditures, Fiscal Year 1976*, SOCIAL SECURITY BULLETIN 40:3–19 (1977).
86. Scitovsky, A., *Changes in the Costs of Treatment of Selected Illnesses, 1951–1965*, AMERICAN ECONOMICS REVIEW 53:1182–90 (1967).
87. Russell, L., *The Diffusion of New Hospital Technologies in the United States*, INTERNATIONAL JOURNAL OF HEALTH SERVICES 6:557–80 (1976).
88. TECHNOLOGY AND THE QUALITY OF HEALTH CARE (R. Egdahl, P. Gertman, eds.) (Aspen Systems Corp., Germantown, Md.) (1978).
89. Fineberg, H. V., Hiatt, H. H., *Evaluation of Medical Practices: The Case of Technology Assessment*, NEW ENGLAND JOURNAL OF MEDICINE 301:1086–91 (1979).
90. Relman, A. S., *Assessment of Medical Practices: A Simple Proposal*, NEW ENGLAND JOURNAL OF MEDICINE 303:153–54 (1980).
91. S. H. ALTMAN, R. J. BLENDON, MEDICAL TECHNOLOGY: THE CULPRIT BEHIND HEALTH CARE COSTS? (Dept. of Health, Education, and Welfare Publication (PHS) 79-3216) (U.S. Government Printing Office, Washington, D.C.) (1979).
92. Moloney, T. W., Rogers, D. E., *Medical Technology: A Different View of the Contentious Debate over Costs*, NEW ENGLAND JOURNAL OF MEDICINE 301:1413–19 (1979).
93. Gaus, C. R., Cooper, B. S., *Controlling Health Technology*, in MEDICAL TECHNOLOGY: THE CULPRIT BEHIND HEALTH CARE COSTS? (S. H. Altman,

R. Blendon, eds.) (Dept. of Health, Education, and Welfare Publication (PHS) 79-3216) (U.S. Government Printing Office, Washington, D.C.) (1979) at 242–52.

94. Marks, R., *Biomedical Research and its Technological Products in the Quality and Cost Problems of Health Practices,* in MEDICAL TECHNOLOGY: THE CULPRIT BEHIND HEALTH CARE COSTS? (S. H. Altman, R. Blendon, eds.) (Dept. of Health, Education, and Welfare Publication (PHS) 79-3216) (U.S. Government Printing Office, Washington, D.C.) (1979) at 235–41.

95. Heyssel, R. M., *Controlling Health Technology: A Public Policy Dilemma,* in MEDICAL TECHNOLOGY: THE CULPRIT BEHIND HEALTH CARE COSTS? (S. H. Altman, R. Blendon, eds.) (Dept. of Health, Education, and Welfare Publication (PHS) 79-3216) (U.S. Government Printing Office, Washington, D.C.) (1979) at 262–72.

96. Bennett, I. L., Jr., *Technology as a Shaping Force,* DAEDALUS 106:125–33 (1977).

97. Blendon, R. J., Moloney, T. W., *Perspectives on the Growing Debate over the Cost of Medical Technologies,* in MEDICAL TECHNOLOGY: THE CULPRIT BEHIND HEALTH CARE COSTS? (S. H. Altman, R. Blendon, eds.) (Dept. of Health, Education, and Welfare Publication (PHS) 79-3216) (U.S. Government Printing Office, Washington, D.C.) (1979) at 10–23.

98. Showstack, J. A., Schroeder, S. A., Matsumoto, M. F., *Changes in the Use of Medical Technologies, 1972–1977: A Study of Ten Inpatient Diagnoses,* NEW ENGLAND JOURNAL OF MEDICINE 306:706–12 (1982).

99. M. FELDSTEIN, A. TAYLOR, THE RAPID RISE OF HOSPITAL COSTS (U.S. Government Printing Office, Washington, D.C.) (1977).

100. NATIONAL COMMISSION ON THE COST OF MEDICAL CARE, REPORT OF THE TASK FORCE ON TECHNOLOGY (American Medical Association, Chicago, Ill.) (vol. 1 1978).

101. Davis, K., *The Role of Technology, Demand and Labor Markets in Determination of Hospital Costs,* in THE ECONOMICS OF HEALTH AND MEDICAL CARE (M. Perlman, ed.) (John Wiley and Sons, Inc., New York, N.Y.) (1974) at 283–301.

102. Waldman, S., *Effect of Changing Technology on Hospital Costs,* SOCIAL SECURITY BULLETIN 35:28–30 (1972).

103. Worthington, N. L., *Expenditures for Hospital Care and Physician's Services: Factors Affecting Annual Charges,* SOCIAL SECURITY BULLETIN 39:3–15 (1975).

104. A. A. SCITOVSKY, N. McCALL, CHANGES IN THE COSTS OF TREATMENT OF SELECTED ILLNESS, 1951–1964–1971 (Dept. of Health, Education, and Welfare Publication (HRA) 77-3161) (U.S. Government Printing Office, Washington, D.C.) (1976).

105. DEPARTMENT OF COMMERCE, BUREAU OF THE CENSUS, STATISTICAL ABSTRACT OF THE U.S., 1981 (U.S. Government Printing Office, Washington, D.C.) (1981).

106. Fineberg, H. V., *Clinical Chemistries: The High Cost of Low-Cost Diagnostic Tests,* in MEDICAL TECHNOLOGY: THE CULPRIT BEHIND HEALTH CARE COSTS? (S. H. Altman, R. Blendon, eds.) (Dept. of Health, Education, and Welfare Publication (PHS) 79-3216) (U.S. Government Printing Office, Washington, D.C.) (1979) at 144–65.

107. Stoughton, W. V., *Medical Costs and Technology Regulation: The Pivotal Role of Hospitals*, in CRITICAL ISSUES IN MEDICAL TECHNOLOGY (B. J. McNeil, E. G. Cravalho, eds.) (Auburn House, Boston, Mass.) (1982) at 37–50.
108. Derzon, R. A., *Influences of Reimbursement Policies on Technology*, in CRITICAL ISSUES IN MEDICAL TECHNOLOGY (B. J. McNeil, E. G. Cravalho, eds.) (Auburn House, Boston, Mass.) (1982) at 139–50.
109. Schroeder, S. A., Showstack, J.A., *Financial Incentives to Perform Medical Procedures and Laboratory Tests: Illustrative Models of Office Practice*, MEDICAL CARE 16:289–98 (1978).
110. Greenberg, B., Derzon, R. A., *Determining Health Insurance Coverage of Technology: Problems and Options*, MEDICAL CARE 19:967–78 (1981).
111. Towery, O. B., Perry, S., *The Scientific Basis for Coverage Decisions by Third-Party Payers*, JOURNAL OF THE AMERICAN MEDICAL ASSOCIATION 245:59–61 (1981).
112. D. ELLIOTT, R. ELLIOTT, THE CONTROL OF TECHNOLOGY (Wykeham Publications Ltd., London, U.K.) (1976).
113. H. E. WENCHEL, A SUMMARY OF THE STUDY OF THE MEDICAL TECHNOLOGY INDUSTRY (Contract 233-79-3011) (National Center for Health Services Research, Hyattsville, Md.) (1981).
114. M. H. COOPER, RATIONING HEALTH CARE (Croom Helm Ltd., London, U.K.) (1977).
115. J. KATZ, A. M. CAPRON, CATASTROPHIC DISEASES: WHO DECIDES WHAT? (Russell Sage Foundation, New York, N.Y.) (1975).
116. Golding, A. M. B., Tosey, D., *The Cost of High-Technology Medicine*, LANCET 2:195–197 (1980).
117. HEALTH: WHAT IS IT WORTH? MEASURES OF HEALTH BENEFITS (S. J. Mushkin, D. W. Dunlop, eds.) (Pergamon Press Ltd., New York, N.Y.) (1979).
118. A. L. COCHRANE, EFFECTIVENESS AND EFFICIENCY: RANDOM REFLECTIONS ON THE NATIONAL HEALTH SERVICE (Nuffield Provincial Hospitals Trust, Burgess and Son Ltd., London, U.K.) (1971).
119. Acton, J., *Measuring the Monetary Value of Lifesaving Programs*, in EMERGENCY MEDICAL SERVICES: RESEARCH METHODOLOGY (Dept. of Health, Education, and Welfare Publication (PHS) 78-3195) (National Center for Health Services Research, Rockville, Md.) (1978).
120. M. W. JONES-LEE, THE VALUE OF LIFE: AN ECONOMIC ANALYSIS (University of Chicago Press, Chicago, Ill.) (1976).
121. Fox, R. C., *Ethical and Existential Developments in Contemporaneous American Medicine: Their Implications for Culture and Society.* MILBANK MEMORIAL FUND QUARTERLY 52:445–83 (1974).
122. R. C. FOX, ESSAYS IN MEDICAL SOCIOLOGY: JOURNEYS INTO THE FIELDS (John Wiley & Sons, Inc., New York, N.Y.) (1979).

Health Care Technology and the Inevitability of Resource Allocation and Rationing Decisions, Part II

Roger W. Evans, Ph.D.

ALLOCATION AND RATIONING OF HEALTH CARE RESOURCES

Of all the resource-shortage crises this nation is expected to confront in the future, the problem of resource distribution is likely to be most acute and problematic in medicine.[23,29,123] Persons will be recognized as in need of, and then denied, benefits that the medical care provision system is capable of providing. Instead of an unidentified mass of persons being denied access to a needed resource, persons whose names have become known to the public will be declared ineligible for a treatment or service they are known to require.[124] Perhaps this scenario is inhumane, but it is undoubtedly a true representation of reality. As already noted, technology now permits to be saved the lives of persons who less than a decade ago would have surely died. Moreover, technology has made it exceedingly difficult to specify at precisely what point life ceases. This has prompted Crane[22] to conclude that both medicine and law are moving toward a "social interpretation" of life.

It should come as no surprise that the resources available to meet the demand for health care are limited.[125-130] Weinstein and Stason,[127] for example, have pointed out that decisions are already being made—physicians allocate their time, hospitals ration beds, fiscal intermediaries devise reimbursement policies—all of which suggest that priorities are being set. This is not to deny the recency of problems associated with resource constraints. Even a few decades ago, before the proliferation of medical technology and the pervasiveness of insurance, constraints on health care resources were largely unheard of. In the past, the distribution of health care resources has been accomplished by implicitly limiting their availability or, when available, restricting people's access to them.[131] Thus, the concepts of availability and accessibility are critical to the problem of resource distribution.[132,133] "Rationing" is the term often used to describe the process of differentially distributing resources. Rationing has become a value-laden term—one that implies that persons are likely to be treated unequally.[134] "Allocation" is another term often used to describe the unequal distribution of resources. While *Webster's New World Dictionary* defines rationing as "a fixed portion; share; allowance," allocation is to "set apart for a specific purpose, to distribute according to a plan."

As suggested by the definitions of rationing and allocation, there is merit in distinguishing between the allocation and the rationing of health care resources. Others have used the terms "macroallocation" and "microallocation" to make a similar distinction.[134,135] Regardless of the terms used, it should be recognized that allocation and rationing differ with regard to temporality and level. First, allocation decisions are likely to precede rationing decisions. Second, allocation is a concept that does not apply well at the level of the individual patient but rather is more appropriately applied at the aggregate or health care program level.

In a period when resources available for health care have become increasingly constrained, attention is directed toward making the provision of health care more efficient. For example, although much attention has recently focused on the enormous cost of the End-Stage Renal Disease Program, the question being addressed is not whether patients should have their Medicare benefits cut off but rather how treatment can be provided at less cost. (The total cost of the kidney program in fiscal year 1982 is expected to be $1.8 billion. Stated in other terms, patients with end-stage renal disease [ESRD], representing less than 0.25 percent of all Medicare part B beneficiaries, now account for more than 9 percent of total Medicare part B expenditures.[136]) Thus, the debate over which type of therapy (primarily home or in-center dialysis) is least costly is again being hotly debated.[137-147] At the same time, there is renewed interest in methods by which donor organ availability can be increased.[148-151] Recent hearings once again have indicated that home dialysis is probably less costly than in-center dialysis but that kidney transplantation is a greater bargain since the cost is not only lower in the long run, but the quality of life of renal transplant recipients is generally thought to be better than that of patients receiving dialysis.[152-155] Since there seems to be room for improving the provision of ESRD services, there is only minimal consideration being given to reduction or discontinuation of benefits that patients with renal disease currently receive. Thus, resources will continue to be allocated to the End-Stage Renal Disease Program, but, in the future, greater attention will focus on the "intraprogram" allocation of resources. It will be expected that the agency responsible for administering the program, the Health Care Financing Administration (HCFA), will write regulations that will maximize the use of those resources made available to the program; that is, the HCFA will be expected to promote the least costly treatment modalities by providing incentives for their adoption.[138]

Should the resources available for health care become increasingly constrained, the Department of Health and Human Services will be put in a position wherein "interprogram" allocation decisions will become necessary. These allocation decisions would concern how to distribute resources across health and, perhaps, social and other publicly financed programs. For example, a question might be raised as to whether the resources currently used to treat kidney disease might better be allocated to prevention activities or to a maternal and child health care program in which the derived benefits are likely to surpass those currently received by patients with ESRD.[55] In the future, competition for the available resources is likely to be great. The high cost of some new technologies might well make their widespread use prohibitive. Should this prove to be the case, it will then be necessary to consider the rationing of resources within health care programs.

Resources are rationed at the individual level, while allocation occurs at the aggregate level. Once it is apparent that all who are in need cannot be treated, the question then becomes one of which potential recipients are going to derive the greatest benefits. Again, this is precisely what occurred during the early years of dialysis, when there was substantial patient selection by physicians or committees. At that time, it was decided that although all patients with ESRD had a terminal condition, some had better prospects for treatment than others.[20,154] The preferred candidates were selected on the basis of a variety of criteria, for example, age, medical suitability, mental acuity, family involvement, criminal record, economic status (income, net worth), employment record, availability of transportation, willingness to cooperate in the treatment regimen, likelihood of vocational rehabilitation, psychiatric status, marital status, educational background, occupation, and future potential.[20,156-158] These criteria served as the basis on which scarce resources were rationed. Similar criteria currently are used to select potential heart transplant recipients and, thus, also serve as a rationing mechanism.[159-162] The decision to extend Medicare benefits to patients with ESRD resolved the rationing problem for the federal government. However, as noted by myself and associates,[20] the federal government "appears to have been more concerned with ridding itself of the moral dilemma of indirectly deciding who could live and who would die in a country of almost unlimited resources" than with simply trying to deal with the more general problem of costly medical care.

Now that the federal government is at least willing to entertain the possibility of differentially allocating resources to health care programs, it inevitably will also have to entertain the need to ration health care resources once interprogram allocation has occurred and the efficient use of available resources is maximized. Should resources be constrained further and no greater efficiency attained, it would become necessary to ration the available resources to certain persons based on some uniform set of guidelines.

The foregoing raises two important questions that have yet to be addressed: (1) On what basis will resource allocation decisions be made? (2) How are criteria for rationing likely to be developed?

ESTABLISHING CRITERIA FOR EXPLICIT RESOURCE ALLOCATION

In the medical literature, one increasingly finds medical procedures, practices, and technology subjected to what is commonly referred to as "cost-effectiveness and cost-benefit analysis."[51,126-130,163-167] Although the two are related, they are different approaches to the assessment of health practices and technology. Nevertheless, both cost-effectiveness analysis (CEA) and cost-benefit analysis (CBA) are presented as tools that can be used by the policymaker to make resource allocation decisions.

A CBA or a benefit-cost analysis requires that both costs and benefits be assigned monetary values.[168] Various methods have been proposed to measure the resource value of health care benefits. These include, for example, expected productivity loss based on discounted future earnings at the age of death or disability.[82,169,170] The benefit-cost framework thus converts decreased deaths and disability into increases in productivity and treats them as the indirect benefits of a health intervention. Thus, indirect benefits are then combined with any direct savings in health resource consumption (the direct benefits) to yield a net value.

A CEA, unlike a CBA, does not require that both costs and benefits be assessed in monetary terms. Instead, the aim of a CEA is to measure benefits in nonmonetary terms using mortality, morbidity, or quality-adjusted life years. To this extent, a CEA preserves a sense of intangible health care benefits whereas a CBA typically notes these but fails to assess them.[168] A CEA is particularly useful for comparing alternative approaches with the treatment of a given medical condition. For example, in-center hemodialysis, home hemodialysis, continuous ambulatory peritoneal dialysis, and kidney transplantation all represent alternative approaches to the treatment of ESRD. A CEA allows one to compare these treatments to determine which provides the greatest benefits at the least cost.[170] Similarly, heart transplantation might be compared with its alternative—traditional medical and surgical management—as approaches to the treatment of end-stage cardiac disease (ESCD).[76] Finally, percutaneous transluminal coronary angioplasty might be compared with coronary artery bypass surgery as alternative approaches to the treatment of atherosclerosis.[171,172] In all these instances, the goal of a CEA is the same—to determine which treatment approach to a given condition yields the greatest benefits at the least cost.

Both CEA and CBA can be applied on a larger scale than described herein. This application is critical to both intraprogram and interprogram allocation decisions. A CEA can be used to compare the benefits derived from various health care programs to determine which program (not specific treatment approach) yields the greatest benefit at the least cost, provided the benefits of each program being compared are expressed in the same terms (M. C. Weinstein, PH.D., written communication, April 14, 1982). For example, kidney dialysis can be compared with heart transplantation to see which has the greatest benefits, with benefits expressed in terms of mortality, morbidity, or quality-adjusted life years. Weinstein describes this process as follows:

> The comparison of cost-effectiveness ratios serves as a basis for allocating resources if the objective is to maximize health benefits. Thus, if kidney dialysis has a cost-effectiveness ratio (relative to the next best alternative for ESRD) of $60,000 per quality-adjusted life year, and cardiac transplant has a cost-effectiveness ratio (relative to the next best alternative for ESCD) of $50,000 per quality-adjusted life year, then resources should be allocated to the latter ahead of the former.

In this case, the proposed interprogram analysis strictly applies to health care programs. Another pertinent example might be to compare the cost of a potential maternal and child health program with the End-Stage Renal Disease Program or a potential ESCD program.

If the goal of the interprogram analysis is to compare the expenditure of health care resources with other socially desirable uses of resources, such as a public assistance program, a cost-benefit analysis is appropriate. Within the CBA framework, all expenditures and benefits are converted to monetary terms, which permits direct comparisons to be made among various diverse programs. The results of such an analysis may indicate that resources should be reallocated from social and other publicly financed programs to support health programs and vice versa. The problem with the CBA framework, however, is the requirement that human lives and quality of life be valued in dollars.[117,127]

Ultimately, the major objective of an interprogram analysis that involves only health programs or health and other publicly financed programs is to ensure that those programs that produce the greatest benefit will be those that receive the greatest support from the federal government. In this regard, it is apparent that, given limited resources and a need to allocate them in the most effective manner possible, a CEA or a CBA allows programs to be ranked according to their effectiveness or benefits derived or both. Weinstein and Stason[127] have summarized how this is done in the case of CEA as follows:

> Alternative programs or services are then ranked from the lowest value of the cost-effectiveness ratio to the highest, and selected from the top until available resources are exhausted. The point on the priority list at which the available resources are exhausted, or at which society is no longer willing to pay the price for the benefits achieved, becomes society's cut-off level of permissible cost per unit effectiveness. Application of this procedure ensures that the maximum health benefit is realized, subject to whatever resource constraint is in effect.

Thus, it is now possible to see that the allocation of health care resources and resources available to other programs as well can be subjected to a formalized set of procedures. By requiring that all assumptions are clearly stated, it is possible to perform the necessary quantitative analyses required to make the appropriate allocation decisions. In those areas where the data are least secure, it is possible to undertake sensitivity analyses to explore further the impact of decisions under differing assumptions.

Table 7 summarizes which type of analysis can be applied to various allocation decisions. If possible to achieve, a CEA should be the method of choice. In only one instance is it likely that a CEA would be inappropriate. This is in the case wherein an interprogram analysis is required to compare health program expenditures and benefits with non-health-related program expenditures and benefits. In this case, it would be necessary to express in monetary terms the benefits derived from the program. If an intraprogram allocation decision is required, a CEA should always be the method of choice, while, in principle, both a CBA and CEA could be applied to making an interprogram health allocation decision.

ESTABLISHING CRITERIA FOR EXPLICIT RATIONING

The resource rationing problem is different from the resource allocation problem. Although, in many respects, allocation decisions set the parameters and constraints within which rationing occurs, it is somewhat more difficult to submit the rationing process to a formalized set of procedures. The literature on clinical decision making, although not solely intended to be a framework for rationing, does provide an excellent framework with which to view rationing.

Once resources have been allocated to programs, and should these not be sufficient to meet the demand of all in need, clinicians are left with the problem of deciding which patients to treat.[173-176] The problems that were faced in the early days of kidney dialysis already have been described, pointing to obvious problems with any system that basically discriminates among people in the distribution of health care resources.[177,178] According to many, all people have a "right to health care" and, in a country as wealthy as the United States, no one should go untreated.[179-185] Yet, people often fail to recognize that with every right there also is an obligation.[186,187] People have a responsibility, an obligation as it were, to care for themselves in a manner that will maximally ensure good health (e.g., eat a good diet and exercise daily). Unfortunately, a vast majority of the population fails to fulfill its end of the "social contract" and chooses to engage in practices and behavior that are known to be detrimental to their health (e.g., excessive smoking, drinking, eating, and failure to exercise). Therefore, it could be argued

Table 7: Applying Cost-Effectiveness and Cost-Benefit Analysis to Program Allocation Decisions

Type of Decision Required	Cost-Effectiveness Analysis (CEA)	Cost-Benefit Analysis (CBA)	Method of Choice
Intraprogram allocation decision	Yes	Yes	CEA
Interprogram health allocation decision	Yes	Yes	CEA
Interprogram health vs. other publicly financed program allocation decision	No	Yes	CBA

that if everyone has a right to health care, then appropriate contracts should be drawn up to ensure that everyone keeps their end of the bargain.[186] This, of course, would require regulatory reform and strict enforcement, something that would be difficult and costly to undertake. Ultimately, however, the limits of the broad humanistic concept of a right to health care must be recognized. Within the context of rationing, those persons who have done the most to preserve their health could conceivably be the first to benefit from the available resources.[187,188]

The problem grows in complexity when it is recognized that the final decision concerning the rationing of resources will be the shared responsibility of the clinician or medical team, the patient, and any other representative of the patient (e.g., family or nearest of kin).[189] It is unlikely that explicit exclusion criteria will be developed that are equally palatable to all involved.[190,191] Thus, any criteria for rationing would be interpreted and practiced by individual clinicians.[192-194] This is consistent with the concept of the "clinical mentality" advanced by Freidson,[195] which suggests that clinicians see each patient as a special case and treat each accordingly. Medical practice is typically occupied with the problems of individuals rather than of aggregates or statistical units. To impose a set of rationing criteria that must be strictly adhered to implies that patients need not be considered as unique individuals but rather as aggregates. This would, in fact, represent a radical restructuring of the process of rendering clinical judgment.[196]

In the final analysis, it is possible to establish some general guidelines on, perhaps, a condition-by-condition basis, to be applied to decide whether a patient should be treated.[197] The problem, however, is that all cases will have to be reviewed individually, with explicit attention given to the manner in which each patient deviates from the guidelines. These decisions are likely to be made when any of the following conditions are met: (1) the treatment is determined to be futile, (2) the patient declines treatment, (3) the quality of the patient's life is unacceptable, or (4) the cost of providing care is too great.[197,198] In evaluating each case, what people decide to do will be subject to considerable variability. What is presented as a formal policy may be informally practiced in a variety of ways. Policy and practice can differ remarkably.

As described here, rationing is the process by which criteria are applied to selectively discriminate among patients who are eligible for resources that have been previously allocated to various programs. Rationing criteria, although conceivably developed at the aggregate level, are likely to be interpreted and implemented at the individual level. Thus, there are two major problems associated with rationing. These are (1) the development of acceptable criteria for withholding treatment on a condition-by-condition basis and (2) identifying that person or those persons who should make the decision not to treat.

Childress,[134] in his discussion of rationing, has distinguished between what he refers to as "rules of exclusion" and "rules of final selection." The first set of rules establishes the pool from which the final selections are made. The final selections are then based on the rules of final selection. Childress[134] provides the following advice: "The best approach to determining the pool for final selection is to forget that the resource is limited and to exclude only those patients whose medical and psychological condition would certainly prevent successful treatment." The rules for final selection, however, are more controversial. Major alternatives include social worth criteria or some form of chance (e.g., randomization, lottery, or "first come, first treated"). Rescher,[123] pursuing this same line of thought, has suggested that there are two biomedical and three social factors relevant to final selection. Relative likelihood of successful treatment and life expectancy are the relevant biomedical factors, while the social factors include family role, potential future contributions, and past services. All of these criteria are difficult to quantify and evaluate.

At this point, it is again important to reiterate that the most critical decisions that must be confronted today are those involving the allocation of resources across health care programs.[117] Once these decisions have been made, it will then become important to consider whether rationing will be necessary and what form it will take. It is precisely at this point that the nature and requirements of clinical decision making will become increasingly subjected to public and professional scrutiny.[198-200] Furthermore, it is at this point that patients and their next of kin will become increasingly involved in the decision-making process, and quantity and quality of life trade-offs will become important.[74,201-203] The decision-making process is well described in the literature.[21,22,128,198,204-211]

RESOURCE ALLOCATION IN PERSPECTIVE

Most discussions of resource allocation and rationing are narrowly focused and lack perspective. Attention is often directed to how health care resources are spent and not how a reallocation of resources from other government programs, such as defense and other publicly financed programs, might produce considerable gains in the health status of the population. Take, for example, the controversy that currently surrounds the End-Stage Renal Disease Program. This program is obviously costly, and the benefits derived by many patients have been reported to be few.[20,212] Policymakers now question whether this program will be allowed to continue in its current form.[20,143]

Unfortunately, excessive attention has probably focused on the kidney program. The problems associated with providing medical care to patients with ESRD is only symptomatic of a more widespread problem—health care costs continue to escalate as a larger number of people increasingly benefit from new and expensive health care technology. However, it must be recognized that other health and social programs are equally costly. For example, in 1981, an estimated 100,000 to 125,000 Americans underwent coronary artery bypass surgery, first performed in 1968, and the numbers continue to rise.[213] Yet those who have the surgery amount to only 0.04 percent of the nation's population. At $2.0 billion per year (a conservative estimate according to Randal), coronary artery bypass surgery accounts for about 1.0 percent of the total annual U.S. health bill.[214,215] The growth in the number of coronary artery bypass procedures performed each year has been substantial. In 1973, it was estimated that 38,000 such procedures were carried out in the United States at a cost in excess of $400 million.[55] Collectively, coronary artery bypass surgery is the most costly operation performed in this country and has boosted private health insurance premiums for the population as a whole.[213]

Interestingly, for most patients, the efficacy of coronary artery bypass surgery is questionable.[56,214-221] There is evidence that the procedure is effective in prolonging the life of patients who suffer from a major blockage of the main trunk of the left coronary artery, but evidence of the efficacy of the procedure on patients with "three-vessel disease" or in whom all three arteries are blocked is less clear. These patients presumably make up 30 percent to 40 percent of the total. Moreover, the rate of return to work among patients who have coronary artery bypass surgery is not impressive.[216,222-227]

The costs associated with neonatal intensive care are also high and are comparable with the costs of ESRD and coronary artery bypass surgery. A recent case study on the costs and effectiveness of neonatal intensive care estimates that the average expenditures per patient in 1978 were about $8,000, with costs for some patients well over $40,000.[228] Since there are no national data on the volume of neonatal intensive care being provided in the United States, only rough estimates can be produced, based on studies with small sample sizes and varying definitions of levels of care. Burdetti and associates provide the following estimates of neonatal intensive care supply and use:

1. Neonatal intensive care unit admissions—6 percent of all live births go to intensive care, accounting for 200,000 admissions each year.
2. Estimated average length of stay—eight to eighteen days per patient.
3. Number of hospitals with neonatal intensive care units—600.
4. Number of intensive care beds—7,500.
5. Total cost of neonatal intensive care—$1.5 billion each year.

Thus, based on the foregoing, questions being asked about the treatment of patients with ESRD could also be asked of coronary artery bypass surgery and neonatal intensive care. Since Medicare finances only a small percentage of these procedures and services (perhaps 20.0 percent nationwide in the case of coronary artery bypass surgery, with Medicaid paying for another 5.0 percent), the amount of publicity they have attracted remains small. In the case of coronary artery bypass procedures, the majority of patients rely on third-party payers, but, even so, their out-of-pocket expenses may equal 20 percent of the total bill.[213]

To provide even greater perspective for this discussion, the current level of defense spending as well as expenditures associated with the federal corrections system should be examined. It is well recognized that the resources devoted to national defense dwarf those available to health and social programs.[229] It is less well recognized, however, that it now costs as much per year to support a convicted felon in the federal correctional system as it does to keep a person alive on home hemodialysis. It seems a paradox that producing and maintaining the means to destroy life and warehousing in correctional facilities people who have outright taken the lives of others continues to absorb enormous resources that might justifiably be used otherwise. Why is it that when health care programs are criticized as being too costly, no attempt is made to put this in perspective by looking at other, less desirable uses of resources?

Table 8 gives budget authority and Table 9 budget outlays as provided in the fiscal year 1983 budget of the U.S. government.[230] National defense expenditures are more than twice those available for government-financed health care programs. The size of the budget for the administration of justice is minuscule when compared with either the budgets for national defense or health; yet, when one examines that portion of the justice budget devoted to corrections, it is not inconsequential, considering how the resources are used. In 1978, the average daily population in federal correctional facilities peaked at 29,347. Today, the average daily population has dropped to approximately 27,000. The cost per person per year (fiscal year 1981) for supporting persons convicted of violating federal laws as well as persons charged with crimes and detained for trial or sentencing is approximately $13,000 ($352 million per year for 27,000 persons). Yet, as the prison population is declining, inflation is driving up the costs of operations to a point where outlays for operating correctional facilities are expected to be about $367 million in 1982 and $386 million in 1983.

Iglehart[7] has recently summarized the proposed budget (fiscal year 1983) for major federal departments and agencies. Figures for defense and military functions and those for health and human services are given in Table 10. In reviewing the total budget, Iglehart concluded that, insofar as research and development funds are concerned, "research in physics, engineering, and other fields with potential military and industrial applications fared considerably better than did medical research."

For fiscal year 1984, the Reagan administration has requested a National Institutes of Health (NIH) budget of $4.1 billion, representing an increase of $73 million, or 1.8 percent over last year's proposal. Once the projected 4.9 percent inflation rate for 1983 is considered, however, the NIH will end up losing this modest gain in terms of real dollars.

Not suprisingly, the Department of Defense (DOD) is expected to fare well in 1984. Since his election, President Reagan has increased annual outlays for the DOD by 33 percent, with plans to increase the DOD budget by another 14 percent in 1984. As of this date, the administration has requested $274 billion for the DOD, with some congressmen indicating that this figure will be reduced by at least $15 billion. Overall, despite pending cuts in the DOD budget, it is still expected to increase by 30.0 percent, reaching a total of $29 billion, or 65 percent of the total U.S. budget for research and development.

In the final analysis, it is apparent that resources directed to health care programs and health-related activities are not excessive when compared with other publicly financed programs of somewhat dubious value.[12] At the same time, it is evident that some health care programs have been unjustly criticized when it is recognized that other medical procedures are equally as costly as those currently receiving careful scrutiny, such as the End-Stage Renal Disease Program. Thus, the following conclusion is unequivocal—resource allocation decisions must be viewed in perspective.

FACING THE INEVITABLE—DEATH AND DYING

As described previously, numerous ethical issues surround the allocation and rationing of health care resources. When not all will benefit, the dilemma becomes one of choosing who will. The ethical problems

Table 8: Budget Authority by Function

Function (Budget Code)	Actual, in Billion Dollars, 1981	Estimates, in Billion Dollars					
		1982	1983	1984	1985	1986	1987
National defense (050)	182.4	218.9	263.0	291.0	338.0	374.9	408.4
Health (550)	68.9	79.2	77.8	81.4	93.6	115.7	128.3
Administration of justice (750)	4.3	4.3	4.5	4.6	4.5	4.6	4.6

Table 9: Budget Outlays by Function

Function (Budget Code)	Actual, in Billion Dollars, 1981	Estimates, in Billion Dollars					
		1982	1983	1984	1985	1986	1987
National defense (050)	159.8	187.5	221.1	253.0	292.1	331.7	364.2
Health (550)	66.0	73.4	78.1	84.9	93.5	102.4	111.9
Administration of justice (750)	4.7	4.5	4.6	4.6	4.5	4.5	4.6

Table 10: Conduct of Research and Development in Defense and Health*

Department or Agency	Obligations, in Billion Dollars			Outlays, in Billion Dollars		
	1981	1982	1983	1981	1982	1983
Defense and military functions	16.5	20.6	24.5	15.7	18.8	22.7
Health and human services	4.0	4.0	4.1	4.0	3.9	4.0

*Data from Inglehart.[7]

inherent in CBA and CEA are by no means resolved.[19,231] It is apparent, however, that should these procedures be applied to resource allocation decisions, this society will become acutely aware of mortality.[232-237]

Historically, within this society, there is a preoccupation with health, almost to the point where death is observed as the ultimate of all evil. Major social surveys of the population have continuously shown that health is highly valued.[238] Interestingly, however, it has become increasingly difficult to define the parameters of health. Even a person's need and ability to interact with others has been designated as "social health."[239-241] Perhaps this is because of the fact that the most commonly accepted definition of health is that provided in the Constitution of the World Health Organization,[242] which states that "health is a state of complete physical, mental, and social well-being and not merely the absence of disease or infirmity." Consequently, at least three types of health are found in the literature—physical health, mental health, and social health. It is now difficult to determine what is and what is not health.

Preoccupation with health is obviously an unacknowledged preoccupation with death and, perhaps, the process of dying. While many people fear death, the overriding concern is with dying, that is, the process by which death comes about. For the most part, this society seems to be fully committed to the preservation of life at all costs, despite the quality of life the afflicted is likely to lead. It has only been in recent years that clinicians and the public have been willing to straightforwardly acknowledge and verbalize their concern with what might be called the "quantity versus quality of life trade-off."[21,22,128,156,164,173,201-203,210,243] Accompanying this, of course, have been open discussions of the value of human life.[78,81,83,244-251] The uncertainty of what follows death has led many to eschew death in favor of living, regardless of the quality of their existence. Recent studies, however, show that persons, when faced with the prospect of a long-term chronic illness, are at least willing to consider the prospects of a shorter but higher quality of life.[128,201,202]

This in itself suggests that people have come to grips with the notion of death. Nevertheless, widely held religious beliefs and convictions would suggest that a large proportion of the population is unwilling to entertain the possibility of voluntary euthanasia or passive suicide as solutions to prolonged suffering.[235] Some religious groups would, in fact, consider life with catastrophic long-term illness an act of God and the illness a test of their religious conviction. In fact, they may believe that illness enhances their ability to demonstrate their religious faith to others in a testimonial fashion.

Over the years, technology has evolved to a point where the determination of death is increasingly problematic.[252-261] In fact, the new understanding of death is largely a consequence of technological advances in life-support systems. The President's Commission has now grappled with the problem of translating the current physiological understanding of death into acceptable statutory language. The Commission was also interested "in the dispute between 'whole brain' and 'higher brain' formulations of death and appraising currently used brain-based tests for death, which have become increasingly varied and sophisticated."[257] A set of guidelines has been established for the determination of death, but these are not accepted by all.[254,255,257]

Thus, the ability of technology to stave off premature death through a variety of means makes it increasingly likely that this society will be unable to fully come to grips with death in a manner that facilitates the withholding of treatment when the expected outcomes are negligible or counterindicative to the well-being of the patient and his or her next of kin. Surprisingly, however, there is considerable interest in hospice care in the United States, which, in effect, suggests that a decision to discontinue vigorous treatment is acceptable.[262-264] As described by Saunders,[262] "The hospice movement sets out to ensure that every person who can no longer benefit from the increasing complexity of the general hospital will have the support he and his family need. The whole family is the unit of care and should also be seen as part of the caring team." By most standards, the hospice concept is not a new innovation; it dates back to as early as 1893, when St Luke's Hospital was established in London.

Perhaps unfortunately, it is rarely the case that the similarity between hospice care and the voluntary withholding of treatment is recognized.[198] The parallel is close, yet it is currently argued that patients, under all circumstances, should receive every extraordinary means of care available to prolong life. Only when society is fully able to come to grips with death and dying is it likely that "policies and procedures for decisions not to treat" not only will be formulated but will also be followed. This period is likely to be hastened as financial constraints force the issue. Putting this in perspective, Manning[236] has stated:

> Somewhere along the way, consciously or unconsciously, explicitly or implicitly, society will have to make some basic decisions about the allocation of economic resources as between human beings of advanced years and those who are younger. . . . We have not begun to consider the violent social dislocation that would be brought about if a large fraction of the population were to be kept alive for significantly longer periods of time.

As noted previously, the problems that must be addressed are essentially ethical or, perhaps, ethical-legal.[189] New medical technology has not only dramatically changed the practice of medicine, but it has also raised a variety of issues with which clinicians are rather uncomfortable. The problem, however, is that these issues are relatively new and must be worked through carefully. Many of the issues surrounding the allocation and rationing of resources are almost metaphysical in nature. There is no clearcut solution to the problems they instill for society. Ethics are relative to time, place, and, perhaps most importantly, culture. The anthropologist Ruth Benedict,[265] in describing the "cultural relativist" perspective on culture, made a profound observation. She stated:

> No man ever looks at the world with pristine eyes. He sees it edited by a definite set of customs and institutions and ways of thinking. Even in his philosophical probings he cannot go behind these stereotypes; his very concepts of the true and the false will still have reference to his particular traditional customs.

The cultural relativist perspective nicely summarizes the problems inherent in making resource allocation and rationing decisions. Even though based on explicit and hopefully rational criteria, any plan that is eventually adopted is certainly debatable from the perspectives of others. To adopt a set of criteria is to make a decision about limiting treatment. On the other hand, to treat all patients with a given disorder or within a given disease category, regardless of derived benefits, necessarily implies the withholding of treatment from patients with other disorders. The question is truly one of priorities. Data can be used to set priorities, but human judgment must be exercised to determine which priorities will hold.

The future is likely to be interesting. The conscious development of explicit allocation criteria, as a first step in the direction of wisely using limited resources, will be controversial. Questions must be raised as to how resources will be allocated not only to health programs but social programs as well. There are certainly many patients with diseases and esoteric medical conditions who could benefit from additional resource allocations. In 1972, it was decided that patients with ESRD would be eligible for Medicare benefits, yet there were and are many other patients with diseases and conditions who could have sustained the prolonged attention of government agencies.

Allocation issues will obviously be submitted to a complex sociopolitical decision-making process. Decisions can be made on the basis of allocation tools such as CEA or CBA, or a grim political battle could be waged between different lobbying groups, each representing the special interests of patients with specific diseases or conditions. In either case, the first decision will be as to which patient groups will receive support (i.e., the resource allocation decision); then, as resources continue to dwindle, allocations will be made within programs and decisions will be made as to how clinicians *might* ration the limited resources made available to them. Increasingly, it is apparent that this scenario approximates the situation of the kidney disease program today. As already noted, people at all levels of government are concerned about the amount spent on the kidney program and are looking for ways to stretch what seem to be increasingly finite resources. In this regard, it could be stated that the "battle" has just begun and that the "war" is yet to be fought.

While the dilemmas created by resource allocation and rationing decisions are undeniable, it would seem that they have and will continue to provide an impetus for a reconsideration of the meaning of death and the essence of life. Reasonably acceptable criteria have been established for the determination of death, yet the very essence of life continues to be elusive. People do seem to be on the verge of seriously valuing their lives, not only in terms of longevity but in terms of quality.[117,201,202]

Although Condorset envisioned that a "period must one day arrive when death will be nothing more than the effect either of extraordinary accidents, or the slow gradual decay of vital powers; and that the duration of the interval between the birth of man and his decay will have no assignable limit," Choron[232] has aptly pointed out that "the postponement of death is not a solution to the problem of the fear of death. ... There still will remain the fear of dying prematurely."

In his treatise on death, Ernst Becker[234] shows that the fear of death is universal and that this fear "haunts the human animal like nothing else; it is a mainspring of human activity—activity designed largely to avoid the fatality of death, to overcome it by denying in some way that it is the final destiny of man." He argues that far too much effort is put into establishing immortality, in his words, into establishing a "formula for triumphing over life's limitations." People have failed to take life and its limitations seriously. He concludes his discourse, as follows, with a challenge for those who have used science to define the very essence of life.[234]

> The problem with all the scientific manipulators is that somehow they don't take life seriously enough; in this sense, all science is "bourgeois," an affair of bureaucrats. I think that taking life seriously means something such as this: that whatever man does on this planet has to be done in the lived truth of the terror of creation, of the grotesque, of the rumble of panic underneath everything. Otherwise it is false. Whatever is achieved must be achieved from within the subjective energies of creatures, without

deadening, with the full exercise of passion, of vision, of pain, of fear, and of sorrow. How do we know that our part of the meaning of the universe might not be a rhythm in sorrow?

Had Becker devoted his attention to an analysis of the full implications of life-prolonging, advanced biomedical technology, it is difficult to speculate what he would have concluded. It is likely, however, that he would have concluded that western society has become too infatuated with the fear of death and has failed to realize the true essence and value of life, despite its length.

COMMENT

I attempted to put modern technology into perspective by noting that technological innovation is in response to the demand created by the increased life expectancy and changing age distribution of the population and the increased prevalence of chronic disease and its concomitant disability. Increasingly, it is recognized that sophisticated medical technology, however, is not without its price. In recent years, it has been argued that technology has been a major contributor to rising health care costs in this country. Whether technology will continue to be viewed as the culprit behind rising health care costs is yet to be seen.

Efforts are now being made to control technology by a more thorough, comprehensive, and ongoing assessment of new, emerging, and existing technological innovations.[51,266-274] In this regard, Relman[90,275] has correctly argued that one effective method of moderating the cost of medical care, while improving its quality, is to initiate "a major new national program of support for the evaluation of medical procedures of all kinds." From his perspective, it is the cost of ignorance associated with medical technology that is too great, not medical progress. In Relman's words, "The cost culprit is not technology per se, but only technology that is ineffective, superfluous, or unsafe."[257,276] In short, the goal of technological assessment should not be to curb the development of technologies but rather to provide the means for an unbiased evaluation of new technology before it becomes too widely diffused in practice. To meet this goal, Bunker and associates[10,11] have proposed the establishment of a private, nonprofit corporation for the collection, analysis, and dissemination of data on medical procedures and for the support of new clinical trials. The Institute for Health Care Evaluation, as they refer to it, would be intended to fill partially the void created by the abolition of the ill-fated National Center for Health Care Technology.[277] This Institute would have neither policy-making nor regulatory functions. At the present time, the HCFA has taken on an increasingly visible role in the assessment and regulation of new health care technology.[278] This role is evidenced by two generic types of policy decisions that the HCFA must make, namely, (1) coverage decisions—whether an item or service is one for which the program can pay—and (2) reimbursement decisions—how much is appropriate to pay for a covered item or service.

Despite Bunker's proposal for an Institute for Health Care Evaluation and the remarkable and noteworthy efforts of the Office of Technology Assessment, the foregoing discussion concludes that technological assessment, although likely to increase the efficiency of the health care provision system, will not be sufficient to wholly resolve impending budget constraints proposed by the Reagan administration. There are, indeed, limitations on the resources that can be allocated to health care programs, although some reallocation decisions would serve to stave off the inevitable. In preparation for the inevitable, plans must be made and techniques developed for the effective allocation and rationing of health care resources. Various suggestions have been offered as to how cost-effectiveness and cost-benefit analytic techniques can be applied to the making of intraprogram and interprogram *allocation* decisions. Clinical decision analysis, although imperfect, is offered as a possible approach to dealing with the resource *rationing* dilemma.

The increasingly apparent need to allocate and ration health care resources has led to a careful scrutiny of medical care costs. Health economists continue to point out that health care costs are almost out of control and that a major solution to this problem is to make the current service provision system more efficient through various competitive strategies, despite the fact that recent reports indicate that competition can have a negative impact on the quality of care patients receive.[279] Taking a differing viewpoint, other commentators have correctly pointed out that the health care industry, employing approximately 4.3 million workers, is the second largest industry in the United States and that reductions in health care through competition or other strategies would serve to displace a large number of persons in this industry.[280] The effect would be dramatic as displaced health care workers "would either displace others from their jobs or go on the welfare rolls. Either way one looks at it, a shrinkage of the health-care industry would create a ripple effect throughout our economy.[280] This has led Kolff to suggest that efforts to control health care costs through careful technology assessment "totally neglects the notion that we should move towards a service oriented economy instead of towards an industrial production directed economy" (W. J. Kolff, M.D., Ph.D, written communication, February 22, 1983). He asks, "What are we to do with our unemployed? Unless we expand our 'services,' there is no solution."

The causes and cure of medical cost inflation are only partially understood and, thus, remain debatable. Jellinek and others,[280-283] however, believe that there are factors other than the "delivery of health care or the marketing of illness" that have led to increased spending in the health care sector. Jellinek[281] believes that the continued rise in health care expenditures is a result of increased alienation and depersonalization associated with post-World War II society. The response of society is to compensate by aggressive attention to the individual when he or she becomes ill. Jellinek[281] summarizes his position as follows:

> Societal willingness to support extraordinarily expensive new medical technology and advanced training, which implicitly communicates a willingness to place a high value on individual human life in contrast to the low value implied by industrial depersonalization, may represent one important form of adjustment of the social contract. The increase in society's expenditures for medical care may constitute a stabilizing force necessary to counter the destabilizing impulses generated by continued economic development.

In the final analysis, however, perhaps Jellinek's[281] assessment of the problem does not go far enough. For example, it seems almost a paradox that defense spending goes unchecked while, at the same time, massive cuts have been made in public health care assistance programs as well as health care research efforts. While public fund-raising efforts may produce the required resources to enable a young child to receive a liver transplant or a middle-aged person to obtain a heart transplant, to date, there remains relatively little public debate over the merits of increased defense expenditures, which obviously pale current health care expenditures.

Unfortunately, the lay public, nevertheless, seems to be either unaware of or has chosen to ignore the key ethical issues implied by resource allocation and rationing decisions. Perhaps not uncharacteristically, people remain willing to come to the aid of identifiable victims of resource scarcity, such as persons in need of organ transplants. At the same time, the lay public finds a special attraction in persons such as artificial heart recipient Barney Clark, who has been honored for "risking his life in order to save it." Thus, in the end, perhaps, the real concern with personal health in today's society is not so much the depersonalization and alienation that many persons feel but rather the fact that destructive forces of an unprecedented magnitude have served to completely threaten human existence.[284-286] Consequently, for many people, the true value of life becomes most apparent either when a person's life is at stake because he or she is denied medical care that is available but in short supply or when the type of medical care required is unavailable. Although often highly publicized by the mass media, each of the patients who fall into these categories serves to underscore the basic dilemma—health care resources are limited.

The inevitability of resource allocation and rationing decisions has been well characterized by Fuchs.[125] In his discussion of the problems of health and medical care, he notes that an economic approach to these is firmly rooted in three fundamental observations of the world. These are as follows: (1) resources are scarce in relation to human wants, (2) resources have alternative uses, and (3) people have different wants, with considerable variation in the relative importance they attach to them. Yet, the basic economic problem identified by Fuchs[125] is "how to allocate scarce resources so as to best satisfy human wants."

While Fuchs places a great deal of emphasis on the economics of resource allocation and provides only cursory attention to the social, ethical, and legal implications of allocation and rationing decisions, the fact is that without economic constraints, most allocation and rationing decisions would be unnecessary except in situations in which the needed resource, natural or otherwise, is severely limited. In instances of the latter, economic resources would not be sufficient to alleviate scarcity. The basic premise of this discussion, therefore, is that constraints on economic resources will necessitate resource-allocation and rationing decisions, which, in turn, will make the confrontation of various social, ethical, and legal issues inescapable. In the future, the major issues confronting not only medicine but this society as a whole will be the social, ethical, and legal implications of resource allocation and rationing, whether framed in terms of distributive justice,[287-292] discrimination against the poor and disadvantaged,[293] or the withholding of treatment from those with catastrophic illness.[197] All of these share a common underlying theme—the need to confront human finality and purposeful existence.[294]

As described herein, the problems associated with the allocation and rationing of scarce medical resources, economic (e.g., health care dollars) or natural (e.g., organs and tissue for transplantation) are, indeed, related to dying as an experience and death as an event. This discriminatory use of resources (and that is basically what allocation and rationing imply) has a lot to do with the fact that persons are eventually denied something they require—in this case, medical care. Schelling[124] underscores the essential ingredient of rationing decisions when he distinguishes between an "individual death/life" and a "statistical death/ life." The two are, in reality, different, and he provides the following example to illustrate his point:

Let a six year-old girl with brown hair need thousands of dollars for an operation that will prolong her life until Christmas, and the post office will be swamped with nickels and dimes to save her. But let it be reported that without a sales tax the hospital facilities of Massachusetts will deteriorate and cause a barely perceptible increase in preventable deaths—not many will drop a tear or reach for their checkbooks.

This distinction is an important one because it highlights the fact that the death of a person is a unique, often private event. Yet, at the local level, the victim and his or her family have an intense interest. In fact, as Schelling[124] notes, if society takes an interest in a local death, it is often because of a general concern that "reasonable efforts are made to conserve life than in whether those efforts succeed."

At this point in time, it is predictable that resource allocation decisions are unlikely to be carefully scrutinized by the public until resource rationing decisions become an inescapable fact of life. When the public is exposed to rationing decisions that it feels are contrary to the interest of the persons involved, despite catastrophic illness, it is likely to call into question the worthiness of allocation decisions. When it becomes apparent that these decisions are based on a mix of medical and social criteria, the latter which the public is much more likely to understand and despise as the basis for differentially valuing human life, the public will become increasingly irritated and resentful.

While selection criteria of any sort are likely to be viewed as unjust, it is a truism that not all people are likely to maximally or optimally benefit from available medical technology. For example, my associates and I[20] have shown how dramatically the extension of Medicare benefits to patients with ESRD affected the composition of the patient population. In particular, indicia of patient rehabilitation, such as employment status, show a decline in the overall status of the patient population.

In the future, decisions must be made concerning which patients will maximally and optimally benefit from expensive health care technology, yet a watchful person must focus on such decisions to ensure that "social worth" will not be the criterion of final determination. The problem, however, is that, in many respects, social and medical criteria are inextricably intertwined. People of low socioeconomic status are likely to be in poorer health with multiple disease conditions, which, in part, reflects poor nutritional habits, detrimental lifestyle, and the historical lack of resources to obtain proper health care. Consequently, if medical criteria were to be the basis on which rationing decisions are made, they might exclude the poor and disadvantaged because health and socioeconomic status are highly interdependent. For example, it is not unusual to find that of those persons with ESRD, those of lower socioeconomic status are likely to have multiple comorbid health conditions such as diabetes, hepatitis, and hypertension. Not only are these patients less desirable candidates for dialysis and transplantation, but they are among the more expensive patients to treat.

Without careful planning and evaluation, the cleavage between the haves and have-nots, as evidenced by formal selection criteria, is likely to become substantial. Those with the financial means may be able to purchase the services they require, while those who are disadvantaged and destitute will be denied care. Claims of a right to health care might well serve as a common goal to bind the disenfranchised.[186,295-302] Specific laws have been promulgated to protect the rights of certain classes of persons; examples include Section 504 of the Rehabilitation Act of 1973, the Age Discrimination Act, and Title VII of the Civil Rights Act. Each of these laws has important implications for resource rationing decisions.

It is highly probable that disclosure of the names, by the media, of persons who have been denied the benefits of medicine will set into motion complex sociopolitical manuevering to reprieve those who have reportedly been treated unjustly by those with authority to make and enforce resource-rationing decisions. Arguments that surround these decisions are likely to be similar to those made in connection with abortion and the withholding of medical treatment.[198-200,303-305] The Quinlin, Saikewicz, and Dinnerstein cases will frequently be cited as precedent setting. Analogies are likely to be made between current events and the events that took place in Nazi Germany. To this end, it will be argued that to set forth criteria that deny people treatment, in effect, represents a devaluation of life. As Carroll[306] has noted:

> Life has become increasingly cheap in our time. Today, Auschwitz and Dachau are museums; Coventry, Dresden, and Hiroshima, vague memories; the deaths several years ago of hundreds of thousands of Indonesians, a footnote to history; race riots in American cities, a subject of study; and war casualties in Vietnam, an object of routine reports.

Moreover, the practice of rationing will bring forth cries that the precedent is now set for the "floodgates to be opened" to the "mass slaughter" of persons whom rationing criteria declare to be of "marginal" value.

The point of the matter, however, is that rationing decisions are already being made.[127] The fact that they are not publicized has prevented them from becoming a social issue, despite the fact that they have attracted the attention of bioethicists.[21,22,307,308] Nevertheless, the future is likely to be filled with accounts of persons who have been refused treatment. Within a society that has failed to come to grips with the meaning of death and the essence of life, rationing decisions will seem unusually cruel. Yet, when these decisions are acknowledged as inescapable, this society, this culture, will be more prepared to deal with the one event that is truly inevitable—death.

REFERENCES

123. Rescher, N., *The Allocation of Exotic Medical Lifesaving Therapy*, ETHICS 79:173–86 (1969).
124. Schelling, T. C., *The Life You Save May Be Your Own*, in PROBLEMS IN PUBLIC EXPENDITURE ANALYSIS (S. B. Chase, Jr., ed.) (The Brookings Institution, Washington, D.C.) (1968) at 127–76.
125. V. R. FUCHS, WHO SHALL LIVE? HEALTH, ECONOMICS, AND SOCIAL CHOICE (Basic Books, New York, N.Y.) (1974).
126. M. C. WEINSTEIN, W. B. STASON, HYPERTENSION: A POLICY PERSPECTIVE (Harvard University Press, Cambridge, Mass.) (1976).
127. Weinstein, M. C., Stason, W. B., *Foundations of Cost-Effectiveness Analysis for Health and Medical Practices*, NEW ENGLAND JOURNAL OF MEDICINE 296:716–21 (1977).
128. M. C. WEINSTEIN, *et al.*, CLINICAL DECISION ANALYSIS (W. B. Saunders Co., Philadelphia, Pa.) (1980).
129. Stason, W. B., Weinstein, M. C., *Allocation of Resources to Manage Hypertension*, NEW ENGLAND JOURNAL OF MEDICINE 296:732–39 (1977).
130. Weinstein, M. C., *Estrogen Use in Postmenopausal Women—Costs, Risks and Benefits*, NEW ENGLAND JOURNAL OF MEDICINE 303:308–16 (1980).
131. Mechanic, D., *The Growth of Medical Technology and Bureaucracy: Implications for Medical Care*, MILBANK MEMORIAL FUND QUARTERLY 55:61–78 (1977).
132. D. MECHANIC, MEDICAL SOCIOLOGY (Free Press, New York, N.Y.) (2nd ed., 1978).
133. L.A. ADAY, R. ANDERSON, DEVELOPMENT OF INDICES OF ACCESS TO MEDICAL CARE (Health Administration Press, Ann Arbor, Mich.) (1975).
134. Childress, J. F., *Rationing of Medical Treatment*, in ENCYCLOPEDIA OF BIOMEDICAL ETHICS (W. T. Reich, ed.) (Oxford University Press, New York, N.Y.) (1979) at 1414–19.
135. J. F. BLUNSTEIN, CONSTITUTIONAL AND LEGAL CONSTRAINTS ON THE RATIONING OF MEDICAL RESOURCES (Prepared for the President's Commission for the Study of Ethical Problems in Medicine and Biomedical and Behavioral Research, Nashville, Tenn.) (October 1981).
136. David, C. K., *Hearings of the U.S. House of Representatives Committee on Governmental Operations, Subcommittee on Intergovernmental Relations and Human Resources*, CONTEMPORARY DIALYSIS 3:23–30 (April 1982).
137. Kusserow, R. P., *Hearings of the U.S. House of Representatives' Committee on*

Governmental Operations, Subcommittee on Intergovernmental Relations and Human Resources, CONTEMPORARY DIALYSIS 59:12–18 (1982).

138. Iglehart, J. K., *Health Policy Report: Funding the End-Stage Renal Disease Program*, NEW ENGLAND JOURNAL OF MEDICINE 306:492–96 (1982).

139. Relman, A. S., *The New Medical-Industrial Complex*, NEW ENGLAND JOURNAL OF MEDICINE 303:963–70 (1980).

140. Rettig, R. A., *The Politics of Health Cost Containment: End-Stage Renal Disease*, BULLETIN OF THE NEW YORK ACADEMY OF MEDICINE 56:115–38 (1980).

141. R. A. RETTIG, IMPLEMENTING THE END-STAGE RENAL DISEASE PROGRAM OF MEDICARE (Rand Publication 2505-HCFA/HEW) (Rand Corporation, Santa Monica, Calif.) (1980).

142. Kolata, G. B., *NMC Thrives Selling Dialysis*, SCIENCE 208:473–76 (1980).

143. Kolata, G. B., *Dialysis after Nearly a Decade*, SCIENCE 208:380–82 (1980).

144. Lowrie, E. G., Hampers, C. L., *The Success of Medicare's End-Stage Renal Disease Program: The Case for Profits and the Private Marketplace*, NEW ENGLAND JOURNAL OF MEDICINE 305:434–38 (1981).

145. Lowrie, E. G., Hampers, C. L., *Proprietary Dialysis and the End-Stage Renal Disease Program*, DIALYSIS AND TRANSPLANTATION 11:191–204 (1982).

146. Hampers, C. L., Hager, E. B., *The Delivery of Dialysis Services on a Nationwide Basis—Can We Afford the Nonprofit System?* DIALYSIS AND TRANSPLANTATION 8:417–23, 442 (1979).

147. Blagg, C. R., Cui bono? *A Response to Drs. Hampers and Hager*, DIALYSIS AND TRANSPLANTATION 8:501–02, 513 (1979).

148. Bart, K. J., Macon, E. J., Humphries, A. L., *A Response to the Shortage of Cadaveric Kidneys for Transplantation*, TRANSPLANTATION PROCEEDINGS 11:455–57 (1979).

149. Bart, K. J., *et al.*, *Increasing the Supply of Cadaveric Kidneys for Transplantation*, TRANSPLANTATION 31:383–87 (1981).

150. Bart, K. J., *et al.*, *Cadaveric Kidneys for Transplantation*, TRANSPLANTATION 31:379–82 (1981).

151. Steinbrook, R. L., *Kidneys for Transplantation*, JOURNAL OF HEALTH POLITICS, POLICY AND LAW 6:504–73 (1981).

152. Simmons, R. G., Schilling, K. J., *Social and Psychological Rehabilitation of the Diabetic Transplant Patient*, KIDNEY INTERNATIONAL SUPPLEMENT 6:S152–58 (1974).

153. R. G. SIMMONS, S. D. KLEIN, R. L. SIMMONS, THE GIFT OF LIFE: THE SOCIAL AND PSYCHOLOGICAL IMPACT OF ORGAN TRANSPLANTATION (John Wiley & Sons, Inc., New York, N.Y.) (1977).

154. Poznanski, E. O., *et al.*, *Quality of Life for Long-Term Survivors of End-Stage Renal Disease*, JOURNAL OF THE AMERICAN MEDICAL ASSOCIATION 239:2343–47 (1978).

155. Guttmann, R. D., *Renal Transplantation:II*, NEW ENGLAND JOURNAL OF MEDICINE 301:1038–48 (1979).

156. R. C. FOX, J. P. SWAZEY, THE COURAGE TO FAIL (University of Chicago Press, Chicago, Ill.) (1974).

157. Abram, H. S., *Dilemmas of Medical Progress,* PSYCHIATRIC MEDICINE 3:51–58 (1972).
158. A. H. KATZ, D. M. PROCTOR, SOCIAL-PSYCHOLOGICAL CHARACTERISTICS OF PATIENTS RECEIVING HEMODIALYSIS TREATMENT FOR CHRONIC RENAL FAILURE: REPORT OF A QUESTIONNAIRE STUDY OF DIALYSIS CENTERS DURING 1967 (The Kidney Disease Program, Division of Chronic Disease Programs, Regional Medical Programs Service, Health Services and Mental Health Administration, Public Health Service, Dept. of Health, Education, and Welfare) (1969).
159. Newman, H. N., *Health Care Financing Administration, Medicare Program: Solicitation of Hospitals and Medical Centers to Participate in a Study of Heart Transplants,* FEDERAL REGISTER 46:7072–75 (1981).
160. Pennock, J. L., *et al., Cardiac Transplantation in Perspective for the Future: Survival, Complications, Rehabilitation, and Cost,* JOURNAL OF THORACIC AND CARDIOVASCULAR SURGERY 83:168–77 (1982).
161. Copeland, J. G., *et al., Cardiac Transplantation, a Two-Year Experience,* HEALTH AND TRANSPLANTATION 1:67–71 (1981).
162. Oyer, P. E., *Cardiac Transplantation: 1980,* TRANSPLANTATION PROCEEDINGS 13:199–206 (1981).
163. OFFICE OF TECHNOLOGY ASSESSMENT, THE IMPLICATIONS OF COST-EFFECTIVENESS: ANALYSIS OF MEDICAL TECHNOLOGY (U.S. Government Printing Office, Washington, D.C.) (1980).
164. J. P. BUNKER, C. F. MOSTELLER, B. A. BARNES, COSTS, RISKS AND BENEFITS OF SURGERY (Oxford University Press, New York, N.Y.) (1977).
165. Fuchs, V. R., *What is CBA/CEA and Why Are They Doing This to Us?* NEW ENGLAND JOURNAL OF MEDICINE 303:937–38 (1980).
166. Lashof, J. C., *et al., The Role of Cost-Benefit and Cost-Effectiveness Analyses in Controlling Health Care Costs,* in CRITICAL ISSUES IN MEDICAL TECHNOLOGY (B. J. McNeil, E. G. Cravalho, eds.) (Auburn House, Boston, Mass.) (1982) at 185–89.
167. K. E. WARNER, B. R. LUCE, COST-BENEFIT AND COST-EFFECTIVENESS ANALYSIS IN HEALTH CARE: PRINCIPLES, PRACTICE, AND POTENTIAL (Health Administration Press, Ann Arbor, Mich.) (1982).
168. H. V. FINEBERG, L. A. PEARLMAN, THE IMPLICATIONS OF COST-EFFECTIVENESS ANALYSIS OF MEDICAL TECHNOLOGY: CASE STUDY #11: BENEFIT-AND-COST ANALYSIS OF MEDICAL INTERVENTIONS: THE CASE OF CIMETIDINE AND PEPTIC ULCER DISEASE, Stock OTA-BP-H-9(11) (Office of Technology Assessment) (1981).
169. Klarman, H. E., *Application of Cost-Benefit Analysis to the Health Services and the Special Case of Technologic Innovation,* INTERNATIONAL JOURNAL OF HEALTH SERVICES 4:325–52 (1974).
170. Evans, R. W., Garrison, L. P., Manninen, D., *The National Kidney Dialysis and Kidney Transplantation Study: Study Description, Statement of Objectives, and Project Significance,* CONTEMPORARY DIALYSIS 3:55–58 (June 1982).
171. Gruntzig, A. R., Senning, A., Siegenthaler, W. E., *Nonoperative Dilation of*

Coronary-Artery Stenosis: Percutaneous Transluminal Coronary Angioplasty, NEW ENGLAND JOURNAL OF MEDICINE 301:61–68 (1979).

172. Levy, R. I., Jesse, M. S., Mock, M. B., *Position on Percutaneous Transluminal Coronary Angioplasty (PTCA),* CIRCULATION 59:613 (1979).

173. Buck, R. W., *Prolonging Life in the Aged,* NEW ENGLAND JOURNAL OF MEDICINE 305:963 (1981).

174. Mazzarella, V., *An Open Letter to my Mother's Nephrologist,* NEW ENGLAND JOURNAL OF MEDICINE 305:175 (1981).

175. Parsons, V., Lock, P., *Triage and the Patient with Renal Failure,* JOURNAL OF MEDICAL ETHICS 6:173–76 (1980).

176. Basson, M. D., *Choosing Among Candidates for Scarce Medical Resources,* JOURNAL OF MEDICINE AND PHILOSOPHY 4:313–33 (1979).

177. Childress, J., *Who Shall Live When Not All Can Live?* SOUNDINGS 43:339–62 (1970).

178. Caplan, A. L., *Kidneys, Ethics, and Politics: Policy Lessons of the ESRD Experience,* JOURNAL OF HEALTH POLITICS, POLICY AND LAW 6:488–503 (1981).

179. Arrow, K. J., *Uncertainty and the Welfare Economics of Medical Care,* AMERICAN ECONOMIC REVIEW 53:941–73 (1963).

180. Mechanic, D., *The Right to Treatment: Judicial Action and Social Change,* in POLITICS, MEDICINE, AND SOCIAL SCIENCE (D. Mechanic, ed.) (Wiley Interscience, New York, N.Y.) (1974) at 227–48.

181. E. A. KRAUSE, POWER AND ILLNESS: THE POLITICAL SOCIOLOGY OF HEALTH AND MEDICAL CARE (Elsevier North-Holland, Inc., New York, N.Y.) (1977).

182. S. P. STRICKLAND, U.S. HEALTH CARE: WHAT'S WRONG AND WHAT'S RIGHT (Universe Books, New York, N.Y.) (1972).

183. H. E. KLARMAN, THE ECONOMICS OF HEALTH (Columbia University Press, New York, N.Y.) (1965).

184. Fried, C., *Equality and Rights in Medical Care,* HASTINGS CENTER REPORT 6:29–34 (1976).

185. Sidel, V., *The Right to Health Care: An International Perspective,* in BIOETHICS AND HUMAN RIGHTS (E. L. Bandman, B. Bandman, eds.) (Little Brown and Co., Boston, Mass.) (1978) at 341–49.

186. Bell, N. K., *The Scarcity of Medical Resources: Are There Rights to Health Care?* JOURNAL OF MEDICAL PHILOSOPHY 4:158–69 (1979).

187. Knowles, J. H., *Responsibility for Health,* SCIENCE 198:1103 (1977).

188. Allegrante, J. P., Green, L. W., *When Health Policy Becomes Victim Blaming,* NEW ENGLAND JOURNAL OF MEDICINE 305:528–29 (1981).

189. MORAL RESPONSIBILITY IN PROLONGING LIFE DECISIONS (D. G. McCarthy, A. S. Moraczewski, eds.) (Pope John XXIII Medical-Moral Research and Education Center, St. Louis, Mo.) (1981).

190. G. R. WINSLOW, TRIAGE AND JUSTICE (University of California Press, Berkeley, Calif.) (1982).

191. Brent, L., *Deciding Who Gets What,* LANCET 1:57 (1983).

192. WHO DECIDES? CONFLICTS OF RIGHTS IN HEALTH CARE (N. K. Bell, ed.) (Humana Press, Clifton, N.J.) (1982).

193. J. F. CHILDRESS, WHO SHOULD DECIDE? PATERNALISM IN HEALTH CARE (Oxford University Press, New York, N.Y.) (1982).

194. F. Harron, J. Burnside, T. Beauchamp, Health and Human Values: Making Your Own Decisions (Yale University Press, New Haven, Conn.) (1982).
195. E. Freidson, Profession of Medicine: A Study of the Sociology of Applied Knowledge (Harper & Row Publishers, Inc., New York, N.Y.) (1967).
196. A. R. Feinstein, Clinical Judgment (Williams & Wilkins Co., Baltimore, Md.) (1967).
197. Lo, B., Jonsen, A. R., *Clinical Decisions to Limit Treatment,* Annals of Internal Medicine 93:764–68 (1980).
198. C. B. Wong, J. P. Swazey, Dilemmas of Dying: Policies and Procedures for Decisions Not to Treat (G. K. Hall Medical Publishers, Boston, Mass.) (1981).
199. Relman, A. S., *The Saikewicz Decision: Judges as Physicians,* New England Journal of Medicine 298:508–09 (1978).
200. Barron, C. H., *Medical Paternalism and the Rule of Law,* American Journal of Law and Medicine 4:337–65 (1979).
201. McNeil, B. J., Weichselbaum, R., Pauker, S. G., *Speech and Survival: Tradeoff Between Quality and Quantity of Life in Laryngeal Cancer,* New England Journal of Medicine 305:982–87 (1981).
202. McNeil, B. J., Pauker, S. G., *Incorporation of Patient Values in Medical Decision Making,* in Critical Issues in Medical Technology (B. J. McNeil, E. G. Cravalho, eds.) (Auburn House, Boston, Mass.) (1982) at 113–26.
203. McNeil, B. J., *et al., On the Elicitation of Preferences for Alternative Therapies,* New England Journal of Medicine 306:1259–62 (1982).
204. H. Faiffa, Decision Analysis: Introductory Lectures on Choices Under Uncertainty (Addison-Wesley Publishing Co., Inc., Reading, Mass.) (1968).
205. R. L. Keeney, H. Raiffa, Decision Making with Multiple Objectives: Preferences and Value Tradeoffs (John Wiley & Sons, Inc., New York, N.Y.) (1976).
206. Brett, A. S., *Hidden Ethical Issues in Clinical Decision Analysis,* New England Journal of Medicine 305:1150–52 (1981).
207. Pauker, S. G., Kassirer, J. P., *The Threshold Approach to Clinical Decision Making,* New England Journal of Medicine 302:1109–17 (1980).
208. Schwartz, W. B., *Decision Analysis: A Look at the Chief Complaints,* New England Journal of Medicine 300:556–59 (1979).
209. Ransoff, D. F., Feinstein, A. R., *Is Decision Analysis Useful in Clincial Medicine?* Yale Journal of Biology and Medicine 49:165–68 (1976).
210. Reich, W. T., *Life: Quality of Life,* in Encyclopedia of Biomedical Ethics (W. T. Reich, ed.) (Oxford University Press, New York, N.Y.) (1979) at 829–40.
211. Eisenberg, J. M., *Sociologic Influences on Decision Making by Clinicians,* Annals of Internal Medicine 90:957–64 (1979).
212. Gutman, R. A., Stead, W. W., Robinson, R. R., *Physical Activity and Employment Status of Patients on Maintenance Dialysis,* New England Journal of Medicine 304:309–13 (1981).

213. Randal, J., *Coronary Artery Bypass Surgery,* HASTINGS CENTER REPORT 12:13–18 (1982).

214. Drunkman, W. B., *et al., Medical Perspectives in Coronary Artery Surgery: A Caveat,* ANNALS OF INTERNAL MEDICINE 81:817–37 (1974).

215. Stoney, W. S., *et al., The Cost of Coronary Bypass Procedures,* JOURNAL OF THE AMERICAN MEDICAL ASSOCIATION 240:2278–80 (1978).

216. Love, J. W., *Employment Status After Coronary Bypass Operations and Some Cost Considerations,* JOURNAL OF THORACIC AND CARDIOVASCULAR SURGERY 80:68–72 (1980).

217. Mundth, E. D., Austen, W. G., *Surgical Measures for Coronary Heart Disease, Part 1,* NEW ENGLAND JOURNAL OF MEDICINE 293:13–19 (1975).

218. *Editorial: Coronary Artery Bypass Surgery,* LANCET 1:841–42 (1976).

219. Kolata, G. B., *Coronary Bypass Surgery: Debate over its Benefits,* SCIENCE 194:1263–65 (1976).

220. Brauwald, E., *Coronary-Artery Surgery at the Crossroads,* NEW ENGLAND JOURNAL OF MEDICINE 297:661–63 (1977).

221. Sanz, G., *et al., Determinants of Prognosis in Survivors of Myocardial Infarction,* NEW ENGLAND JOURNAL OF MEDICINE 306:1065–70 (1982).

222. Hammermeister, K. E., *et al., Effect of Surgical Versus Medical Therapy on Return to Work in Patients with Coronary Artery Disease,* AMERICAN JOURNAL OF CARDIOLOGY 44:105–11 (1979).

223. Rimm, A. A., *et al., Changes in Occupation After Aortocoronary Vein-Bypass Operation,* JOURNAL OF THE AMERICAN MEDICAL ASSOCIATION 236:361–64 (1976).

224. Wallwork, J., Potter, B., Caves, P. K., *Return to Work After Coronary Artery Surgery for Angina,* BRITISH MEDICAL JOURNAL 2:1680–81 (1978).

225. Frick, M. H., Harjola, P. T., Valle, M., *Work Status After Coronary Bypass Surgery,* ACTA MEDICA SCANDINAVICA 206:61–64 (1979).

226. Barnes, G. K., *et al., Changes in Working Status of Patients Following Coronary Bypass Surgery,* JOURNAL OF THE AMERICAN MEDICAL ASSOCIATION 238:1259–62 (1977).

227. Blumlein, S. L., *et al., Changes in Occupation After Coronary Arteriography,* SCANDINAVIAN JOURNAL OF REHABILITATION MEDICINE 9:79–83 (1977).

228. P. BURDETTI, *et al.,* NEONATAL INTENSIVE CARE (U.S. Government Printing Office, Washington, D.C.) (1982).

229. Hiatt, H. H., *Sounding Board: The Physician and National Security,* NEW ENGLAND JOURNAL OF MEDICINE 307:1142–45 (1982).

230. OFFICE OF THE PRESIDENT, THE BUDGET OF THE UNITED STATES GOVERNMENT: FISCAL YEAR, 1983 (House Document 97–124) (U.S. Government Printing Office, Washington, D.C.) (1982).

231. Tancredi, L. R., Barsky, A. J., *Technology and Health Care Decision Making— Conceptualizing the Process for Societal Informed Consent,* MEDICAL CARE 12:845–58 (1974).

232. J. CHORON, DEATH AND MODERN MAN (Collier Bros., New York, N.Y.) (1964).

233. DEATH IN CONTEMPORARY AMERICA: NEW MEANINGS OF DEATH (H. Feifel, ed.) (McGraw-Hill Book Co., New York, N.Y.) (1977).

234. E. BECKER, THE DENIAL OF DEATH (Free Press, New York, N.Y.) (1973).
235. D.C. MAGUIRE, DEATH BY CHOICE (Schocken Books, Inc., New York, N.Y.) (1973).
236. Manning, B., *Legal and Policy Issues in the Allocation of Death,* in THE DYING PATIENT (O. G. Brim, Jr., *et al.,* eds.) (Russell Sage Foundation, New York, N.Y.) (1970) at 253–74.
237. R. M. VEATCH, DEATH, DYING, AND THE BIOLOGICAL REVOLUTION (Yale University Press, New Haven, Conn.) (1976).
238. A. CAMPBELL, P. E. CONVERSE, W. L. RODGERS, THE QUALITY OF AMERICAN LIFE (Russell Sage Foundation, New York, N.Y.) (1976).
239. C. A. DONALD, *et al.,* CONCEPTUALIZATION AND MEASUREMENT OF HEALTH FOR ADULTS IN THE HEALTH INSURANCE SURVEY: SOCIAL HEALTH (Publication R-1987/4-HEW) (Rand Corporation, Santa Monica, Calif.) (vol. 4, 1978).
240. Renne, K. S., *Measurement of Social Health in a General Population Survey,* SOCIAL SCIENCE RESEARCH 3:25–44 (1974).
241. Russell, R. D., *Social Health: An Attempt to Clarify this Dimension of Well-Being,* INTERNATIONAL JOURNAL OF HEALTH EDUCATION 74:74–82 (1973).
242. *Constitution of the World Health Organization,* in THE FIRST TEN YEARS OF THE WORLD HEALTH ORGANIZATION (Palais des Nations, World Health Organization, Geneva, Switzerland) (1958).
243. Sackett, D. L., Torrance, G. W., *The Utility of Different Health States as Perceived by the General Public,* JOURNAL OF CHRONIC DISEASES 31:697–704 (1978).
244. Dorfman, N. S., *The Social Value of Saving a Life,* in HEALTH: WHAT IS IT WORTH? MEASURES OF HEALTH BENEFITS (S. J. Mushkin, D. Dunlop, eds.) (Pergamon Press, New York, N.Y.) (1979) at 61–68.
245. Lipscomb, J., *The Willingness-to-Pay Criterion and Public Program Evaluation in Health,* in HEALTH: WHAT IS IT WORTH? MEASURES OF HEALTH BENEFITS (S. J. Mushkin, D. Dunlop, eds.) (Pergamon Press, New York, N.Y.) (1979) at 91–139.
246. Clarke, E. H., *Social Valuation of Life- and Health-Saving Activities by the Demand-Revealing Process,* in HEALTH: WHAT IS IT WORTH? MEASURES OF HEALTH BENEFITS (S. J. Mushkin, D. Dunlop, eds.) (Pergamon Press, New York, N.Y.) (1979) at 69–90.
247. Fischer, G. W., *Willingness to Pay for Probabilistic Improvements in Functional Health Status,* in HEALTH: WHAT IS IT WORTH? MEASURES OF HEALTH BENEFITS (S. J. Mushkin, D. Dunlop, eds.) (Pergamon Press, New York, N.Y.) (1979) at 167–202.
248. Ware, J. E., Jr., Young, J., *Issues in the Conceptualization and Measurement of Value Placed on Health,* in HEALTH: WHAT IS IT WORTH? MEASURES OF HEALTH BENEFITS (S. J. Mushkin, D. Dunlop, eds.) (Pergamon Press, New York, N.Y.) (1979) at 141–66.
249. G. MOONEY, THE VALUATION OF HUMAN LIFE (Macmillan Publishers Ltd., London, U.K.) (1977).
250. A. J. CULYER, THE POLITICAL ECONOMY OF SOCIAL POLICY (Martin Robertson and Co. Ltd., Oxford, England) (1980).
251. Culyer, A. J., *Assessing Cost-Effectiveness,* in RESOURCES FOR HEALTH: TECH-

NOLOGY ASSESSMENT FOR POLICY MAKING (H. D. Banta, ed.) (Praeger Publishers, New York, N.Y.) (1982).

252. Beecher, H. J., *A Definition of Irreversible Coma: Report of the Ad Hoc Committee of the Harvard Medical School to Examine the Definition of Brain Death*, JOURNAL OF THE AMERICAN MEDICAL ASSOCIATION 205:337–40 (1968).

253. Mohandas, A., Chou, S. N., *Brain Death: A Clinical and Pathological Study*, JOURNAL OF NEUROSURGERY 35:211–18 (1971).

254. PRESIDENT'S COMMISSION FOR THE STUDY OF ETHICAL PROBLEMS IN MEDICINE AND BIOMEDICAL AND BEHAVIORAL RESEARCH: DEFINING DEATH: MEDICAL, LEGAL AND ETHICAL ISSUES IN THE DETERMINATION OF DEATH (U.S Government Printing Office, Washington, D.C.) (1981).

255. President's Commission for the Study of Ethical Problems in Medicine and Biomedical and Behavioral Research, *Guidelines for the Determination of Death*, JOURNAL OF THE AMERICAN MEDICAL ASSOCIATION 246:2184–86 (1981).

256. Bernat, J. L., Culver, C. M., Gert, B., *On the Definition and Criterion of Death*, ANNALS OF INTERNAL MEDICINE 94:389–94 (1981).

257. Bernat, J. L., Culver, C. M., Gert, B., *Defining Death in Theory and Practice*, HASTINGS CENTER REPORT 12:5–9 (1982).

258. Stahlman, M. T., Cotton, R. B., *Defining Death: Which Way? A Reply*, HASTINGS CENTER REPORT 12:44 (1982).

259. Capron, A. M., Lyn, J., *Defining Death: Which Way?* HASTINGS CENTER REPORT 12:43–44 (1982).

260. Parisi, J. E., *et al.*, *Brain Death with Prolonged Somatic Survival*, NEW ENGLAND JOURNAL OF MEDICINE 306:14–16 (1982).

261. Nagle, C. E., *Brain Death with Prolonged Somatic Survival*, NEW ENGLAND JOURNAL OF MEDICINE 306:1361 (1982).

262. Saunders, C., *Hospice Care*, AMERICAN JOURNAL OF MEDICINE 65:726–28 (1978).

263. THE MANAGEMENT OF TERMINAL DISEASE (C. Saunders, ed.) (Edward Arnold [Publishers] Ltd., London, U.K.) (1978).

264. Smith, D. H., Granbois, J. A., *The American Way of Hospice*, HASTINGS CENTER REPORT 12:8–10 (1982).

265. R. BENEDICT, PATTERNS OF CULTURE (Houghton Mifflin Co., Boston, Mass.) (1934).

266. CRITICAL ISSUES IN MEDICAL TECHNOLOGY (B. J. McNeil, E. G. Cravalho, eds.) (Auburn House, Boston, Mass.) (1982)

267. REPORT OF A WORKING PARTY OF THE COUNCIL FOR SCIENCE AND SOCIETY: EXPENSIVE MEDICAL TECHNIQUES (Council for Science and Society, London, U.K.) (1982).

268. *Editorial: Expensive Medical Techniques*, LANCET 1:279–80 (1983).

269. Omenn, G. S., Ball, J. R., *The Role of Health Technology Evaluation: A Policy Perspective*, in HEALTH CARE TECHNOLOGY EVALUATION PROCEEDINGS, COLUMBIA, MISSOURI, 1978 (J. Goldman, ed.) (Springer-Verlag, New York, N.Y.) (1978) at 5–32.

270. Sun, M., *Fishing for a Forum on Health Policy*, SCIENCE 219:37–38 (1983).

271. Perry, S., *Technology Assessment Proposed*, HEALTH AFFAIRS 1:123–28 (1982).

272. Perry, S., *Special Report: The Brief Life of the National Center for Health Care Technology*, NEW ENGLAND JOURNAL OF MEDICINE 307:1095–1100 (1982).

273. RESOURCES FOR HEALTH: TECHNOLOGY ASSESSMENT FOR POLICY MAKING (H. D. Banta, ed.) (Praeger Publishers, New York, N.Y.) (1982).

274. Evans, R. W., Anderson, A., Perry, B., *The National Heart Transplantation Study: An Overview*, HEART TRANSPLANTATION 2:85–87 (1982).

275. Relman, A. S., *The New Medical-Industrial Complex*, NEW ENGLAND JOURNAL OF MEDICINE 303:963–70 (1980).

276. Blumenthal, D., Feldman, P., Zeckhauser, R., *Misuse of Technology: A Symptom, Not the Disease*, in CRITICAL ISSUES IN MEDICAL TECHNOLOGY (B. J. McNeil, E. G. Cravalho, eds.) (Auburn House, Boston, Mass.) (1982) at 163–74.

277. Relman, A. S., *An Institute for Health-Care Evaluation*, NEW ENGLAND JOURNAL OF MEDICINE 306:669–70 (1982).

278. Schaeffer, L. D., *Role of the HCFA in the Regulation of New Medical Technologies*, in CRITICAL ISSUES IN MEDICAL TECHNOLOGY (B. J. McNeil, E. G. Cravalho, eds.) (Auburn House, Boston, Mass.) (1982) at 151–61.

279. OFFICE OF TECHNOLOGY ASSESSMENT, MEDICAL TECHNOLOGY PROPOSALS TO INCREASE COMPETITION IN HEALTH CARE (U.S. Government Printing Office, Washington, D.C.) (1982).

280. Le Maitre, G. D., *Medical Cost Inflation*, NEW ENGLAND JOURNAL OF MEDICINE 307:1649 (1982).

281. Jellinek, P. S., *Yet Another Look at Medical Cost Inflation*, NEW ENGLAND JOURNAL OF MEDICINE 307:496–97 (1982).

282. Jellinek, P. S., *Medical Cost Inflation*, NEW ENGLAND JOURNAL OF MEDICINE 307:1649–50 (1982).

283. Lee, B., *Medical Cost Inflation*, NEW ENGLAND JOURNAL OF MEDICINE 307:1649 (1982).

284. Weinberger, C. W., *Shattuck Lecture—Remarks by the Secretary of Defense to the Massachusetts Medical Society, May 1982*, NEW ENGLAND JOURNAL OF MEDICINE 307:765–68 (1982).

285. Relman, A. S., *Physicians, Nuclear War, and Politics*, NEW ENGLAND JOURNAL OF MEDICINE 307:744–45 (1982).

286. Caldicott, H. M., Walker, P. F., *Preventing Nuclear War: The Secretary of Defense Replies to his Critics*, NEW ENGLAND JOURNAL OF MEDICINE 308:338–39 (1983).

287. J. A. RAWLS, THEORY OF JUSTICE (Harvard University Press, Cambridge, Mass.) (1971).

288. Soltan, K. E., *Empirical Studies of Distributive Justice*, ETHICS 92:673–91 (1982).

289. Branson, R., *Theories of Justice and Health Care*, in ENCYCLOPEDIA OF BIOETHICS (W. T. Reich, ed.) (Free Press, New York, N.Y.) (1978) at 630–37.

290. Daniels, N., *Health Care Needs and Distributive Justice*, PHILOSOPHY OF PUBLIC AFFAIRS 10:146–79 (1981).

291. Feinberg, J., *Justice*, in ENCYCLOPEDIA OF BIOETHICS (W. T. Reich, ed.) (Free Press, New York, N.Y.) (1978) at 802–10.

292. READING RAWLS: CRITICAL STUDIES ON RAWLS' 'A THEORY OF JUSTICE' (N. Daniels, ed.) (Basic Books, Inc., Publishers, New York, N.Y.) (1975).

293. F. F. PIVEN, R. A. CLOWARD, REGULATING THE POOR: THE FUNCTIONS OF PUBLIC WELFARE (Vintage Books, New York, N.Y.) (1971).
294. Jonsen, A. R., *Purposefulness in Human Life*, WESTERN JOURNAL OF MEDICINE 125:5–7 (1976).
295. Englehardt, H. T., Jr., *Rights to Health Care: A Critical Approach*, JOURNAL OF MEDICINE AND PHILOSOPHY 4:113–17 (1979).
296. Beauchamp, T. L., Faden, R. R., *The Right to Health and the Right to Health Care*, JOURNAL OF MEDICINE AND PHILOSOPHY 4:118–31 (1979).
297. Childress, J. F., *A Right to Health Care?* JOURNAL OF MEDICINE AND PHILOSOPHY 4:132–47 (1979).
298. Siegler, M., *A Right to Health Care: Ambiguity, Professional Responsibility and Patient Liberty*, JOURNAL OF MEDICINE AND PHILOSOPHY 4:148–57 (1979).
299. Veatch, R. M., *Just Social Institutions and the Right to Health Care*, JOURNAL OF MEDICINE AND PHILOSOPHY 4:170–73 (1979).
300. Daniels, N., *Rights to Health Care and Distributive Justice: Programmatic Worries*, JOURNAL OF MEDICINE AND PHILOSOPHY 4:174–91 (1979).
301. Ruddick, W., *Doctors' Rights and Work*, JOURNAL OF MEDICINE AND PHILOSOPHY 4:192–203 (1979).
302. McCullough, L. B., *Rights, Health Care, and Public Policy*, JOURNAL OF MEDICINE AND PHILOSOPHY 4:204–15 (1979).
303. Curran, W. J., *The Saikewicz Decision*, NEW ENGLAND JOURNAL OF MEDICINE 298:499–500 (1978).
304. Relman, A. S., *The Saikewicz Decision: A Medical Viewpoint*, AMERICAN JOURNAL OF LAW AND MEDICINE 4:233–37 (1979).
305. Glantz, L. H., Swazey, J. P., *Decisions Not to Treat: The Saikewicz Case and its Aftermath*, FORUM ON MEDICINE 2:22–32 (1979).
306. Carroll, C., *The Ethics of Heart Transplantation*, JOURNAL OF THE NATIONAL MEDICAL ASSOCIATION 62:14–20 (1970).
307. A. R. JONSEN, M. SIEGLER, W. J. WINSLADE, CLINICAL ETHICS: A PRACTICAL APPROACH TO ETHICAL DECISIONS IN CLINICAL MEDICINE (Macmillan Publishing Co., Inc., New York, N.Y.) (1982).
308. C. M. CULVER, B. GERT, PHILOSOPHY IN MEDICINE: CONCEPTUAL AND ETHICAL ISSUES IN MEDICINE AND PSYCHIATRY (Oxford University Press, New York, N.Y.) (1982).

The Prostitute, the Playboy, and the Poet: Rationing Schemes for Organ Transplantation

George J. Annas, J.D., M.P.H.

In the public debate about the availability of heart and liver transplants, the issue of rationing on a massive scale has been credibly raised for the first time in United States medical care. In an era of scarce resources, the eventual arrival of such a discussion was, of course, inevitable.[1] Unless we decide to ban heart and liver transplantation, or make them available to everyone, some rationing scheme must be used to choose among potential transplant candidates. The debate has existed throughout the history of medical ethics. Traditionally it has been stated as a choice between saving one of two patients, both of whom require the immediate assistance of the only available physician to survive.

National attention was focused on decisions regarding the rationing of kidney dialysis machines when they were first used on a limited basis in the late 1960s. As one commentator described the debate within the medical profession:

> Shall machines or organs go to the sickest, or to the ones with most promise of recovery; on a first come, first served basis; to the most "valuable" patient (based on wealth, education, position, what?); to the one with the most dependents; to women and children first; to those who can pay; to whom? Or should lots be cast, impersonally and uncritically?[2]

In Seattle, Washington, an anonymous screening committee was set up to pick who among competing candidates would receive the life-

Reprinted with the permission of the author and the *American Journal of Public Health* 75(2) (February 1985). Copyright 1985, *American Journal of Public Health* 0090-0036/85 $1.50.

saving technology. One lay member of the screening committee is quoted as saying:

> The choices were hard. . . . I remember voting against a young woman who was a known prostitute. I found I couldn't vote for her, rather than another candidate, a young wife and mother. I also voted against a young man who, until he learned he had renal failure, had been a ne'er-do-well, a real playboy. He promised he would reform his character, go back to school, and so on, if only he were selected for treatment. But I felt I'd lived long enough to know that a person like that won't really do what he was promising at the time.[3]

When the biases and selection criteria of the committee were made public, there was a general negative reaction against this type of arbitrary device. Two experts reacted to the "numbing accounts of how close to the surface lie the prejudices and mindless cliches that pollute the committee's deliberations," by concluding that the committee was "measuring persons in accordance with its own middle-class values." The committee process, they noted, ruled out "creative nonconformists" and made the Pacific Northwest "no place for a Henry David Thoreau with bad kidneys."[4]

To avoid having to make such explicit, arbitrary, "social worth" determinations, the Congress, in 1972, enacted legislation that provided federal funds for virtually all kidney dialysis and kidney transplantation procedures in the United States.[5] This decision, however, simply served to postpone the time when identical decisions will have to be made about candidates for heart and liver transplantation in a society that does not provide sufficient financial and medical resources to provide all "suitable" candidates with the operation.

There are four major approaches to rationing scarce medical resources: the market approach; the selection committee approach; the lottery approach; and the "customary" approach.[1]

THE MARKET APPROACH

The market approach would provide an organ to everyone who could pay for it with their own funds or private insurance. It puts a very high value on individual rights, and a very low value on equality and fairness. It has properly been criticized on a number of bases, including that the transplant technologies have been developed and are supported with public funds, that medical resources used for transplantation will not be available for higher priority care, and that financial success alone is an insufficient justification for demanding a medical procedure. Most telling is its complete lack of concern for fairness and equity.[6]

A "bake sale" or charity approach that requires the less financially fortunate to make public appeals for funding is demeaning to the individuals involved, and to society as a whole. Rationing by financial ability says we do not believe in equality, but believe that a price can and should be placed on human life and that it should be paid by the individual whose life is at stake. Neither belief is tolerable in a society in which income is inequitably distributed.

THE COMMITTEE SELECTION PROCESS

The Seattle Selection Committee is a model of the committee process. Ethics Committees set up in some hospitals to decide whether or not certain handicapped newborn infants should be given medical care may represent another.[7] These committees have developed because it was seen as unworkable or unwise to explicitly set forth the criteria on which selection decisions would be made. But only two results are possible, as Professor Guido Calabrezi has pointed out: either a pattern of decision-making will develop or it will not. If a pattern does develop (e.g., in Seattle, the imposition of middle-class values), then it can be articulated and those decision "rules" codified and used directly, without resort to the committee. If a pattern does not develop, the committee is vulnerable to the charge that it is acting arbitrarily, or dishonestly, and therefore cannot be permitted to continue to make such important decisions.[1]

In the end, public designation of a committee to make selection decisions on vague criteria will fail because it too closely involves the state and all members of society in explicitly preferring specific individuals over others, and in devaluing the interests those others have in living. It thus directly undermines, as surely as the market system does, society's view of equality and the value of human life.

THE LOTTERY APPROACH

The lottery approach is the ultimate equalizer which puts equality ahead of every other value. This makes it extremely attractive, since all comers have an equal chance at selection regardless of race, color, creed, or financial status. On the other hand, it offends our notions of efficiency and fairness since it makes *no* distinctions among such things as the strength of the desires of the candidates, their potential survival, and their quality of life. In this sense it is a mindless method of trying to solve society's dilemma which is caused by its unwillingness or inability to spend enough resources to make a lottery unnecessary. By making this macro spending decision evident to all, it also undermines society's view of the pricelessness of human life. A first-come, first-served system is a type of natural lottery since referral to a transplant program is generally random in time. Nonetheless, higher income groups have quicker access to referral networks and thus have an inherent advantage over the poor in a strict first-come, first-served system.[8,9]

THE CUSTOMARY APPROACH

Society has traditionally attempted to avoid explicitly recognizing that we are making a choice not to save individual lives because it is too expensive to do so. As long as such decisions are not explicitly acknowledged, they can be tolerated by society. For example, until recently there was said to be a general understanding among general practitioners in Britain that individuals over age fifty-five suffering from end-stage kidney disease not be referred for dialysis or transplant. In 1984, however, this unwritten practice became highly publicized, with figures that showed a rate of new cases of end-stage kidney disease treated in Britain at forty per million (versus the U.S. figure of eighty per million) resulting in 1500–3000 "unnecessary deaths" annually.[10] This has, predictably, led to movements to enlarge the National Health Service budget to expand dialysis services to meet this need, a more socially acceptable solution than permitting the now publicly recognized situation to continue.

In the United States, the customary approach permits individual physicians to select their patients on the basis of medical criteria or clinical suitability. This, however, contains much hidden social worth criteria. For example, one criterion, common in the transplant literature, requires an individual to have sufficient family support for successful aftercare. This discriminates against individuals without families and those who have become alienated from their families. The criterion may be relevant, but it is hardly medical.

Similar observations can be made about medical criteria that include I.Q., mental illness, criminal records, employment, indigency, alcoholism, drug addiction, or geographical location. Age is perhaps more difficult, since it may be impressionistically related to outcome. But it is not medically logical to assume that an individual who is forty-nine years old is necessarily a better medical candidate for a transplant than one who is fifty years old. Unless specific examination of the characteristics of older persons that make them less desirable candidates is undertaken, such a cut off is arbitrary, and thus devalues the lives of older citizens. The same can be said of blanket exclusions of alcoholics and drug addicts.

In short, the customary approach has one great advantage for society and one great disadvantage: it gives us the illusion that we do not have to make choices; but the cost is mass deception, and when this deception is uncovered, we must deal with it either by universal entitlement or by choosing another method of patient selection.

A Combination of Approaches

A socially acceptable approach must be fair, efficient, and reflective of important social values. The most important values at stake in organ transplantation are fairness itself, equity in the sense of equality, and the value of life. To promote efficiency, it is important that no one receive a transplant unless they want one and are likely to obtain significant benefit from it in the sense of years of life at a reasonable level of functioning.

Accordingly, it is appropriate for there to be an initial screening process that is based exclusively on medical criteria designed to measure the probability of a successful transplant, that is, one in which the patient survives for at least a number of years and is rehabilitated. There is room in medical criteria for social worth judgments, but there is probably no way to avoid this completely. For example, it has been noted that "in many respects social and medical criteria are inextricably intertwined" and that therefore medical criteria might "exclude the poor and disadvantaged because health and socioeconomic status are highly interdependent."[11] Roger Evans gives an example. In the End-Stage Renal Disease Program, "those of lower socioeconomic status are likely to have multiple comorbid health conditions such as diabetes, hepatitis, and hypertension" making them both less desirable candidates and more expensive to treat.[11]

To prevent the gulf between the haves and have-nots from widening, we must make every reasonable attempt to develop medical criteria that are objective and independent of social worth categories. One minimal way to approach this is to require that medical screening be reviewed and approved by an ethics committee with significant public representation, filed with a public agency, and made readily available to the public for comment. In the event that more than one hospital in a state or region is offering a particular transplant service, it would be most fair and efficient for the individual hospitals to perform the initial medical screening themselves (based on the uniform, objective criteria), but to have all subsequent nonmedical selection done by a method approved by a single selection committee composed of representatives of all hospitals engaged in the particular transplant procedure, as well as significant representation of the public at large.

As this implies, after the medical screening is performed, there may be more acceptable candidates in the "pool" than there are organs or surgical teams to go around. Selection among waiting candidates will then be necessary. This situation occurs now in kidney transplantation, but since the organ matching is much more sophisticated than in hearts and livers (permitting much more precise matching of organ and recipient), and since dialysis permits individuals to wait almost indefinitely for an organ without risking death, the situations are not close enough to permit use of the same matching criteria. On the other hand, to the extent that organs are specifically tissue- and size-matched and fairly distributed to the best-matched candidate, the organ distribution system itself will resemble a natural lottery.

When a pool of acceptable candidates is developed, a decision about who gets the next available, suitable organ must be made. We must choose between using a conscious, value-laden, social worth selection criterion (including a committee to make the actual choice), or some type of random device. In view of the unacceptability and arbitrariness of social worth criteria being applied, implicitly or explicitly, by committee, this method is neither viable nor proper. On the other hand, strict adherence to a lottery might create a situation where an individual who has only a one-in-four chance of living five years with a transplant (but who could survive another six months without one) would get an organ before an individual who could survive as long or longer, but who will die within days or hours if he or she is not immediately transplanted. Accordingly, the most reasonable approach seems to be to allocate organs on a first-come, first-served basis to members of the pool but permit individuals to "jump" the queue if the second level selection committee believes they are in immediate danger of death (but still have a reasonable prospect for long-term survival with a transplant) and the person who would otherwise get the organ can survive long enough to be reasonably assured that he or she will be able to get another organ.

The first come, first served method of basic selection (after a medical screen) seems the preferred method because it most closely approximates the randomness of a straight lottery without the obviousness of making equity the only promoted value. Some unfairness is introduced by the fact that the more wealthy and medically astute will likely get into the pool first, and thus be ahead in line, but this advantage should decrease sharply as public awareness of the system grows. The possibility of unfairness is also inherent in permitting individuals to jump the queue, but some flexibility needs to be retained in the system to permit it to respond to reasonable contingencies.

We will have to face the fact that should the resources devoted to organ transplantation be limited (as they are now and are likely to be in the future), at some point it is likely that significant numbers of individuals will die in the pool waiting for a transplant. Three things can be done to avoid this: (1) medical criteria can be made stricter, perhaps by adding a more rigorous notion of "quality" of life to longevity and prospects for rehabilitation; (2) resources devoted to transplantation and organ procurement can be increased; or (3) individuals can be persuaded not to attempt to join the pool.

Of these three options, only the third has the promise of both conserving resources and promoting autonomy. While most persons medically eligible for a transplant would probably want one, some would not—at least if they understood all that was involved, including the need for a lifetime commitment to daily immunosuppression medications, and periodic medical monitoring for rejection symptoms. Accordingly, it makes public policy sense to publicize the risks and side effects of transplantation, and to require careful explanations of the procedure be given to prospective patients before they undergo medical screening. It is likely that by the time patients come to the transplant center they have made up their minds and would do almost anything to get the transplant. Nonetheless, if there are patients who, when confronted with all the facts, would voluntarily elect not to proceed, we enhance both their own freedom and the efficiency and cost-effectiveness of the transplantation system by screening them out as early as possible.

Conclusion

Choices among patients that seem to condemn some to death and give others an opportunity to survive will always be tragic. Society has developed a number of mechanisms to make such decisions more acceptable by camouflaging them. In an era of scarce resources and conscious cost containment, such mechanisms will become public, and they will be usable only if they are fair and efficient. If they are not so perceived, we will shift from one mechanism to another in an effort to continue the illusion that tragic choices really do not have to be made, and that we can simultaneously move toward equity of access, quality of services, and cost containment without any challenges to our values. Along with the prostitute, the playboy, and the poet, we all need to be involved in the development of an access model to extreme and expensive medical technologies with which we can live.

NOTES

1. G. CALABRESI, P. BOBBITT, TRAGIC CHOICES (Norton, New York, N.Y.) (1978).
2. Fletcher, J., *Our Shameful Waste of Human Tissue,* in THE RELIGIOUS SITUATION (D. R. Cutler, ed.) (Beacon Press, Boston, Mass.) (1969) at 223–52.
3. *Quoted in* R. FOX, J. SWAZEY, THE COURAGE TO FAIL (University of Chicago Press, Chicago, Ill.) (1974) at 232.
4. Sanders, D., and Dukeminier, J., *Medical Advance and Legal Lag: Hemodialysis and Kidney Transplantation,* UCLA LAW REVIEW 15:357 (1968).
5. Rettig, R. A., *The Policy Debate on Patient Care Financing for Victims of End Stage Renal Disease,* LAW AND CONTEMPORARY PROBLEMS 40:196 (1976).
6. PRESIDENT'S COMMISSION FOR THE STUDY OF ETHICAL PROBLEMS IN MEDICINE, SECURING ACCESS TO HEALTH CARE (U.S. Government Printing Office, Washington, D.C.) (1983) at 25.
7. Annas, G. J., *Ethics Committees on Neonatal Care: Substantive Protection or Procedural Diversion?* AMERICAN JOURNAL OF PUBLIC HEALTH 74:843–45 (1984).
8. Bayer, R., *Justice and Health Care in an Era of Cost Containment: Allocating Scarce Medical Resources,* SOCIAL RESPONSIBILITY 9:37–52 (1984).
9. Annas, G. J., *Allocation of Artificial Hearts in the Year 2002:* Minerva v. National Health Agency, AMERICAN JOURNAL OF LAW AND MEDICINE 3:59–76 (1977).
10. *Commentary: UK's Poor Record in Treatment of Renal Failure,* LANCET (July 7, 1984) at 53.
11. Evans, R., *Health Care Technology and the Inevitability of Resource Allocation and Rationing Decisions, Part II,* JOURNAL OF THE AMERICAN MEDICAL ASSOCIATION 249:2208, 2217 (1983).

Shattuck Lecture:
Allocating Scarce Medical Resources
and the Availability
of Organ Transplantation

H. Tristram Engelhardt, Jr., Ph.D., M.D.

SOME MORAL PRESUPPOSITIONS

THE PROBLEM

Some controversies have a staying power because they spring from un-avoidable moral and conceptual puzzles. The debates concerning trans-plantation are a good example. To begin with, they are not a single controversy. Rather, they are examples of the scientific debates with heavy political and ethical overlays that characterize a large area of pub-lic policy discussions.[1] The determination of whether or not heart or liver transplantation is an experimental or nonexperimental procedure for which it is reasonable and necessary to provide reimbursement is not simply a determination on the basis of facts regarding survival rates or the frequency with which the procedure is employed. Nor is it a purely moral issue.[2]

It is an issue similar to that raised regarding the amount of pol-lutants that ought to be considered safe in the work place. The question cannot be answered simply in terms of scientific data, unless one pre-sumes that there will be a sudden inflection in the curve expressing the relationship of decreasing parts per billion of the pollutant and the in-

Presented at the Annual Meeting of the Massachusetts Medical Society, May 12, 1984. Reprinted with permission from the *New England Journal of Medicine* (July 5, 1984). Co-pyright 1984, the Massachusetts Medical Society.

cidence of disease or death, after which very low concentrations do not contribute at all to an excess incidence of disability or death. If one assumes that there is always some increase in death and disability due to the pollutant, one is not looking for an absolutely safe level but rather a level at which the costs in lives and health do not outbalance the costs in jobs and societal vexation that most more stringent criteria would involve. Such is not a purely factual judgment but requires a balancing of values. Determinations of whether a pollutant is safe at a particular level, of whether a procedure is reasonable and necessary, of whether a drug is safe, of whether heart and liver transplantations should be regarded as nonexperimental procedures are not simply factual determinations. In the background of those determinations is a set of moral judgments regarding equity, decency, and fairness, cost-benefit trade-offs, individual rights, and the limits of state authority.

Since such debates are structured by the intertwining of scientific, ethical and political issues, participants appeal to different sets of data and rules of inference, which leads to a number of opportunities for confusion. The questions that cluster around the issue of providing for the transplantation of organs have this distracting heterogeneity. There are a number of questions with heavy factual components, such as, "Is the provision of liver transplants an efficient use of health care resources?" and "Will the cost of care in the absence of a transplant approximate the costs involved in the transplant?" To answer such questions, one will need to continue to acquire data concerning the long-term survival rates of those receiving transplants.[3-8] There are, as well, questions with major moral and political components, which give public-policy direction to the factual issues. "Does liver or heart transplantation offer a proper way of using our resources, given other available areas of investment?" "Is there moral authority to use state force to redistribute financial resources so as to provide transplantations for all who would benefit from the procedure?" "How ought one fairly to resolve controversies in this area when there is important moral disagreement?"

These serious questions have been engaged in a context marked by passion, pathos, and publicity. George Deukmejian, governor of California, ordered the state to pay for liver transplantation for Koren Crosland, and over $265,000 was raised through contributions from friends and strangers to support the liver transplantation of Amy Hardin of Cahokia, Illinois.[9] Charles and Marilyn Fiske's testimony to the Subcommittee on Investigations and Oversight of the House Committee on Science and Technology provided an example of how fortuitous publicity can lead to treatment[10]—in this case, to their daughter Jamie's receiving payment through Blue Cross of Massachusetts by agreement on

October 1, 1982,[11] along with contingency authorization for coverage
for liver-transplantation expenses through the Commonwealth of Massachusetts on October 29, 1982.[12] The proclamation by President
Reagan of a National Organ Donation Awareness Week, which ran from
April 22 through 28, further underscored the public nature of the issues
raised.[13] In short, several serious and difficult moral and political dilemmas have been confronted under the spotlight of media coverage and
political pressures.[14-17] What is needed is an examination of the moral
and conceptual assumptions that shape the debate, so that one can have
a sense of where reasonable answers can be sought.

WHY DEBATES ABOUT ALLOCATING RESOURCES
GO ON AND ON

The debates concerning the allocation of resources to the provision of
expensive, life-saving treatment such as transplantation have recurred
repeatedly over the past two decades and show no promise of abating.[18-
21] To understand why that is the case, one must recall the nature of the
social and moral context within which such debates are carried on.
Peaceable, secular, pluralist societies are by definition ones that renounce
the use of force to impose a particular ideology or view of the good life,
though they include numerous communities with particular, often divergent, views of the ways in which men and women should live and use
their resources. Such peaceable, secular societies require at a minimum
a commitment to the resolution of disputes in ways that are not fundamentally based on force.[22] There will thus be greater clarity regarding
how peaceably to discuss the allocation of resources for transplantation
than there will be regarding the importance of the allocation of resources itself.[23] The latter requires a more concrete view of what is
important to pursue through the use of our resources than can be de-
cisively established in general secular terms. As a consequence, it is
clearer that the public has a right to determine particular expenditures
of common resources than that any particular use of resources, as for
the provision of transplantation, should be embraced.

This is a recurring situation in large-scale, secular, pluralist states.
The state as such provides a relatively neutral bureaucracy that tran-
scends the particular ideological and religious commitments of the communities it embraces, so that its state-funded health care service (or its
postal service) should not be a Catholic, Jewish, or even Judeo-Christian
service. This ideal of a neutral bureaucracy is obviously never reached.
However, the aspiration to this goal defines peaceable, secular, pluralist

societies and distinguishes them from the political vision that we inherited from Aristotle and which has guided us and misguided us over the past two millennia. Aristotle took as his ethical and political ideal the city-state with no more than 100,000 citizens, who could then know each other, know well whom they should elect, and create a public consensus.[24,25] It is ironic that Aristotle fashioned this image as he participated in the fashioning of the first large-scale Greek state.

We do not approach the problems of the proper allocations of scarce resources within the context of a city-state, with a relatively clear consensus of the ways in which scarce resources ought to be used. Since the Reformation and the Renaissance, the hope for a common consensus has dwindled, and with good cause. In addition, the Enlightenment failed to provide a fully satisfactory secular surrogate. It failed to offer clearly convincing moral arguments that would have established a particular view of the good life and of the ways in which resources ought to be invested. One is left only with a general commitment to peaceable negotiation as the cardinal moral canon of large-scale peaceable, secular, pluralist states.[26]

As a result, understandings about the proper use of scarce resources tend to occur on two levels in such societies. They occur within particular religious bodies, political and ideological communities, and interest groups, including insurance groups. They take place as well within the more procedurally oriented vehicles and structures that hold particular communities within a state. The more one addresses issues such as the allocation of scarce resources in the context of a general secular, pluralist society, the more one will be pressed to create an answer in some procedurally fair fashion, rather than hope to discover a proper pattern for the distribution of resources to meet medical needs. However, our past has left us with the haunting and misguided hope that the answer can be discovered.

There are difficulties as well that stem from a tension within morality itself: a conflict between respecting freedom and pursuing the good. Morality as an alternative to force as the basis for the resolution of disputes focuses on the mutual respect of persons. This element of morality, which is autonomy-directed, can be summarized in the maxim, Do not do unto others what they would not have done unto themselves. In the context of secular pluralist ethics, this element has priority, in that it can more clearly be specified and justified. As a result, it sets limits to the moral authority of others to act and thus conflicts with that dimension of morality that focuses on beneficence, on achieving the good for others. This second element of morality may be summarized in the maxim, Do to others their good. The difficulty is that the achievement of the good will require the cooperation of others who may claim a right to be respected in their nonparticipation. It will require as well deciding what goods are to be achieved and how they are to be ranked. One might think here of the conflict between investing communal resources in liver and heart transplantations and providing adequate general medical care to the indigent and near indigent. The more one respects freedom, the more difficult it will be for a society to pursue a common view of the good. Members will protest that societal programs restrict their freedom of choice, either through restricting access to programs or through taxing away their disposable income.

The problem of determining whether and to what extent resources should be invested in transplantation is thus considerable. The debate must be carried on in a context in which the moral guidelines are more procedural than supplied with content. Moreover, the debate will be characterized by conflicting views of what is proper to do, as well as by difficulties in showing that there is state authority to force the participation of unwilling citizens. Within these vexing constraints societies approach the problem of allocating scarce medical resources and in particular of determining the amount of resources to be diverted to transplantation. This can be seen as a choice among possible societal insurance mechanisms. As with the difficulty of determining a safe level of pollutants, the answer with respect to the correct level of insurance will be as much created as discovered.

INSURANCE AGAINST THE NATURAL AND SOCIAL LOTTERIES

Individuals are at a disadvantage or an advantage as a result of the outcomes of two major sets of forces that can be termed the natural and social lotteries.[27,28] By the natural lottery I mean those forces of nature that lead some persons to be healthy and others to be ill and disabled through no intention or design of their own or of others. Those who win the natural lottery do not need transplantations. They live long and healthy lives and die peacefully. By the social lottery I mean the various interventions, compacts, and activities of persons that, with luck, lead to making some rich and others poor. The natural lottery surely influences the social lottery. However, the natural lottery need not conclusively determine one's social and economic power, prestige, and advantage. Thus, those who lose at the natural lottery and who are in need of heart and liver transplantation may still have won at the social lottery by having either inherited or earned sufficient funds to pay for a transplantation. Or they may have such a social advantage because their case receives sufficient publicity so that others contribute to help shoulder the costs of care.

An interest in social insurance mechanisms directed against losses at the natural and social lotteries is usually understood as an element of beneficence-directed justice. The goal is to provide the amount of coverage that is due to all persons. The problem in such societal insurance programs is to determine what coverage is due. Insofar as societies provide all citizens with a minimal protection against losses at the natural and the social lotteries, they give a concrete understanding of what is due through public funds. At issue here is whether coverage must include transplantation for those who cannot pay.

However, there are moral as well as financial limits to a society's protection of its members against such losses. First and foremost, those limits derive from the duty to respect individual choices and to recognize the limits of plausible state authority in a secular, pluralist society. If claims by society to the ownership of the resources and services of persons have limits, then there will always be private property that individuals will have at their disposal to trade for the services of others, which will create a second tier of health care for the affluent. Which is to say, the more it appears reasonable that property is owned neither totally societally nor only privately, and insofar as one recognizes limits on society's right to constrain its members, two tiers of health care services will by right exist: those provided as a part of the minimal social guarantee to all and those provided in addition through the funds of those with an advantage in the social lottery who are interested in investing those resources in health care.

In providing a particular set of protections against losses at the social and natural lotteries, societies draw one of the most important societal distinctions—namely, between outcomes that will be socially recognized as unfortunate and unfair and those that will not be socially recognized as unfair, no matter how unfortunate they may be. The Department of Health and Human Services, for instance, in not recognizing heart transplantation as a nonexperimental procedure, removed the provision of such treatment from the social insurance policy. The plight of persons without private funds for heart transplantation, should they need heart transplantation, would be recognzied as unfortunate but not unfair.[29-31] Similarly, proposals to recognize liver transplantation for children and adults as nonexperimental are proposals to alter the socially recognized boundary between losses at the natural and social lotteries that will be understood to be unfortunate and unfair and those that will simply be lamented as unfortunate but not seen as entitling the suffering person to a claim against societal resources.[32]

The need to draw this painful line between unfortunate and unfair outcomes exists in great measure because the concerns for beneficence do not exhaust ethics. Ethics is concerned as well with respecting the freedom of individuals. Rendering to each his or her due also involves allowing individuals the freedom to determine the use of their private energies and resources. In addition, since secular pluralist arguments for the authority of peaceable states most clearly establish those societies as means for individuals peaceably to negotiate the disposition of their communally owned resources, difficulties may arise in the allocation of scarce resources to health care in general and to transplantation in particular. Societies may decide to allocate the communal resources that would have been available for liver and heart transplantation to national defense or the building of art museums and the expansion of the national park system. The general moral requirement to respect individual choice and procedurally fair societal decisions will mean that there will be a general secular, moral right for individuals to dispose of private resources, and for societies to dispose of communal resources, in ways that will be wrong from a number of moral perspectives. As a result, the line between outcomes that will count as unfortunate and those that will count as unfair will often be at variance with the moral beliefs and aspirations of particular ideological and moral communities encompassed by any large-scale secular society.

Just as one must create a standard of safety for pollutants in the work place by negotiations between management and labor and through discussions in public forums, one will also need to create a particular policy for social insurance to cover losses at the natural and social lotteries. This will mean that one will not be able to discover that any particular investment in providing health care for those who cannot pay is morally obligatory. One will not be able to show that societies such as that of the United Kingdom, which do not provide America's level of access to renal dialysis for end-stage renal disease, have made a moral mistake.[33,34] Moral criticism will succeed best in examining the openness of such decisions to public discussion and control.

It is difficulties such as these that led the President's Commission for the Study of Ethical Problems in Medicine and Biomedical and Behavioral Research to construe equity in health care neither as equality in health care nor as access to whatever would benefit patients or meet their needs. The goal of equality in health care runs aground on both conceptual and moral difficulties. There is the difficulty of understanding whether equality would embrace equal amounts of health care or equal amounts of funds for health care. Since individual health needs differ widely, such interpretations of equality are fruitless. Attempting to understand equality as providing health care only from a predetermined list of services to which all would have access conflicts with the personal liberty to use private resources in the acquisition of additional care not on the list. Construing equity as providing all with any health care that would benefit them would threaten inordinately to divert resources to health care. It would conflict as well with choices to invest resources in alternative areas. Substituting "need" for "benefit" leads to similar difficulties unless one can discover, among other things, a notion of need that would not include the need to have one's life extended, albeit at considerable cost.

The commission, as a result, construed equity in health care as the provision of an "adequate level of health care." The commission defined adequate care as "enough care to achieve sufficient welfare, opportunity, information, and evidence of interpersonal concern to facilitate a reasonably full and satisfying life."[35] However, this definition runs aground on the case of children needing liver transplants and other such expensive health care interventions required to secure any chance of achieving "a reasonably full and satisfying life." There is a tension in the commission's report between an acknowledgment that a great proportion of one's meaning of "adequate health care" must be created and a view that the lineaments of that meaning can be discovered. Thus, the commission states that "[i]n a democracy, the appropriate values to be assigned to the consequences of policies must ultimately be determined by people expressing their values through social and political processes as well as in the marketplace."[36] On the other hand, the commission states that "adequacy does require that everyone receive care that meets standards of sound medical practice."[37] The latter statement may suggest that one could discover what would constitute sound medical practice. In addition, an appeal to a notion of "excessive burdens" will not straightforwardly determine the amount of care due to individuals, since a notion of "excessiveness" requires choosing a particular hierarchy of costs and benefits.[38] Neither will an appeal to excessive burdens determine the amount of the tax burden that others should bear,[39] since there will be morally determined upper limits to taxation set by that element of property that is not communal. People, insofar as they have private property in that sense, have the secular moral right, no matter how unfeeling and uncharitable such actions may appear to others, not to aid those with excessive burdens, even if the financial burdens of those who could be taxed would not be excessive.

Rather, it would appear, following other suggestions from the commission, that "adequate care" will need to be defined by considering, among other things, professional judgments of physicians, average current use, lists of services that health maintenance organizations and others take to be a part of decent care, as well as more general perceptions of fairness.[40] Such factors influence what is accepted generally in a society as a decent minimal or adequate level of health care. As reports considering the effects of introducing expensive new technology suggest, there is a danger that treatments may be accepted as part of "sound medical practice" before the full financial and social consequences of that acceptance are clearly understood. Much of the caution that has surrounded the development of liver and heart transplantation has been engendered by the experience with renal dialysis, which was introduced with overly optimistic judgments regarding the future costs that would be involved.

Even if, as I have argued, the concrete character of "rights to health care" is more created as an element of societal insurance programs than discovered and if the creation is properly the result of the free choice of citizens, professional and scientific bodies will need to aid in the assessment of the likely balance of costs and benefits to be embraced with the acceptance of any new form of treatment as standard treatment, such as heart and liver transplantation. A premature acceptance may lead to cost pressures on services that people will see under mature consideration to be more important. At that point it may be very difficult to withdraw the label of "standard treatment" from a technologic approach that subsequent experience shows to be too costly, given competing opportunities for the investment of resources. On the other hand, new technologic developments may offer benefits worth the cost they will entail, such as the replacement by computerized tomography of pneumoencephalography. But in any event, there is no reason to suppose that there is something intrinsically wrong with spending more than 10.5 percent of the gross national product on health care.

Is Transplantation Special?

All investments in expensive life-saving treatment raise a question of prudence. Could the funds have been better applied elsewhere? Will the investment in expensive life-saving treatment secure an equal if not greater decrease in morbidity and mortality than an investment in improving the health care of the millions who lack health care insurance or have only marginal coverage? If the same funds were invested in prenatal health care or the treatment of hypertension, would they secure a greater extension of life and diminution of morbidity for more people? When planning for the rational use of communal funds, it is sensible to seek to maximize access and contribution to the greatest number of people as a reasonable test of what it means to use communal resources for the common good. However, not everything done out of the common purse need be cost-effective. It is unclear how one could determine the cost-effectiveness of symphony orchestras or art museums. Societies have a proclivity to save the lives of identifiable individuals while failing to come to the aid of unidentified, statistical lives that could have been saved with the same or fewer resources. Any decision to provide expensive life-saving treatment out of communal funds must at least frankly acknowledge when it is not a cost-effective choice but instead a choice made because of special sympathies for those who are suffering or because of special fears that are engendered by particular diseases.

The moral framework of secular, pluralist societies in which rights to health care are more created than discovered will allow such choices as morally acceptable, even if they are less than prudent uses of resources. It will also be morally acceptable for a society, if it pursues expensive life-saving treatment, to exclude persons who through their own choices increase the cost of care. One might think here of the question whether active alcoholics should be provided with liver transplants. There is no invidious discrimination against persons in setting a limit to coverage or in precluding coverage if the costs are increased through free choice. However, societies may decide to provide care even when the costs are incurred by free decision.

Though none of the foregoing is unique to transplantation, the issue of transplantation has the peculiarity of involving the problem not only of the allocation of monetary resources and of services but of that of organs as well. In a criticism of John Rawls' *Theory of Justice,* which theory attempts to provide a justification for a patterned distribution of resources that would redound to the benefit of the least-well-off class, Robert Nozick tests his readers' intuitions by asking whether societal rights to distribute resources would include the right to distribute organs as well.[41] He probably chose this as a test case because our bodies offer primordial examples of private property. The example is also forceful, given the traditional Western reluctance, often expressed in religious regulations, to use corpses for dissection. There is a cultural reluctance to consider parts of the body as objects for the use of persons. No less a figure than Immanuel Kant argued for a position that would appear to preclude the sale or gift of a body part to another.[42] This view of Kant's, one should note, is very close to the traditional Roman Catholic teaching that one has a duty to God regarding one's self not to alter one's body except to preserve health.[43]

The concern to have a sufficient supply of organs for transplantation has expressed itself in recent political proposals and counterproposals regarding the rights of individuals to sell their organs, the provision of federal funds for the support of organ procurement, the study of the medical and legal issues that procurement may raise, and even the taking of organs from cadavers by society with the presumption of consent unless individuals have indicated the contrary.[44-49] It will be easier to show that persons have a right to determine what ought to be done with their bodies, even to the point of making donor consent decisive independently of the wishes of the family, than to show that society may presume consent. A clarification of policy, to make donor decisions definitive, would be in accord with the original intentions of the Uniform Act of Donation of Organs and would ease access to needed organs. It would not impose on people the burden of having to announce to others that they do not want their organs used for transplantation. The more one presumes that organs are not societal property, the more difficult it is to justify shifting the burden to individuals to show that they do not want their organs used. If sufficient numbers of organs are not available, it will be unfortunate, but from the point of view of general secular morality, not unfair. Free individuals will have valued other goals (e.g., having an intact body for burial) more highly than the support of transplantation. One will have encountered again one of the recurring limitations on establishing and effecting a general consensus regarding the ways in which society ought to respond to the unfortunate deliverances of nature.

LIVING WITH THE UNFORTUNATE, WHICH IS NOT UNFAIR

Proposals for the general support of transplantation are thus restricted by various elements of the human condition. There is not simply a limitation due to finite resources, making it impossible to do all that is conceivably possible for all who might marginally benefit. There are restrictions as well that are due to the free decisions of both individuals and societies. Individuals will often decide in ways unsympathetic to transplantation programs that would involve the use of their private resources, including their organs. Insofar as one takes seriously respect for persons, one must live with the restrictions that result from numerous free choices. One may endeavor to educate, entice, and persuade people to participate. However, free societies are characterized by the commitment to live with the tragedies that result from the decisions of free individuals not to participate in the beneficent endeavors of others.

There are then also the restrictions due to the inability to give a plausible account of state authority that would allow the imposition of a concrete view of the good life. Secular, pluralist societies are more neutral moral frameworks for negotiation and creation of ways to use their common resources than modes for discovering the proper purpose for those resources. If societies freely decide to give a low priority to transplantation and invest instead in generally improving health care for the indigent in the hope of doing greater good, there will be an important sense in which they have acted within their right, even if from particular moral perspectives that may seem wrongheaded.

These reflections on the human condition suggest that we will need in the future to learn to live with the fact that some may receive expensive life-saving treatment while others do not, because some have the luck of access to the media, the attention of a political leader, or sufficient funds to purchase care in their own right. The differences in need, both medical and financial, must be recognized as unfortunate. They are properly the objects of charitable response. However, it must be understood that though unfortunate circumstances are always grounds for praiseworthy charity, they do not always provide grounds, by that fact, for redrawing the line between the circumstances we will count as unfortunate but not unfair and those we will count as unfortunate and unfair. To live with circumstances we must acknowledge as unfortunate but not unfair is the destiny of finite men and women who have neither the financial nor moral resources of gods and goddesses. We must also recognize the role of these important conceptual and moral issues in the fashioning of what will count as reasonable and necessary care, safe and efficacious procedures, nonexperimental treatment, or standard medical care. Though we are not gods and goddesses, we do participate in creating the fabric of these "facts."

NOTES

1. SCIENTIFIC CONTROVERSIES (H. T. Engelhardt, Jr., A. L. Caplan, eds.) (Cambridge University Press, London, U.K.) (in press).
2. Newman, H., *Medicare Program: Solicitation of Hospitals and Medical Centers to Participate in a Study of Heart Transplants*, FEDERAL REGISTER 46:7072–75 (January 22, 1981).
3. Copeland, J. G., *et al.*, *Heart Transplantation: Four Years' Experience with Conventional Immunosuppression*, JOURNAL OF THE AMERICAN MEDICAL ASSOCIATION 251:1563–66 (1984).
4. DeVries, W. C., *et al.*, *Clinical Use of the Total Artificial Heart*, NEW ENGLAND JOURNAL OF MEDICINE 310:273–78 (1984).

5. Dummer, J. S., *et al.*, *Early Infections in Kidney, Heart, and Liver Transplant Recipients on Cyclosporin*, TRANSPLANTATION 36:259–67 (1983).
6. Shunzaburo, I., Byers, W. S., Starzl, T. E., *Current Status of Hepatic Transplantation*, SEMINAR OF LIVER DISEASE 3:173–80 (1983).
7. Starzl, T. E., *et al.*, *Evolution of Liver Transplantation*, HEPATOLOGY 2:614–36 (1982).
8. Van Thiel, D. H., *et al.*, *Liver Transplantation in Adults*, HEPATOLOGY 2:637–40 (1982).
9. Wessel, D., *Transplants Increase, and So Do Disputes over Who Pays Bills*, Wall Street Journal 73:1, 12 (April 12, 1984).
10. Sprito, T. H., *Letter of October 29, 1982*, in ORGAN TRANSPLANTS: HEARINGS BEFORE THE SUBCOMMITTEE ON INVESTIGATIONS AND OVERSIGHT, 98TH CONGRESS, 1ST SESSION (U.S. Government Printing Office, Washington, D.C.) (1983) at 226.
11. Litos, P. A., *Letter of October 1, 1982*, in ORGAN TRANSPLANTS: HEARINGS BEFORE THE SUBCOMMITTEE ON INVESTIGATIONS AND OVERSIGHT, 98TH CONGRESS, 1ST SESSION (U.S. Government Printing Office, Washington, D.C.) (1983) at 227.
12. Fiske, C., Fiske, M., *Statements of Charles and Marilyn Fiske, and Daughter Jamie, Liver Transplant Patient*, in ORGAN TRANSPLANTS: HEARINGS BEFORE THE SUBCOMMITTEE ON INVESTIGATIONS AND OVERSIGHT, 98TH CONGRESS, 1ST SESSION (U.S. Government Printing Office, Washington, D.C.) (1983) at 212–18.
13. Gunby, P., *Organ Transplant Improvements, Demands Draw Increasing Attention*, JOURNAL OF THE AMERICAN MEDICAL ASSOCIATION 251:1521–23, 1527 (1984).
14. Gunby, P., *Media-Abetted Liver Transplants Raise Questions of Equity and Decency*, JOURNAL OF THE AMERICAN MEDICAL ASSOCIATION 249:1973–74, 1980–82 (1983).
15. Iglehart, J. K., *Transplantation: The Problem of Limited Resources*, NEW ENGLAND JOURNAL OF MEDICINE 309:123–28 (1983).
16. Iglehart, J. K., *The Politics of Transplantation*, NEW ENGLAND JOURNAL OF MEDICINE 310:864–68 (1984).
17. Strauss, M. J., *The Political History of the Artificial Heart*, NEW ENGLAND JOURNAL OF MEDICINE 310:332–36 (1984).
18. AD HOC TASK FORCE ON CARDIAC REPLACEMENT, CARDIAC REPLACEMENT: MEDICAL, ETHICAL, PSYCHOLOGICAL, AND ECONOMIC IMPLICATIONS (U.S. Government Printing Office, Washington, D.C.) (1969).
19. ARTIFICIAL HEART ASSESSMENT PANEL, THE TOTALLY IMPLANTABLE ARTIFICIAL HEART (DHEW Publication No. (NIH) 74-191) (National Institutes of Health, Bethesda, Md.) (1973).
20. Leaf, A., *The MGH Trustees Say No to Heart Transplants*, NEW ENGLAND JOURNAL OF MEDICINE 302:1087–88 (1980).
21. B. A. Barnes, *et al.*, FINAL REPORT OF THE TASK FORCE ON LIVER TRANSPLANTATION IN MASSACHUSETTS (Blue Cross and Blue Shield, Boston, Mass.) (1983).
22. Engelhardt, H. T., Jr., *Bioethics in Pluralist Societies*, PERSPECTIVES OF BIOLOGICAL MEDICINE 26:64–78 (1982).

23. Engelhardt, H. T., Jr., *The Physician-Patient Relationship in a Secular, Pluralist Society,* in THE CLINICAL ENCOUNTER (E. E. Shelp, ed.) (D. Reidel, Dordrecht, Holland) (1983) at 253–66.

24. *Aristotle, Nicomachaean Ethics,* ix 10.1170b.

25. *Aristotle, Politics,* vii 4.1326b.

26. H. T. ENGELHARDT, BIOETHICS: AN INTRODUCTION AND CRITIQUE (Oxford University Press, New York, N.Y.) (1986).

27. J. RAWLS, A THEORY OF JUSTICE (Belknap Press, Cambridge, Mass.) (1971).

28. R. NOZICK, ANARCHY, STATE, AND UTOPIA (Basic Books, New York, N.Y.) (1974).

29. Newman, H., *Exclusion of Heart Transplantation Procedures from Medicare Coverage,* FEDERAL REGISTER 45:52296 (1980).

30. Knox, R. A., *Heart Transplants: To Pay or Not to Pay,* SCIENCE 209:570–72, 574–75 (1980).

31. Evans, R. W., Anderson, A., Perry, B., *The National Heart Transplantation Study: An Overview,* HEART TRANSPLANTATION 2(1):85–87 (1982).

32. Consensus Conference, *Liver Transplantation,* JOURNAL OF THE AMERICAN MEDICAL ASSOCIATION 250:2961–64 (1983).

33. *Who Shall Be Dialysed?* LANCET 1:717 (1984).

34. H. J. AARON, W. B. SCHWARTZ, THE PAINFUL PRESCRIPTION: RATIONING HOSPITAL CARE (Brookings Institution, Washington, D.C.) (1984).

35. PRESIDENT'S COMMISSION FOR THE STUDY OF ETHICAL PROBLEMS IN MEDICINE AND BIOMEDICAL AND BEHAVIORAL RESEARCH, SECURING ACCESS TO HEALTH CARE (U.S. Government Printing Office, Washington, D.C.) (vol. 1, 1983) at 20.

36. *Supra* note 35, at 37.

37. *Supra* note 35, at 37.

38. *Supra* note 35, at 42–43.

39. *Supra* note 35, at 43–46.

40. *Supra* note 35, at 37–47.

41. R. NOZICK, ANARCHY, STATE, AND UTOPIA (Basic Books, New York, N.Y.) (1974) at 206–07.

42. I. KANT, KANTS WERKE: AKADEMIC TEXTAUSGABE (Walter de Gruyter, Berlin, Germany) (vol. 6, 1968) at 423.

43. G. KELLY, MEDICO-MORAL PROBLEMS (Catholic Hospital Association, St. Louis, Mo.) (1958) at 245–52.

44. Caplan, A. L., *Organ Transplants: The Costs of Success,* HASTINGS CENTER REPORT 13(6):23–32 (1983).

45. Kolata, G., *Organ Shortage Clouds New Transplant Era,* SCIENCE 221:32–33 (1983).

46. Overcast, T. D., *et al., Problems in the Identification of Potential Organ Donors: Misconceptions and Fallacies Associated with Donor Cards,* JOURNAL OF THE AMERICAN MEDICAL ASSOCIATION 251:1559–62 (1984).

47. Prottas, J. M., *Encouraging Altruism: Public Attitudes and the Marketing of Organ Donation,* MILBANK MEMORIAL FUND QUARTERLY 61:278–306 (1983).

48. U.S. Congress, House. To amend the public health service act to authorize financial assistance for organ procurement organizations, and for other purposes. *By:* Gore A. *98th Congress, 1st Session.* H. Rept. 4080 (1983).
49. U.S. Congress, Senate. To provide for the establishment of a task force on organ procurement and transplantation and an organ procurement and transplantation registry, and for other purposes. *By:* Hatch O. *98th Congress, 1st Session.* S. Rept. 2048 (1983).

The Other Victim

Tom Regan

Like most people, my heart broke when Baby Fae died. It was no good my telling myself that thousands of babies die every day. Baby Fae was special. A member of our extended family, she was a child of the nation. When she died, we all grieved.

Others on this occasion will be drawn to debate the ethics of her treatment. I shall not here defend, only voice, my conviction that she was not treated fairly, that her interests were not uppermost in the aspirations of her principal caregivers. On this occasion I am pulled in another direction. For, unlike some people, my heart broke twice during Baby Fae's public struggle. There were two victims, in my view, not just one, though, like the proverbial black cat in the dark room, the other victim was easy to overlook.

In grieving Baby Fae's death, we were on familiar ground. She was somebody, a distinct individual with an unknown but partly imaginable future. If we allowed ourselves, we could share her first taste of ice cream, feel the butterflies in her stomach before the third grade play, endure her braces. When we consider the other victim, the baboon, the landscape changes. That lifeless corpse, the still beating heart wrenched from the uncomprehending body: for some people that death marks the end, not of somebody, but of some *thing*. A member of some species. A model. A tool. A token of a type. After all, there were no braces, there was no junior prom in that brute creature's future.

Lack of empathy for the baboon is not easily improved upon. Even to note its absence or, more boldly, to suggest the appropriateness of our grieving over "its" death will meet with stiff incredulity in some quarters. When the choice is between a baby and a baboon, can there be any question? Really?

Reprinted from the *Hastings Center Report*, February 1985, by permission of the Hastings Center and the author.

However natural it may seem to answer "no," I think we must answer "yes." It is true that Goobers (though seldom used, this was the baboon's name) had a quite different potential, a quite different future form of life than Baby Fae. But no one, surely, will seriously question whether the duration and quality of his life mattered to that animal. Surely no one will seriously suggest that it was a matter of indifference to Goobers whether he kept his heart or had it transferred to another. Are we not yet ready to see that creatures such as baboons not only are alive, they have a life to live?

The weary charges of "anthropomorphism" will fill the air. Baboons feel pain, it may be allowed. But their sentience exhausts their psychology. A twinge of discomfort here, maybe a warm stroke of pleasure there; that about does it.

This sparse view of baboon psychology will not stand up under the weight of our best thinking, neither philosophical nor scientific. Baboons not only feel pain, they prefer to avoid it, remember what it is like, intentionally seek to avoid it, fear its source. To describe and explain baboon behavior in such mentalistic terms is intelligible, confirmable, and defensible. As Darwin saw, and as we should see, the psychology of such creatures differs from ours in degree, not in kind. Like us, Goobers was somebody, a distinct individual. He was the experiencing subject of a life, a life whose quality and duration mattered to him, independently of his utility to us.

Suppose this is true. Where does it take us morally? Everything depends on how firm the moral status of experiencing subjects-of-a-life is believed to be. You are such a subject, and so am I. Morally, I do not believe that you exist for me, as my resource, to be used by me to forward my own or, for that matter, someone else's interests. And, of course, I do not believe that I exist as your resource either. Just as I would violate your right to be treated with respect if I forced my will on you in the name of promoting my own or anyone else's welfare, so you would do the same to me if you treated me similarly. This sort of strict equality between us, viewed as experiencing subjects-of-a-life, is, I believe, the fundamental precept in terms of which the morality of all our interactions ultimately must be gauged.

I would appeal to this precept to defend my opposition to using a healthy Baby Fae's heart to save the life of a sick Goobers. She did not exist as his resource. But I would insist upon equal treatment for Goobers. He did not exist as her resource either. Those people who seized his heart, even if they were motivated by their concern for Baby Fae, grievously violated Goobers's right to be treated with respect. That he could do nothing to protest, and that many of us failed to recognize the transplant for the injustice that it was, does not diminish the wrong, a wrong settled before Baby Fae's sad death. Fundamental moral wrongs are not alterable by future results. Or past intentions.

What, then, can we do when, as is certain, we face other Baby Faes whose life hangs by a thread? Morally and medically, we must do everything we may, balancing, as best we can, the vital interests present in health care contexts such as these against those we find in others. With limited resources, we cannot, alas, do everything it would be good to do. What we must not do, either now or in the future, is violate the rights of some in order to benefit others. Our gains must be well-gotten not ill-gotten. One measure of our medical progress will be the number of Baby Faes we are able to keep alive. But our resolve not to kill future Goobers will be one measure of our moral growth.

Clinical Urgency and Media Scrutiny

Keith Reemtsma, M.D.

I would like to comment on two questions that the Baby Fae case raises. First, when is it proper to move from the experimental laboratory to the operating room with new procedures? Second, what is the proper role of public information in cases such as this?

There is a widespread misperception that medical treatments and surgical procedures are easily classified as either experimental or accepted. In fact, all treatments have an element of experimentation, and new surgical procedures are based on extrapolations from prior work. Baby Fae was not the first baby to have a heart transplant nor the first person to receive a vital organ from a nonhuman primate.

When does a surgeon decide to apply a new operation to a patient? There is no simple answer to this question, but the decision is based on balancing, on the one hand, the experimental evidence suggesting the procedure may succeed, and, on the other, the clinical urgency—including alternative approaches. As the Baby Fae case shows, answers to these questions rarely are unambiguous. There is no single standard that permits a surgeon to guarantee that a laboratory experiment on an animal will be successful in a human. And there are mountains of evidence that procedures may succeed in humans that were unsuccessful in animals. For example, in the 1950s, open-heart surgery was never proved to be consistently successful in animals before it was applied to humans.

What was the a priori evidence that a primate heart might succeed in Baby Fae? There is evidence from the 1963–64 studies that primate kidneys may function for months in humans. And Baby Fae had two

Reprinted from the *Hastings Center Report,* February 1985, by permission of the Hastings Center and the author.

advantages: as a newborn, she might have been more likely to accept a graft (although this is far from certain), and she received immunosuppressive drugs that were superior to those available two decades ago. These factors, and the clinical urgency, can be used to make a persuasive case for the physicians taking care of Baby Fae.

The second area for comment is the role of public information in the Baby Fae case. Science and news are, in a sense, asymmetrical and sometimes antagonistic. News emphasizes the uniqueness, the immediacy, the human interest in a case such as this. Science emphasizes verification, controls, comparisons, and patterns. Such scientific studies may not be possible in time for an afternoon press conference, and the uncertainties that scientists express may be misinterpreted as a lack of candor.

In evaluating the place of public information in the Baby Fae case, I believe the patient's and family's right to privacy takes precedence over the public's right to know, and I have sympathy for physicians and administrators who are involved in situations such as this. In 1963, when I began the work on cross-species transplants in humans, I made a rule that no public information would be given before the patient left the hospital and a scientific report was prepared and submitted. I do not know whether that was the proper approach or whether it would be either desirable or possible now. But it is probably fortunate that the early results in open-heart surgery were not subjected to the moment-to-moment scrutiny we saw in the Baby Fae case.

Medical scientists, many of whom lead cloistered lives, have been slow to understand that operations such as Baby Fae's are as much a part of today's news as airline hijackings, Central American revolutions, and the Super Bowl. Scientists who do this kind of work must expect the glare of publicity that goes with such news. They must be ready for the most intense scrutiny and criticism. And they must accept the journalistic corollary to Gresham's law: sensationalism drives out thoughtful reporting.

In our society it is inevitable that cases such as Baby Fae will attract attention. And recent events suggest that scientists are accepting the need for public information. I have found that most journalists involved in work of this type are responsible professionals who are trying to explain complex medical events to the public in understandable terms. Most scientists and journalists seem aware of their responsibilities to patients and the public.

The lessons from the Baby Fae case are still being learned. But I would hope that this case does not precipitate additional restrictions, rules, or guidelines, either in the scientific or journalistic communities.

One great advantage of our system of scientific and journalistic freedom is that we have numerous self-correcting mechanisms. These will prove more effective and less crippling than additional governmental restrictions.

Was There Any Real Hope for Baby Fae?

Richard A. McCormick

Among the ethical issues raised by the Baby Fae case are the quality of consent, the expertise of the practitioners, other available options, the introduction of expensive and untested technology, and the priorities and economics of medicine. Here I want to highlight four concerns, the last three really spinoffs of the first.

First, was there any realistic therapeutic hope in this case—any hope of a reasonable benefit for Baby Fae in terms of remedy and survival? Nothing in the history of previous xenografts indicates that there was. Even after the advent of cyclosporin—the drug used to control transplant rejection—the question remains urgent because so little is known about appropriate dosage and reactions in infants.

If there was no realistic therapeutic hope (when the chips are down that judgment must be left to the experts), then the Loma Linda procedure was straightforward nonbeneficial (to the infant) experimentation, a use of the infant for the advance of science.*

But is that not justified at times? Yes, Paul Ramsey notwithstanding, I believe it is—but under the glaring proviso that the procedure involves minimum or no risk, discomfort, or inconvenience. Surely no one would regard the implantation of a baboon heart as in this category. Therefore, absent any realistic therapeutic hope, we have here an instance of violation of a basic canon of medical practice, the requirement of informed consent. For no one may legitimately consent that an infant be used in this way.

Dr. James Hardy, an expert in primate heart transplants, stated: "I don't think people outside the transplant field can appreciate what

Reprinted from the *Hastings Center Report*, February 1985, by permission of the Hastings Center and the author.

this will do for research." (*Newsweek,* November 12, 1984). Maybe yes, maybe no. But "people outside the transplant field" will and should insist that those within this field make this their first question: What will this do for Baby Fae?

Second, while there is no insuperable ethical obstacle to cross-species grafts to benefit humans (pace the Humane Society,) still, special concerns would arise when the transplanted organ is the heart. True, the heart is only a pump. But that is an abstract anatomical statement. More important, do people think of it that way only? Ask the poets, the novelists, the mystics, lovers . . . anyone. Concretely, if the patient survives, how would she be viewed by other people, and eventually and most importantly, by herself? Would she be so medically signalized, at least early on, that a social bracketing would stamp her early years? What effects would this have?

I use the phrase "special concerns," not "insuperable obstacles" because if baboon heart transplants to humans became both successful and common, a kind of public self-education and adjustment would accompany the process and such concerns would very likely dissipate apace. But did the Loma Linda team weigh such concerns seriously enough? Or did they dismiss them too lightly, believing that there was no real hope for Baby Fae? If the latter, that underlines my first point.

Third, I am concerned about the quality of disclosure. Charles Krauthammer is correct (*Time,* December 3, 1984) in arguing that this is not the central issue. But it will not go away as easily as he thinks. Clearly Loma Linda wanted this venture widely publicized. But just as clearly, details (and by that I do not refer to the family's identity) crucial to an ethical assessment were not available (for example, the team's attitudes to past failures involving xenografts and their realistic therapeutic hopes in this instance). This creates the nagging suspicion that a fuller disclosure might have revealed the sheerly and nonbeneficially experimental nature of the attempt. What human beings feel entitled to do to other human beings is a matter of grave public concern. A good test of one's appreciation of this is the willingness to endure and survive public scrutiny.

My fourth and final point concerns the twenty-three member IRB. I would love to have a tape of the session that approved Bailey's baboon transplant. And not one, but five such transplants, and that with no possible knowledge of the outcome of the first, and with nothing but past failures to bolster their hopes. The issue raised is, of course, the ethics of ethics committees. I mean in no way to impugn the sincerity or integrity of Loma Linda's IRB. I mean only to suggest that ethics too is a public enterprise. While there may be vast areas of pluralism in that enterprise, I would wager that that pluralism dissolves when we are tempted to identify the celebrity of certain patients in a kind of public sacrament (TRB, "Celebrity Surgery," *The New Republic,* December 17, 1984)—(which we surely need to bolster our corporate consciousness about the sanctity of life)—with a kind of absoluteness of the research imperative—which we surely do not need.

The Need for a New Partnership

Albert Gore, Jr.

There were many lessons learned in the extraordinary attempt to save the life of Baby Fae, but one lesson stands above all of the rest: the need for a new partnership between society and the medical profession, to create a sustained dialogue about the increasingly difficult bioethical issues confronting us.

To promote this partnership, I plan to reexamine a way I see to create such a medical-societal partnership in the upcoming 99th Congress. During the last Congress I sponsored legislation that would have created an independent advisory commission as a forum for discussions of biomedical ethics. Unfortunately, after passing both houses of Congress, it fell just short of enactment into law.

Baby Fae's struggle brought out the defenders of the dignity of man, the rights of animals, and the public's right to know. But what was right for Baby Fae?

Traditionally, a physician's first duty is to his patient. The Hippocratic oath says "First, do no harm." This limits a physician's response to only that which will help the patient.

With that in mind, we need to consider the role of Dr. Bailey as Baby Fae's physician. Dr. Bailey's specialty is the heart xenograft. He is a very capable medical scientist who prepared for the heart xenograft with seven years of painstaking research on animals.

Baby Fae's ailment, hypoplastic left heart syndrome (HLHS), is a condition for which a therapy has not yet been developed. This is the tragedy of Baby Fae and the hundreds like her born each year. It is a tragedy that Dr. Bailey has said so moved him during his year of training

Reprinted from the *Hastings Center Report*, February 1985, by permission of the Hastings Center and the author.

in Toronto that he has devoted much of his professional career to developing the heart xenograft.

When the doctors at Loma Linda called back Baby Fae's mother, had they suddenly found a new reason to believe Baby Fae's life might really be saved or had they found a patient who could provide valuable medical knowledge for the treatment of other infants with HLHS? I think it was the latter and this makes me uneasy.

I would like to think that the doctors at Loma Linda were only trying everything possible to save the life of a patient, but the facts do not support this conclusion.

There are four paths to choose from for infants born with HLHS. The most common is to allow the patient to die. That was the initial decision made for Baby Fae. There are also three treatments: the heart xenograft, the human heart transplant, and a surgical procedure developed by Dr. Norwood in Philadelphia.

I am satisfied, after speaking with the medical experts, that each procedure is highly experimental. The two cardiac replacement procedures hold the most promise for successfully treating HLHS infants, and of the two, a human heart transplant is ever so slightly less experimental than the xenograft. Yet the doctors at Loma Linda never sought a human heart.

Over the past two years, I have worked successfully to pass legislation in Congress that will help solve the current organ shortage. Infants born with HLHS, however, present an organ shortage problem that will not very likely be solved.

In HLHS infants, medical science is forced to align two extremely small windows of opportunity. First, there is a very brief amount of time—a few days, if not hours—during which something can be done to save the lives of these infants. This must be matched with the very rare occurrence of finding an infant donor. Organ donations result from trauma deaths, which are quite unusual in infants. It is also extremely unlikely that an infant would be declared brain dead in as short a time as is available for organ donation to be successful. So the likelihood of aligning these two small windows of opportunity is practically nonexistent.

Still, as unlikely as finding a human heart was, not even to attempt to find one says a lot about the motivations of her doctors. During the six days while Dr. Bailey was waiting for the result of the tissue matching tests, it would have taken only a few minutes to begin a nationwide search for a suitable donor. The search may not have found a donor and the xenograft may have then become Baby Fae's best chance, but I would have felt more comfortable knowing that the sequence of steps taken was in the order that was first best for Baby Fae.

Questions such as these point to the need for a new partnership. Cases such as Baby Fae involve more than questions of medical science, they involve societal questions of medical ethics, resource allocation, and health care policy, and for answers they require a new decision-making process that has as its cornerstone public participation. The enormous impact decisions made today will have in shaping our health care delivery system for future generations makes it imperative that society's views be melded with the facts of medical science.

While a physician's scientific expertise plays an essential role in the decision-making process, we must, through our institutions and our laws, develop the means by which society can collectively provide the guidance needed to make these decisions.

Important events like Baby Fae help to reopen and provide renewed momentum for development of a new partnership. I want to encourage broad participation in this discussion.

Clinical Problems
in the Use
of Brain-Death Standards

Peter McLaren Black, M.D., Ph.D.

A twenty-year-old woman is brought to the emergency room, after being found on the side of the road. She has fixed 8-mm pupils, no extraocular movements, no corneal response, no gag or cough reflex; she makes no response to any stimulus and is not breathing spontaneously. Her blood pressure is palpable at 60 mm Hg, with a pulse rate of forty beats per minute. In the emergency room, she is resuscitated with intubation, central venous line placement, and administration of volume and pressor agents. An emergency computed tomography (CT) scan shows early cerebral edema but no cerebral hematoma. Twenty-four and forty-eight hours later, there is no change in her neurologic findings. Her physician requests a neurologic consultation. The consultant establishes the absence of any brain-stem reflexes and asks for an EEG. This shows no activity; her barbiturate level is zero. The neurologic consultant wishes to declare the patient brain dead and to consider organ transplantation. Her family believes she might still survive and does not wish her to be declared dead. Her physician has to decide the appropriate course of action.

This composite case illustrates three of the problems a physician may have to face when dealing with brain death: (1) the concept of brain death as death, (2) the criteria for the diagnosis of brain death, and (3) the responsibilities of the clinician toward the patient and toward the patient's family when brain-death criteria have been met. These three questions involve practical problems for a physician but are also philosophical questions, because they are not susceptible to resolution by empirical data alone. Decision making here is a paradigm for decision making in medicine in general and requires a combination of practical and moral judgment regarding the proper care of individual patients.

THE CONCEPT OF BRAIN DEATH

Before this century, physicians used the absence of respiratory and cardiac function as the major criteria for death. It is only within the last twenty years that irreversible loss of brain function has been suggested as an alternative criterion for death. This suggestion, however, has been widely accepted in the United States. In twenty-five states, it is law, and in many others, it has been accepted in courtroom decisions.[1,2] The National Conference of Commissioners and Uniform State Laws, for example, has recently approved "The Uniform Brain-Death Act." This proposal states the following:

> For medical and legal purposes, an individual with irreversible cessation of functioning of the brain, including the brain stem, is dead. Determinations of death under this act should be made in accordance with reasonable medical standards.[1]

This proposal is intended to be a guideline for state legislatures who wish to pass uniform statutes for the declaration of brain death.

These legislative and judicial actions sanction a concept of death based on the irreversible absence of brain function. They, therefore, shift the emphasis from the heart to the brain as the central organ in the determination of death. What is the basis for doing so? More importantly, what reasons might a physician have for accepting brain death as the equivalent of death?

One possible argument for developing an explicit brain-death definition is that, perhaps, this kind of definition has been implicit in all previous traditional criteria. By this reasoning, the heart, liver, lungs, and other organs do not themselves define a living human being. Rather, some kind of ability to function as an integrated whole is necessary. This requires at least brain-stem activity.

The concept of brain death, therefore, may reflect our understanding of what makes a human being alive. As technologic advances have allowed for artificial support of bodily function, it has been necessary to reexamine our understanding of what functions are ultimately relevant to human life. In this respect, the brain-death standard for death can be seen as an intellectual refinement of what life means.

A second reason for the development of brain-death criteria involves the moral more than the intellectual realm. To appreciate this reason, consider the various comatose states. They include conditions in which a patient does not communicate with an observer but may moan, move about, open his eyes, look around and appear "almost awake," to states in which there is almost no response to any internal or external stimulus, not even the stimulus to breathe spontaneously. The state called brain death is at the lowest end of this continuum. It was initially, in fact, called "coma depassé" because it seemed to be "beyond coma"—a state just short of death itself as it was then understood.[1] There is no eye movement, no pupil response, no cough or gag reflex, no arm or leg movement, and no respiratory drive. There is no electrical activity discernible on EEG with any manipulation of patient or equipment. If ventilation is discontinued, cardiac arrest will follow.

All the comatose states present problems to the physician because their outcome is uncertain. A diagnosis of brain death, however, seems to portend a more certain prognosis. Patients who fit brain-death criteria seem to have cardiac arrest within a few weeks, despite all the support possible.[1,3] A recent article has reported one case of more prolonged somatic survival.[4]

However, on the whole, patients with brain death represent a group with a totally hopeless outlook who require substantial nursing and respiratory support to be maintained.

One moral attitude toward this group would be to say that it warrants passive euthanasia, that is, the withdrawal of life support so that the patient may die passively. This is one medical response to situations in which the outcome is hopeless and the physician's treatment is entirely ineffective. A different alternative is to declare that patients who fulfill brain-death criteria are, in fact, already dead. There is no medical or social obligation to continue support in dead patients. It would be appropriate to stop ventilatory and other assistance. These two different positions may lead to the same end, the withdrawal of treatment and the cessation of the patient's heartbeat and lung function. However, these two positions are based on different reasons—the first depends on the absence of an obligation of a physician to perform useless actions; the second depends on a redefinition of what criteria should be used in situations in which death has occurred. In the latter case, we are, in effect, making a moral decision by making a definition. We are asserting that total brain destruction—even if ventilation and heartbeat are being maintained by machines—is really being dead. It broadens the definition of death to include patients once thought to be living.

There is one advantage to using the definitional approach rather than the passive euthanasia approach to resolve the dilemma of how to deal with patients without neurologic function.

Such a stance avoids any explicit discussion of euthanasia at all. The problem of withdrawing support in hopelessly ill patients is a difficult one in medicine. Some persons have argued that its varied possibilities create a slippery slope in which no boundaries can be developed for preventing widespread euthanasia. The brain-death concept avoids the problem of mercy killing or allowing patients to die. It simply removes, by definition, a certain group of patients from the living. Those patients with total brain destruction will be declared dead, and, therefore have no need for ventilatory or other support.

To return to the question of why we should have a diagnosis called brain death and why it should be considered death, brain death results from our technologic ability to keep heart and lungs functioning in a body without any brain function. There is no hope of neurologic recovery from such a state at the present time. If the brain stem and cortex have been physically destroyed, they will not function again. Brain death recognizes the reality of this situation.

CRITERIA FOR BRAIN DEATH

In defining death, the medical profession is faced with a problem common to definitions. How does it know that it is defining what should be defined? For the practicing physician, this question becomes a question of the accuracy of the criteria used to describe a dead brain.

There seem to be three approaches to validating brain-death definitions. One is authority, based on clinical expertise and judgment. The combined medical organizations of the United States might simply declare that, henceforth, a certain set of clinical findings will be accepted as constituting brain death. This is what the Conference of Royal Colleges and Faculties of Great Britain did in 1977, when it promulgated criteria for diagnosing brain death.[5] This document was based on the concept of brain-stem death and its accurate clinical diagnosis. It demonstrates the problems and advantages of declaring criteria for brain death without data supporting each criterion. When the British television show, "Panorama," criticized these criteria, gaps were apparent in the scientific support for specific points. These gaps are now being filled in by retrospective information. The advantage of such criteria, of course, is that they provide uniformity within a given social group.

A consensual definition of death has recently been proposed by the President's Commission for the Study of Ethical Problems in Medicine and Biomedical and Behavioral Research.[6] Their guidelines suggest that both brain-stem and cortical functions must be absent and that reversible causes of coma must be excluded from the diagnosis. Thus,

(1) the cause of the coma must be established and be sufficient to account for the loss of brain functions, (2) the possibility of recovery of any brain functions must be excluded, specifically by excluding sedative drugs or neuromuscular blocking agents, and (3) the cessation of all functions must persist for an appropriate period.

These criteria are remarkably broad; they do not specify which tests are absolutely necessary and which are not. Even then, however, they may have the disadvantage of freezing the diagnosis at the point achieved when the pronouncement is made. Moreover, because they are primarily based on authority, they may have little foundation in hard scientific data to support them in the face of criticism. The extent to which this is the case would depend on the quality of the information used by authorities in their promulgation of criteria.

A second approach is to use clinical studies to develop criteria for brain death. This has several potential problems. No single center has enough experience with brain death to establish valid answers to the questions that need answers; the concept of a clinical study to determine criteria for death has moral and practical difficulties; and most important, it is not entirely clear what such a clinical study should be trying to show. As an example, consider the cooperative study of cerebral death conducted by the National Institutes of Health between 1972 and 1975.[7] This study involved 9 hospitals and 503 patients and had several problems. It used the death of a patient within three months of entry into the hospital as a sign that brain death had occurred. Study leaders could show that a flat EEG, an absence of brain-stem reflexes, and the absence of demonstrable drug levels in the blood were all correlated highly with cardiac death within three months. However, in the end, it was impossible to be sure that failure of survival was a result of the inevitability of cardiac arrest and not the effect of physicians giving up support of the patient. Furthermore, survival for three months is longer than most physicians would expect after brain-death criteria had been met. A major problem with the study therefore involved the clinical endpoint of using death within three months as a validating touchstone for brain death.

All clinical studies validating brain death by failure of survival or cardiac death have the same major flaw. Unless one can be certain that brain destruction in humans leads to inevitable cardiac arrest, such studies will always have the stigma of the self-fulfilling prophecy about them. Moreover, they may suffer from the wrong philosophical concept of brain death. To say someone is brain dead is not just to say he is going to be heart dead; brain death should be able to stand independently as a diagnosis.

A third verifying principle in brain-death criteria is the demonstration in the clinical setting of actual physical destruction of the brain. This has been both supported and opposed by physicians.[8,9] Destruction can be shown by direct examination, for example, by the neurosurgeon in the operating room or with a CT scan showing an intracerebral hematoma so massive that there is no hope of recovery. Alternatively, it may be implied by clinical testing. Angiography, for example, may show nonfilling of cerebral vessels with the presumption that infarction of the entire brain will follow obstruction of its blood flow. Monitoring of intracranial pressure may demonstrate an intracerebral pressure higher than the systolic arterial pressure. Again, this implies that no flow can occur. When these conditions prevail for twenty-five minutes or more in a normothermic patient, extensive irreversible brain destruction will result. This approach tries to predict the presence of widespread or complete destruction of the brain, not failure of clinical survival.

In philosophical terms, it is more satisfying to have as the touchstone of brain death some method of demonstrating that there has been massive brain destruction rather than to have failure of clinical survival. However, at this time, it seems that most physicians and laypersons believe failure of survival is the appropriate touchstone.

DIFFICULT PROBLEMS A PRACTITIONER MAY FACE IN DECLARING BRAIN DEATH

This section discusses two problems in the current and practical treatment of patients with widespread brain injury. They are (1) where to nurse a patient who is being considered for a diagnosis of brain death and (2) what to do if the family does not want support to be stopped even after brain death has been declared.

PROBLEM 1

From the practical viewpoint, a patient who seems about to fulfill brain-death criteria belongs in an intensive care unit (ICU). In fact, only an ICU of some sophistication can support such a patient with ventilatory assistance, intravenous alimentation, accurate recording of input and output, heating and cooling blankets, arterial and central venous pressure catheters, intracranial pressure monitors, and other monitoring equipment that optimum care requires.

To expend ICU time and money on a patient who is almost certainly going to die may seem paradoxical and wasteful, however. In the cost-benefit ratio analysis of intensive care use, a patient potentially brain dead does not rank highly. In terms of human dignity, however, he deserves maximum care until it is perfectly clear there is no hope for survival. The point at which brain death is declared is the point at which survival appears to be impossible. An argument can, therefore, be made that until a patient suspected of being brain dead actually meets formal brain-death criteria, he should attain the highest level of care that can be given to him considering the demands for space.

PROBLEM 2

A more difficult problem arises when the family does not wish support terminated in a family member as in the earlier case. Here the physician may be left with a difficult decision. Jonsen et al.[10] have outlined four levels of decision making in medicine: (1) decision by medical indications, (2) decision by patient preferences, (3) decision by quality of life factors, and (4) decision by external factors (these include family wishes). The decision to declare brain death is based best on medical indications. When a patient is dead, he should be declared dead. In fact, however, there is still enough controversy and uncertainty about brain death as an entity that the physician may feel uncomfortable when faced with families that do not want their son or daughter moved out of the ICU. For this reason, it seems important to have a clear idea of the purpose of brain death and its goals as one tries to deal with it in daily practice. The physician may decide that the family's opinion and input in the matter should be ignored and then may turn the ventilator off to allow cardiac death, despite the family's wish. This is certainly legal in states where a brain-death statute exists. Even where there has not been legislative approval of the brain-death criterion, the general practice in medicine has been to accept brain death as a criterion of death. No one asks the family whether a relative can be declared dead once his heart has stopped beating; perhaps the same kind of demonstration of medical authority should accompany the declaration of brain death. However, in practice, there may be a variety of responses to the situation where a family does not want death declared. The most common response is to maintain minimal support but to continue ventilatory assistance. Death then supervenes either from cardiac causes or from dehydration and infection.

COMMENT

These two problems exemplify many more that the practitioner may find himself facing in dealing with brain death, problems that make the case at the beginning of this article a typical kind of case study. The problems presented herein require not only a knowledge of facts about the diagnosis of brain death but also some understanding of the philosophical background for this concept. They illustrate the importance of philosophical concerns in medicine even regarding a diagnosis that seems to be as straightforward and well accepted as brain death.

REFERENCES

1. Black, P.M., *Brain Death,* NEW ENGLAND JOURNAL OF MEDICINE 299:338–44, 393–401 (1978).
2. Veith, F. J., *et al.,* *Brain Death: I. A Status Report of Medical and Ethical Considerations,* JOURNAL OF THE AMERICAN MEDICAL ASSOCIATION 238:1651–55 (1977).
3. Becker, D. P., *et al.,* *An Evaluation of the Definition of Cerebral Death,* NEUROLOGY 20:459–62 (1970).
4. Parisi, J. E., *et al.,* *Brain Death with Prolonged Somatic Survival,* NEW ENGLAND JOURNAL OF MEDICINE 306:14–16 (1982).
5. Conference of Royal Colleges and Faculties of the United Kingdom, *Diagnosis of Brain Death,* LANCET 2:1069–70 (1976).
6. *Guidelines for the Determination of Death: Report of the Medical Consultants on the Diagnosis of Death to the President's Commission on the Study of Ethical Problems in Medicine and Biomedical and Behavioral Research,* JOURNAL OF THE AMERICAN MEDICAL ASSOCIATION 246:2184–86 (1981).
7. *An Appraisal of the Criteria of Cerebral Death: A Summary Statement,* JOURNAL OF THE AMERICAN MEDICAL ASSOCIATION 237:982–86 (1977).
8. Byrne, P.A., O'Reilly, S., Quay, P. M., *Brain Death: An Opposing Viewpoint,* JOURNAL OF THE AMERICAN MEDICAL ASSOCIATION 242:1985–90 (1979).
9. Veith, F. J., Tendler, M. D., *In Response to an Opposing Viewpoint on Brain Death,* JOURNAL OF THE AMERICAN MEDICAL ASSOCIATION 243:180–89 (1979).
10. A. R. JONSEN, M. SIEGLER, W. J. WINSLADE, CLINICAL ETHICS (MacMillan Publishing Co., Inc., New York, N.Y.) (1982).

An NIH Panel's Early Warnings

Harold P. Green

In 1972 and 1973, I chaired the Artificial Heart Assessment Panel, a ten-member body constituted by the unit of the National Institutes of Health (NIH), then known as the National Heart and Lung Institute (NHLI). The composition of this panel was remarkable: it consisted of two lawyers, two economists, three physicians (one a psychiatrist, one a cardiologist, and one a heart-lung specialist), a sociologist, a political scientist, and a priest-ethicist, none of whom had any previous knowledge of the artificial heart program or technology. The panel was charged with "detailing the economic, ethical, legal, medical, psychiatric, and social implications of a totally implantable artificial heart" and submitting "recommendations concerning desirable courses of development and use of such a device in man." Its final report was submitted in September 1973.

Some ten years later, an artificial heart was implanted in Dr. Barney Clark at the University of Utah. The implantation was successful in that he lived for several weeks thereafter. However, the device implanted in Barney Clark bears little resemblance to the one that was the subject of our panel's consideration. Dr. Clark's artificial heart was powered by a rather large, cumbersome, noisy piece of machinery outside his body; it was connected to the implanted artificial heart through leads inserted into his body through the skin and flesh.

A PLUTONIUM-POWERED HEART

On the other hand, our panel was asked to consider a device, including the energy source, that would be totally implanted within the recipient's

Reprinted from the *Hastings Center Report*, October 1984, by permission of the Hastings Center and the author.

body. The implanted energy source would be a capsule containing 53 grams of Plutonium 238. The entire device was designed by the paternalistic NHLI to provide the maximum benefits for its recipients. It would operate reliably and trouble-free, without any dependence on external machinery for a period of at least ten years. The recipient would be free to come and go, to work, to play, to travel as he or she pleased, and to lead an essentially normal and fully productive life.

We were told that clinical experimental implantations were likely within the next several years. We were also told to assume that all technical problems such as biocompatibility of materials had been overcome; that the device would in fact function as advertised; and that implantations would be made in patients whose cardiac condition would otherwise lead to imminent death or whose cardiac condition necessarily involved a very low quality of continuing life.

We estimated that when the totally implantable artificial heart was fully available, about 50,000 candidates would be eligible for implantation each year; and that, accordingly, these 50,000 individuals could then look forward to an active and productive life for an additional ten-year period (unless, of course, they died sooner because of some noncardiac condition or event).

The totally implantable artificial heart had been under development with NIH funding in one form or another since the late 1950s. In the mid-1960s funding support substantially increased for the purpose of rapidly developing a practical device for clinical use. A parallel, probably competing, program, under the auspices of the Atomic Energy Commission, had probably reached a comparable stage of development by 1973. Total NIH expenditures on development of the implantable artificial heart are difficult to isolate from expenditures for development of other devices, such as the left-ventricular assist device, but were probably approaching $100 million by the mid-1970s.

Based on the assumption that all research and development costs were written off, the panel estimated that the costs of manufacturing the device itself would range from $1,500 to $6,000, while the medical costs for surgery and subsequent treatment would range from $15,000 to $25,000. Thus, the aggregate of these costs would probably fall between $17,000 and $31,000. If the plutonium-powered artificial heart were used, the value of the plutonium would probably add an additional $10,000 to $25,000. Remember that these figures were based on the 1973 dollar. In retrospect, for various reasons, these estimates appear to be quite low. It probably would have been more realistic if the panel had flatly projected aggregate costs of at least $50,000 to $60,000 (in 1973 dollars) per implantation. The panel believed that, since the totally implantable artificial heart had been developed at government expense, the device should be broadly available to any candidate without regard to ability to pay. It seemed inevitable that there would be extraordinary political pressures, similar to those in the case of kidney dialysis and transplants, for the government to ensure that anyone in need of an artificial heart would get one. The potential costs of 50,000 devices at $50,000 per implantation amount to a staggering $2.5 billion per year, again in 1973-dollars.

Risks to Recipients and Others

Unfortunately, the plutonium-powered artificial heart involved other cost and risk considerations. Emanations of radiation from the implanted fuel cell were likely to produce leukemia, and possibly solid tumors, in recipients if they lived long enough. Moreover, even though (we assumed) the recipient would not die of cardiac disease, a relatively unobnoxious form of death, there was a greatly increased statistical possibility that he or she would die a much more unpleasant death as a consequence of cancer or stroke. The panel did not regard these costs to the recipients as unacceptable, since the patient, with informed consent based on full and candid disclosure, could make his or her own judgment as to the balance between benefits and risks. To further complicate the matter, however, the plutonium-powered artificial heart could adversely affect the health of others. For example, it would be medically imprudent for the recipient to sleep in the same bed as his or her spouse because exposure to the radiation would tend to cause leukemia in the spouse. Were the recipient to become pregnant, the fetus would be at considerable risk; there would be some risk to the fetus even if the male parent carried the plutonium.

Furthermore, emanations of radiation from the body of the recipient could have adverse somatic or genetic consequences to the community. Social or occupational associates of the recipient and fellow travelers on public conveyances would be exposed to small amounts of radiation. As one authority on the effects of radiation on life wrote the panel, "My main worry about a Plutonium 238 powered heart pump is that one day on a trans-Pacific flight, economy class, I will be seated between two of them."

The catalog of difficulties with the plutonium fuel source did not end there, however. The very high intrinsic monetary value of the implanted 53 grams of Plutonium 238, and the utility of this material for military or terrorist purposes, would make the recipient of such a device a prime target for murder. Indeed, these considerations mandated that the plutonium fuel cell be removed from the bodies of the recipients upon their death so that the material could be recycled for use in other candidates and kept out of the hands of grave-robbers.

Perhaps the panel's most important conclusion was that the nuclear-powered artificial heart should not be implanted to extend the lives of specific individuals if there was even a very low statistical probability that persons other than the recipient might be injured as a consequence. Accordingly, the panel recommended against implantation of such a device in a human being until it had been demonstrated that other persons would not be injured. At the same time the panel saw no problem with continuing to experiment on animals with the nuclear-powered device. Indeed, it might have favored limited experimental use on human beings except for its belief that it would be impossible to hold the line against broad clinical use if the experiment proved successful from the recipient's standpoint.

A BATTERY-POWERED ALTERNATIVE

The panel's conclusions about the nuclear-powered device were made somewhat easier by the possibility of a battery-powered alternative. In that device the batteries would be implanted as the fuel source and periodically recharged, perhaps three or four times a day, across the intact skin. The recharging device would plug into an ordinary electric outlet or could be carried about in an attaché case. Such a device would obviously be less satisfactory from the standpoint of the recipient, since he or she would be dependent for life upon recharging the battery from external sources. In addition, rechargeable batteries have a limited life, and the recipient would probably have to undergo surgery at least once or twice during the ten-year period in order to replace the batteries. The panel judged that the lesser benefits to the recipients were preferable to the imposition of risks on other individuals.

Although the question of the plutonium energy source dominated the panel's deliberations and report, the panel also explored more fundamental social and ethical issues. This exploration was, however, inhibited by the requirement that we base our considerations on the optimistic assumptions we were given, and avoid discussing *whether* development and clinical use of an artificial heart was desirable. Also, remember that all our discussions were intensified and exacerbated by the plutonium energy source problem.

In general, the panel concluded that if the optimistic assumptions were realized, the benefits of the artificial heart to society would be immense. Significantly, however, we did not attempt to quantify their benefits in monetary terms. At the same time, we observed, perhaps cautioned, that successfully accomplishing the objectives of the artificial heart program would open the door to more "goal-directed, technologically sophisticated solutions to public health problems." We expressed concern about a number of implications arising from the higher costs of clinical applications of the artificial heart: the impact on financing (including government funding) mechanisms and "the potentially enormous commitment" of health resources to this single form of therapy. The panel also cautioned that the values assigned to extension of life must be weighed against the quality of the extended life, particularly in the case of older recipients. It worried that demand for implantation of the device would outstrip supply, necessitating forms of rationing; it rejected any use, even implicit, of social worth criteria.

It is not clear how the panel's report affected the subsequent evolution of the government's artificial heart programs. What is clear is that development of the plutonium-powered artificial heart was slowed down and ultimately terminated. It also became clear that many of the assumptions on which the panel was asked to proceed were unrealistically optimistic. For example, the problem of compatibility of the materials used in the artificial heart with human tissue and blood has not yet been resolved. In any event, the government is no longer funding to any substantial extent development of an artificial heart per se, although it does continue to support research and development on devices such as the left ventricular assist device, the results of which are directly applicable to artificial heart technology. The artificial heart implanted in Barney Clark was essentially a product of a private enterprise.

The facts that I have recited raise a substantial question about the allocation of economic resources for medical purposes. In retrospect, one must seriously question the commitment of millions, let alone hundreds of millions, or billions of dollars per year for high-technology medical fixes for a relatively small number of patients with serious cardiac disease. This is particularly true when there is substantial doubt as to the quality of life that the recipient of an artificial heart will enjoy. By all accounts, although Barney Clark is reported to have said that his postoperative condition was preferable to the alternative, it is difficult to believe that continuing life while being tethered to a power source could be particularly enjoyable over the long term. Even if the device were the totally implantable one that the Artificial Heart Assessment Panel considered, there is still reason to believe that the quality of life of the recipients would not be very satisfactory.

I am not opposed to the artificial heart per se or to entirely private decisions between physician and patient to implant an artificial heart. The autonomy of the patient to seek and obtain an artificial heart should be respected. Rather, I question paternalistic government support for the funding of development, manufacture, and implantation of the artificial heart. Such government encouragement, in my view, pushes the practice of medicine into enormously expensive and, worse still, highly uneconomical directions: in the case of the plutonium-powered device, the direction is also highly dubious.

One does not have to agree with Governor Richard Lamm of Colorado that we all have a duty to die to question the massive commitment of resources to prolong life as an end in itself. One might feel differently if our society first addressed the problem of the miserably low quality of life faced by the growing proportion of older people.

As I look back on the work of the panel, I believe that it made three major contributions. First, it demonstrated that a broadly interdisciplinary group of nonexperts could comprehend and effectively cope with the potential impact of a relatively narrow piece of technology. Second, it demonstrated that technology assessment and cost-benefit analysis could be performed meaningfully in qualitative rather than quantitative terms. Third, it rejected the utilitarian concept where society's (that is, the government's) role was to create a technology that might actively, albeit perhaps insignificantly, harm the health of the larger community in order to confer great good on a relatively few persons. A majority of the panel firmly believed that under no circumstances is it a legitimate function of government to cause risk of injury to members of the community generally in order to extend the productive lives of specific individuals.

However, NIH has not implemented one of the panel's most important recommendations: the establishment of a permanent, broadly interdisciplinary, and representative group of public members to monitor further steps and to participate in the formulation of guidelines and policies for the artificial heart. Review of artificial heart developments today is in the hands of an essentially expert committee with only token participation by the kinds of "soft" disciplines that comprised the Artificial Heart Assessment Panel in 1972 and 1973. This probably reflects a judgment that the technological imperative should not be thwarted by the musings of those who are concerned with the broader social, ethical, and policy considerations.

The Artificial Heart: Questions to Ask, and Not to Ask

Samuel Gorovitz, Ph.D.

Harold Green has provided a comprehensive view of what the problems associated with an artificial heart program seemed to be just a decade ago. It is always instructive to look back at the predictions that attend the early days of a technological advance, and to compare them with the subsequent unfolding of events. In some fields—computer technology being the most visible example—progress has outstripped all but the most wildly optimistic expectations. In other areas, such as the development of new weapon systems, costs are notoriously underestimated, while performance chronically lags far behind even the most solemn promises. The artificial heart program seems to lie somewhere between these two extremes, and it is not obvious how we should decide whether or not it merits our support. The issues do involve matters of social policy and ethical choice.

It is no surprise that autonomy has been the central notion in the effort by writers in medical ethics and others to curb the excesses of medical paternalism. Until recently, discussions of ethical issues in the practice of medicine were physician-centered, emphasizing the obligations the physicians bore to do what would be best for their patients. In that climate of paternalism, a heavy dose of respect for autonomy was needed as an antidote to historically grounded conventions of practice that simply did not fit the changing contexts of modern medical care.

One of the central features of that changing context was the development of new medical capacities that greatly increased the possibility of divergence between the values of the physician and those of the patient. Once physicians could accomplish more than their patients might

Reprinted from the *Hastings Center Report*, October 1984, by permission of the Hastings Center and the author.

want them to, it became crucial to acknowledge the place of independent judgment on the part of patients in the making of medical decisions. This led to a shift in focus to a patient-centered medical ethics, with a resulting emphasis on rights rather than on obligations (although the notion that physicians, too, might have rights was largely ignored).

I certainly agree that it is time for a more explicit emphasis on broader values than simple respect for autonomy. But I see this as a natural evolution in our thinking about ethical matters in medicine, not as a radical change. It may be fashionable at the moment to attack autonomy, but it is better to assess it with a balanced perspective, acknowledging that it is still too little regarded in many medical settings.

Consider what respect for autonomy is all about. Roughly speaking, it is the view that each person should have the right, within broad (and arguable) limits, to pursue his or her own aspirations without impediment. In endorsing that value, however, we ought to remember that our aspirations are fundamentally interpersonal. We do not live in isolation; our structures of knowledge, our characters and personalities, our language, and the formation of the concepts in which our aspirations are cast are all inherently social. This is not merely to say that the lives we lead as individuals are typically intertwined with the lives of others. The point goes much deeper. What and who we are is itself a product of that connectedness with our backgrounds and our environments. It is in this context that autonomy is advocated as a value, and that advocacy in no way denies the fundamentally social nature of moral choice.

HELPING ONE, HARMING MANY

There is, however, a familiar tension between certain kinds of individual interests and certain social values. At least since Garrett Hardin's discussion of the inevitable clash between individual freedom and limited resources—what he called the "tragedy of the commons"—it has been clear that a series of choices by individual agents in a community, each of which is to the advantage of the agent in question—for example, the farmer, the manufacturer, or the patient—may have collective effects that work to the disadvantage of the entire community.

In considering the issues that surround the prospect of further development of an artificial heart, it is important to distinguish the question of whether an artificial heart is beneficial therapy for a particular patient from the very different question of whether an artificial heart program is a wise choice for support by the community. The answer is unclear at both levels; it is not obvious, for example, that Barney Clark was well served by the treatment he received, nor is it clear that even if he were, the program constitutes a wise social choice.

Roger Evans, writing about the economic constraints on high-technology medical care, offers some gloomy predictions.[1] He distinguishes between resource allocation and resource rationing—the former being the determination of a level of support for a program; the latter being the determination of which subset of those in need will receive benefits provided by the program. He then argues: "It is now apparent that both resource allocation and resource rationing decisions will become inevitable. . . . The demand for health care will doubtlessly outstrip available resources. . . . Persons will be recognized as in need of, and then denied, benefits that the medical care system is capable of providing."

These unpleasant conclusions are followed by a discussion of criteria for allocation and rationing, including the suggestion that the availability of health care be based in part not on medical need but on some measure of worthiness:

> Ultimately . . . the limits of the broad humanistic concept of a right to health care must be recognized. Within the context of rationing, those persons who have done the most to preserve their health could conceivably be the first to benefit from the available resources.

With these discomforting observations as background, consider a few aspects of the program to develop an artificial heart. Pierre Galletti argues that "fear of an imminent major impact on health care services and costs is not justified."[2] Yet the *New York Times* worries that a successful artificial heart program would cost $3 billion per year (assuming 34,000 recipients annually), and conjectures that "there may well be more sensible ways to spend that kind of money." Barton Bernstein projects the cost in the range of $1.6 to $6.6 billion per year, and calls for "a probing public dialogue about the costs—economic and social—of developing this device."[3]

Thus, substantial dispute exists about just what is at stake economically. I shall not address that dispute. I agree, however (apart from one misgiving, noted below), with Bernstein's call for a probing dialogue about both the economic and the social issues. Given that the debate will continue about the relative costs and benefits of an artificial heart program, a few points ought to be borne in mind in any effort to reach a conclusion about the merits of any program of development concerning an expensive, high-technology medical capacity.

QUESTIONS TO ASK

First, whether an artificial heart benefits a particular patient is not solely a medical question. Physicians can assess the extent to which the treatment fulfills their aspirations, but the patient's independent assessment is crucial, as Dr. Robert Jarvik has pointed out in discussing Dr. Clark's case. This is so precisely because the aspirations of patient and physician can easily diverge in a case of this sort, and a due regard for the autonomy of the patient requires us to guard against mistaking physicians' goals for those of the patient.

Second, assuming genuine benefit to individual patients, the issue of whether the program is worth pursuing raises new and thoroughly nonmedical questions. Not that medical judgments are irrelevant. They have great bearing. But they are not decisive; they are merely important data in the context of a social policy debate.

Third, it is a clear inferential error to conclude that a program is good on the grounds that each instance of treatment can be reasonably expected to be good, considered separately. We need to make such judgments, instead, on the basis of collective concerns. And that is something we do not yet know very well how to do.

Fourth, even if it were clear that a program of artificial heart treatment was generally worth pursuing, serious problems of social justice would remain regarding the distribution of costs and benefits. Despite the increasing role of for-profit corporations in the development programs, it is still the case, and will long remain the case, that most of the investment in mechanical heart assist and replacement devices of all sorts has come from public funds. Yet small men and most women are excluded from potential direct benefit, since none of the presently envisioned devices are small enough to fit them. Large males are the only potential recipients.

Fifth, many of those involved professionally in live organ transplantation argue that the practice is a stopgap stage in medical progress. Artificial organs, they hold, will ultimately solve all the problems of availability and rejection, making the replacement of failed organs a more secure and straightforward procedure. At the same time, some commentators have argued that artificial hearts should be thought of as a stopgap stage in medical progress, until the problems associated with transplantation can be dealt with more effectively. The frequent juxtaposition of these incompatible assertions should cast suspicion on both.

Sixth, as Gerald Dworkin has noted, by making something possible, we sometimes unwittingly make it necessary.[4] The availability of an artificial heart will have as one consequence a coercive pressure on patients to pursue that remedy and on families to provide it. Neither may be able to muster the temerity, in the face of a vital crisis, to challenge the assumption that what can be done should be done. Yet one can easily imagine an unexpressed preference all around for spurning such heroic efforts. I do not want to make too much of this point, nor to suggest that it is a conclusive objection to the development of any new capacity. But it is a significant, and often inadequately recognized, consequence of progress.

AND QUESTIONS BETTER UNASKED

Seventh, there is a tradition that values the raising of questions, even where we do not yet have any clear sense of how to answer them. This is a typical and worthy part of the philosopher's stock-in-trade. Anticipating the questions we may have to face in the future is always good, we are tempted to think, and the harder they will be to answer, the greater the value of raising them early.

But some questions are better unasked, and surely better unanswered. Here is an example: in the face of severe fiscal uncertainty, some of the senior administrators of my university once felt the need to engage in contingency planning. The word came down; department heads were to state explicitly what they would do in the event of budget cuts of various degrees of stringency. Answering the question as it was asked would have meant identifying those faculty members who were in greatest peril. The only tolerable response to the inquiry was a flat refusal to comply. To identify particular faculty members as most dispensable would be to incur damage, of a potentially lasting sort, needlessly.

I thought of that episode as I contemplated the prospect of rationing artificial hearts within a population of medically qualified patients desirous of that treatment. Whom would we deny—people older than some chronological maximum? Those who had engaged in culpable behavior, such as smoking? (What of the beef-eater, the sedentary, or the workaholic?) Those who failed a test of social utility. Those not wealthy enough to meet high costs? These are familiar questions; some of them were faced in the early days of renal dialysis. They are also destructive questions, for to answer them at all, even on the most tentative basis, is to devalue categories of people with scant justification. We have been able to set these questions aside in the case of renal dialysis, but only by adopting a very costly program of federal funding. It seems highly questionable whether the same strategy can work in the case of artificial hearts. We may, therefore, be unable in the end, as Roger Evans fears, to avoid such questions. But until we are unable to avoid them, it may be best to keep on trying.

Finally, aesthetic criteria are fine for making aesthetic judgments. And they surely play a role in science, both in respect to what motivates scientific inquiry, and sometimes—though perhaps not properly—even in the assessment of theories. (Recall that Dirac chastized Schrödinger for losing confidence in his wave equation when the equation seemed to conflict with experimental data. Dirac's grounds were that Schrödinger should have known that an equation so beautiful had to be right.) Aesthetic criteria offer a perilous basis, however, for making judgments about what policies to adopt in respect to health care or about the choice of interventions in a particular case. Granted, good medical care has an aesthetic dimension in the sense that well-being has an aesthetic dimension, which physicians must take into account in planning and assessing interventions. But that is a question of the aesthetic merit of the result (Is the scar as little disfiguring as it could be? Is the reconstruction appealing to the patient?) The aesthetics of the process are another matter. An elegant intervention, from the point of view of medical technique, may be an "ugly" violation of the patient's values.

Consider Barney Clark once again. One can argue that his story is grotesque, an ugly assault on a gullible, desperate, vulnerable, and ill-chosen patient. One can argue that it is a story with great dramatic appeal, and hence with substantial literary merit. Or one can argue that it is a beautiful example of a stage in the process of scientific progress. But no such considerations are relevant to the question of what our policy should be regarding support for an artificial heart program, or even to assessing whether Barney Clark's treatment was justified. Medical care is not provided for the aesthetic satisfaction of witnesses or of health care providers, and it should not be evaluated as if it were.

None of these considerations is decisive with respect to artificial hearts; indeed, most of them do not point in any clear policy direction. Taken together, they surely do not favor any particular resolution to the quandaries we face and will face as we contemplate this developing technology. They are simply some of the considerations we will need to keep in mind as we struggle to keep pace with the impact of high technology on medical care.

References

1. Evans, R. W., *Health Care Technology and the Inevitability of Resource Allocation and Rationing Decisions, I, II,* JOURNAL OF THE AMERICAN MEDICAL ASSOCIATION 249:2047–53 (1983); 249:2208–19 (1983).
2. Galletti, P. M., *Replacement of the Heart with a Mechanical Device,* NEW ENGLAND JOURNAL OF MEDICINE 310:312–14 (1984).
3. Bernstein, B. J., *The Artificial Heart: Is It a Boon or a High-Tech Fix?* THE NATION 7–12 (January 22, 1983).
4. Dworkin, G., *Is More Choice Better than Less?* in MIDWEST STUDIES IN PHILOSOPHY: SOCIAL AND POLITICAL PHILOSOPHY (P. French, T. Uehling, Jr., H. Wettstein, eds.) (University of Minnesota Press, Minneapolis, Minn.) (vol. 7 1982).

Appendixes

APPENDIX A

Executive Summary of the Report of the National Task Force on Organ Transplantation

In response to widespread public interest and involvement in the field of organ transplantation, the Congress enacted the National Organ Transplant Act of 1984 (PL 98-507). In addition to prohibiting the purchase of organs, the act provided for the establishment of grants to organ procurement agencies (OPAs) and a national organ-sharing system. This act also established a twenty-five member Task Force on Organ Transplantation representing medicine, law, theology, ethics, allied health, the health insurance industry, and the general public. The Office of the Surgeon General of the Public Health Service, the National Institutes of Health (NIH), the Food and Drug Administration (FDA), and the Health Care Financing Administration (HCFA) were also represented.

The mandate given to the Task Force was to conduct comprehensive examinations of the medical, legal, ethical, economic, and social issues presented by human organ procurement and transplantation and to report on these issues within one year. In addition, we were asked to assess immunosuppressive medications used to prevent rejection and to report on our findings within seven months; this report also was to include a series of recommendations, including recommending a means of assuring that individuals who need such medications can obtain them.

During the twelve months following its organizational meeting on February 11, 1985, the Task Force met in public session on nine occasions and held two public hearings. We were supported by staff from the Office of Organ Transplantation and by consultants from HFCA and other agencies and organizations. Data were obtained through surveys, literature reviews, commissioned studies, consultations, and public testimony. Five workgroups were established within the Task Force to address each of the mandated issues identified by Congress and to prepare presentations and recommendations for consideration by the full membership.

As required by the act, the Task Force completed an assessment of immunosuppressive medications and the costs of these therapies, and submitted its report and recommendations to the Secretary and the Congress on October 21, 1985. Briefly, we found that the new immunosuppressive regimens, although expensive, proved to be cost-saving due to improvement in outcome; therefore, the Task Force recommended that the federal government establish a mechanism to provide immunosuppressive drugs to recipients otherwise unable to pay for these drugs, when Medicare paid for the transplantation procedure.

In this final report, the Task Force summarizes its arguments on the issues identified as major concerns by the Congress, and presents a series of recommendations for consideration of federal and state legislators, public health officials, the organ and tissue transplantation community, organized medicine, nursing, and the NIH.

ORGAN AND TISSUE DONATION AND PROCUREMENT

The serious gap between the *need* for organs and tissues and the *supply* of donors is common to all programs in organ transplantation, as well as to tissue banking and transplantation. The Task Force believes that substantial improvements in organ donation would ensue through new, innovative, and expanded programs in public and professional education and the coordination of efforts of the many organizations and agencies that engage in these activities. In particular, we support both the enactment of legislation in states that have not clarified determination of death based on irreversible cessation of brain function (the Uniform Determination of Death Act), and the enactment of legislation requiring implementation of routine hospital policies and procedures to provide the next-of-kin with the opportunity to donate organs and tissues. In addition, we found both a serious lack of uniform standards of accountability and quality assurance in organ and tissue procurement and a spectrum of effectiveness of procurement activities. Therefore, the Task Force supports the development both of minimum performance and certification standards, and of monitoring mechanisms.

RECOMMENDATIONS

1. The Task Force recommends that the Uniform Determination of Death Act be enacted by the legislatures of states that have not adopted this or a similar act.
2. The Task Force recommends that each state medical association

develop and adopt model hospital policies and protocols for the determination of death based upon irreversible cessation of brain function that will be available to guide hospitals in developing and implementing institutional policies and protocols concerning brain death.

3. The Task Force recommends that states enact legislation requiring coroners and medical examiners to give permission for organ and tissue procurement when families consent unless the surgical procedure would compromise medicolegal evidence. The Task Force further recommends that states enact legislation that (1) requires coroners and medical examiners to develop policies that facilitate the evaluation of all non-heart-beating cadavers under their jurisdiction for organ and tissue donation, and (2) provides the next-of-kin with the opportunity to consider postmortem tissue donation. The Task Force further recommends that coroners develop agreements with local tissue banks to help implement these policies.

4. The Task Force recommends that all health professionals involved in caring for potential organ and tissue donors voluntarily accept the responsibility for identifying these donors and for referring such donors to appropriate organ procurement organizations.

5. The Task Force recommends that hospitals adopt routine inquiry/required request policies and procedures for identifying potential organ and tissue donors and for providing next of kin with appropriate opportunities for donation.

6. The Task Force recommends that the Joint Commission on the Accreditation of Hospitals develop a standard that requires all acute care hospitals both to have an affiliation with an organ procurement agency and to have formal policies and procedures for identifying potential organ and tissue donors and for providing next of kin with appropriate opportunities for donation. The Task Force further recommends that the Department of Defense and the Veterans Administration require their hospitals to have routine inquiry policies.

7. The Task Force recommends that the Health Care Financing Administration incorporate into the Medicare conditions of participation for hospitals certified under subpart U of the Code of Federal Regulations, a condition that requires hospitals to have routine inquiry policies.

8. The Task Force recommends that all state legislatures formulate, introduce, and enact routine inquiry legislation.

9. The Task Force recommends that the Commission for Uniform State Laws develop model legislation that requires acute care hospitals

to develop an affiliation with an organ procurement agency and to adopt routine inquiry policies and procedures.

10. The Task Force recommends that a study of the potential donor pool be conducted using data available through the National Hospital Discharge Survey, supplemented by regional retrospective hospital record reviews.

11. The Task Force recommends that living donors be fully informed about the risks of kidney donation. Health care professionals must guarantee that the decision to donate is entirely voluntary. In the case of all living donors, special emphasis should be placed on histocompatibility.

12. The Task Force recommends that educational efforts aimed at increasing organ donation among minority populations be developed and implemented, so that the donor population will come to more closely resemble the ethnic profile of the pool of potential recipients.

13. The Task Force recommends that at the regional level, single consortia, composed of public, private, and voluntary groups that have an interest in education on organ and tissue donation develop, coordinate, and implement public and professional education to supplement, but not replace, activities undertaken by local programs.

14. The Task Force recommends that a single organization, such as the American Council on Transplantation, composed of public, private, and voluntary groups that are national in scope and have an interest in education for organ and tissue donation, develop and coordinate broad-scale public and professional educational programs and materials on the national level. This umbrella organization would both develop and distribute model educational materials for use by national and local organizations and plan, coordinate, and develop national efforts using nationwide electronic and print media.

15. The Task Force recommends establishment of a national educational program, similar to the High Blood Pressure Education Program of NIH's National Heart, Lung, and Blood Institute, aimed at increasing organ donation. This program should include development both of curricula and instructional materials for use in primary and secondary schools throughout the nation, and of programs directed to special target populations, for example, minority groups, family units, and churches.

16. The Task Force recommends that medical and nursing schools incorporate curricula focusing on organ and tissue procurement and transplantation.

17. The Task Force recommends that the Accreditation Council of

Graduate Medical Education, the body responsible for accrediting residency programs, include requirements for exposure to organ and tissue donation and transplantation in relevant graduate medical education programs, such as emergency and critical care medicine and the neurological sciences.

18. The Task Force recommends that each appropriate medical and nursing specialty board require demonstration of knowledge of organ and tissue donation and transplantation for board certification.

19. The Task Force recommends that all professional associations of physicians and nurses involved in caring for potential organ and tissue donors (especially neurosurgeons; trauma surgeons; emergency physicians; and critical care, emergency room, and trauma team nurses), establish programs to educate and encourage their members both to participate in the referral of donors and to cooperate in the organ donation process.

20. The Task Force recommends that organizations of physician specialists who frequently come in contact with organ and tissue donors should establish mechanisms, such as a committee on transplantation, to facilitate communication and cooperation with physicians in the transplantation specialties.

21. The Task Force recommends that a national registry of human organ donors not be established.

22. The Task Force recommends that professional peer group organizations, for example, the North American Transplant Coordinators Organization (NATCO), establish mechanisms for certification of non-physician organ and tissue procurement specialists and standards for evaluation of performance at regular intervals.

23. The Task Force recommends that the Health Care Financing Administration certify no more than one organ procurement agency in any standard metropolitan statistical area or existing organ donor referral area, whichever is larger.

24. The Task Force recommends that the Health Care Financing Administration use the criteria developed by the Association of Independent Organ Procurement Agencies as a guideline to develop consistent certification standards for independent organ procurement agencies and hospital-based organ procurement agencies.

25. The Task Force recommends that the Health Care Financing Administration establish minimal performance productivity standards as part of a recertification process that could be conducted at regular

intervals. Such standards should address procurement activity, organizational structure and programs, staff training and competence, and fiscal accountability.

26. The Task Force recommends that the Health Care Financing Administration collect uniform data on organ procurement activities of all organ procurement agencies, including, at a minimum, the number of kidneys procured, kidneys transplanted, kidneys procured but not transplanted, kidneys exported abroad, and relevant cost data. (The data could be collected through the Organ Procurement Transplantation Network or from each organ procurement agency.)

27. The Task Force recommends that the Health Care Financing Administration require all organ procurement agencies to have, as a minimum, a form of governance that would be similar to that described for the national Organ Procurement and Transplantation Network, that is, it should include adequate representation from each of the following categories: transplant surgeons from participating transplant centers, transplant physicians from participating transplant centers, histocompatibility experts from the affiliated histocompatibility laboratories, representatives of the organ procurement agencies, and members of the general public. Representatives of the general public should have no direct or indirect professional affiliation with the transplant centers or the organ procurement agency. Not more than 50 percent of the board of directors may be surgeons or physicians directly involved in transplantation, and at least 20 percent should be members of the general public. Where the governing boards of existing organ procurement agencies differ from this composition, it is desirable that those boards be modified over a maximum of two years to achieve this distribution. The Task Force believes that all organ procurement agency boards should consider immediate steps to include public representatives.

28. The Task Force recommends that appropriate peer organizations develop standards to certify tissue banks and conduct performance evaluations at regular intervals. Such standards should include assessment of quality and quantity of performance, organizational structure and programs, staff training and competency, and fiscal responsibility.

29. The Task Force recommends that formal cooperative agreements be established among eye, skin, and bone banks.

30. The Task Force recommends that all organ procurement agencies evaluate all potential donors for multiple organ and tissue donation.

31. The Task Force recommends that organ procurement agencies and tissue banks enter into formal agreements for collaborative programs to educate the public and health professionals and to coordinate

donor identifications, discussions with next of kin, and the procurement process.

Organ Sharing

The Task Force believes that establishment of a unified national system of organ sharing that encompasses a patient registry and coordinates organ allocation and distribution will go far in assuring equity and fairness in the allocation of organs. In addition, a national network organization, through adoption of agreed-upon standards and policies, may serve as the vehicle both for improving matching of donors and recipients and for improving access of groups at special disadvantage (the sensitized and small pediatric recipients); thus, the outcome of organ transplantation in this country will surely improve. The development of a national network will permit the gathering and analysis of comprehensive data and, through the establishment of a scientific registry, will facilitate the exchange of new information vital to progress in the field. We assisted the Office of Organ Transplantation in developing specifications for a model network, and urge that the National Organ Procurement and Transplantation Network be established promptly; in addition, we urge Congress to appropriate the funds necessary to initiate the development of the scientific registry.

RECOMMENDATIONS

1.   The Task Force recommends that a single national system for organ sharing be established; that its participants agree on and adopt uniform policies and standards by which all will abide; and that its governance include a broad range of viewpoints, interests, and expertise, including the public.

2.   The Task Force recommends regional centralization of histocompatibility testing where it is geographically feasible, and standardization of key typing reagents and crossmatching techniques.

3.   The Task Force recommends that organ sharing be mandated for perfectly matched (HLA A, B, and DR) donor-recipient pairs and for donors and recipients with zero antigen mismatches (assuming that at least one antigen has been identified at each locus for both donor and recipient).

4.   To increase the rate of transplantation in the highly sensitized patient group by increasing the effective size of the donor pool, the Task Force recommends that a system of serum sharing and/or allocation of

organs based on computer-determined prediction of a negative cross-match, be developed.

5.   Because of the limited local and regional donor pools available to small pediatric patients, the Task Force recommends implementation of a national organ-sharing system that provides pediatric extrarenal transplant patients access to a national pool of pediatric donors.

6.   The Task Force recommends that blood group "O" organs be transplanted only into blood group "O" recipients.

7.   The Task Force recommends that the national organ-sharing network, when established, conduct ongoing reviews of organ procurement activities, particularly organ discard rates, and develop mechanisms to assist those agencies and programs with high discard rates. In the meantime, the Task Force recommends that the Health Care Financing Administration conduct a study to identify why procured kidneys are not transplanted and why the discard rates vary widely from one organ procurement program to another.

8.   The Task Force recommends that the national network establish a method for systematic collection and analysis of data related to both kidney and extrarenal organ procurement and transplantation. Further, to provide an ongoing evaluation of the scientific and clinical status of organ transplantation, the Task Force recommends that a scientific registry of the recipients of kidney and extrarenal organ transplants be developed and administered through the national network, and urges the Congress to appropriate funds to initiate this activity.

9.   The Task Force recommends that the Congress appropriate funds to establish a national End-Stage Renal Disease (ESRD) registry that would combine a renal transplant registry with a dialysis registry. The Task Force further recommends that the national organ-sharing network be represented on any committee responsible for management and data analysis of a national ESRD registry.

EQUITABLE ACCESS TO ORGAN TRANSPLANTATION

The process of selecting patients for transplantation, both in the formation of the waiting list and in the final selection for allocation of the organ, is generally fair and for the most part has succeeded in achieving equitable distribution of organs. However, the Task Force believes that these processes must be defined by each center and by the system as a whole, and that the standards for patient selection and organ allocation must be based solely on objective medical criteria that are applied fairly and are open to public examination. Moreover, as vital participants in the process, the public must be included in developing these standards and in implementing the policies. We recognized the complex conflict between need for an organ (medical urgency) and the probability of success of the transplant, and did not presume to make recommendations in this sphere; rather, we believe that a thoughtful process of development of policies for organ allocation, which takes into account both medical utility and good stewardship, must take place within a broadly representative group.

The Task Force condemns commercialization of organ transplantation and the exploitation of living unrelated donors. The Task Force also addressed the difficult problem of offering organ transplantation to nonimmigrant aliens. When transplantable organs are scarce, we have recommended that no more than 10 percent of all cadaveric kidney transplants in any center be performed in nonimmigrant aliens and that extrarenal transplants be offered only when no suitable recipient who is a resident of this country can be found. The Task Force also concluded that equitable access of patients to extrarenal organ transplantation is impeded unfairly by financial barriers, and recommends that all transplant procedures that are efficacious and cost-effective be made available to patients, regardless of their ability to pay, through existing public and private health insurance or, as a last resort, through a publicly funded program for patients who are without insurance, Medicare, or Medicaid who could not otherwise afford to obtain the organ transplant.

RECOMMENDATIONS

1.   The Task Force recommends that donated organs be considered a resource to be used for the community good; the public must participate in the decisions on how this resource can be used to best serve the public interest.

2.   The Task Force recommends that health professionals provide unbiased, timely, and accurate information to all patients who could possibly benefit from organ transplantation so that they can make informed choices about whether they want to be evaluated and placed on a waiting list.

3.   The Task Force recommends that information be published annually for patients and physicians on the graft and patient-survival data by transplant center. A clear explanation of what the data represent should preface the presentation of data. A strong recommendation should be made in the publication that each patient discuss with his or

her attending physician the circumstances of medical suitability for transplantation and where that patient may best be served.

4. The Task Force recommends that selection of patients both for waiting lists and for allocation of organs be based on medical criteria that are publicly stated and fairly applied. The Task Force also recommends that the criteria be developed by a broadly representative group that will take into account both need and probability of success. Selection of patients otherwise equally medically qualified should be based on length of time on the waiting list.

5. The Task Force recommends that selection of patients for transplants not be subject to favoritism, discrimination on the basis of race or sex, or ability to pay.

6. The Task Force recommends that organ-sharing programs designed to improve the probability of success be implemented in the interests of justice and the effective and efficient use of organs, and that the effect of mandated organ sharing be constantly assessed to identify and rectify imbalances that might reduce access of any group.

7. The Task Force recommends that nonimmigrant aliens not comprise more than 10 percent of the total number of kidney transplant recipients at each transplant center, until the Organ Procurement and Transplantation Network has had an opportunity to review the issue. In addition, extrarenal organs should not be offered for transplantation to a nonimmigrant alien unless it has been determined that no other suitable recipient can be found.

8. The Task Force recommends that as a condition of membership in the Organ Procurement Transplantation Network (OPTN), each transplant center be required to report every transplant or organ procurement procedure to the OPTN. Moreover, transplantation procedures should not be reimbursed under Medicare, Medicaid, CHAMPUS, and other public payers, unless the transplant center meets payment, organ-sharing, reporting, and other guidelines to be established by the OPTN or another agency administratively responsible for the development of such guidelines. Failure to comply with these guidelines will require that the center show cause why it should not be excluded from further organ sharing through the OPTN.

9. The Task Force recommends that exportation and importation of donor organs be prohibited except when distribution is arranged or coordinated by the Organ Procurement and Transplantation Network and the organs are to be sent to recognized national networks. Even then, when an organ is to be exported from the United States, documentation must be available to demonstrate that all appropriate efforts

have been made to locate a recipient in the United States and/or Canada. The Task Force has every expectation that these international organ-sharing programs will be reciprocal.

10. The Task Force recommends that the practice of soliciting or advertising for nonimmigrant aliens and performing a transplant for such patients, without regard to the waiting list, cease.

11. The Task Force recommends that transplanting kidneys from living unrelated donors should be prohibited when financial gain rather than altruism is the motivating factor.

12. To the extent that federal law does not prohibit the intrastate sale of organs, the Task Force recommends that states prohibit the sale of organs from cadavers or living donors within their boundaries.

13. The Task Force recommends that private and public health benefit programs, including Medicare and Medicaid, should cover heart and liver transplants, including outpatient immunosuppressive therapy that is an essential part of posttransplant care.

14. The Task Force recommends that a public program be set up to cover the costs of people who are medically eligible for organ transplants but who are not covered by private insurance, Medicare, or Medicaid, and who are unable to obtain an organ transplant due to lack of funds.

DIFFUSION OF ORGAN TRANSPLANTATION TECHNOLOGY

The number of organ transplant centers in this country is rapidly increasing. As the technical aspects of the procedures have been mastered and patient management is better understood and standardized, it is not surprising that diffusion of this technology has taken place. The issue of designating centers for reimbursement purposes requires careful consideration of many factors, including cost, criteria for facilities, resources, staffing, and the training and experience of personnel. After lengthy debate, the Task Force has agreed with the widely accepted principle within surgery that the volume of surgical procedures performed is positively associated with outcomes and inversely related to cost, and believes that this principle applies to organ transplantation procedures as well. Therefore, we recommend that a minimum-volume criterion be enforced, together with other criteria defining the minimal requirements for both institutional and professional support and outcome of transplantation procedures. In the context of scarcity of donor organs, we strongly support regulating diffusion of transplantation technology.

RECOMMENDATIONS

1. The Task Force recommends that transplant centers be designated by an explicit, formal process using well-defined, published criteria.

2. The Task Force recommends that the Health Care Financing Administration designate centers to perform kidney, heart, and liver transplants, and that the centers be evaluated against explicit criteria to ensure that only those institutions with requisite capabilities are allowed to perform the procedures.

3. The Task Force recommends that the Health Care Financing Administration adopt minimum criteria for kidney, heart, and liver transplant centers that address facility requirements, staff experience, training requirements, volume of transplants to be performed each year, and minimum patient and graft survival rates.

RESEARCH IN ORGAN TRANSPLANTATION

Organ transplantation continues to evolve and improve at a fast pace. Strong research programs in basic and applied clinical sciences have been vital to this fortunate development. As is clearly evident in the concerns of the public that resulted in the enactment of the National Organ Transplant Act, research is also needed in the social, ethical, economic, and legal aspects of organ donation and transplantation. The Task Force acknowledges the important role played by the NIH in transplantation research, and encourages the NIH to coordinate the free flow of information regarding transplant-related research through an interinstitutional council on transplantation. Moreover, we strongly urge that research on all aspects of transplantation be fostered, encouraged, and funded. Therein lies the future of transplantation.

RECOMMENDATIONS

1. The Task Force recommends that basic research continue to receive high priority.

2. The Task Force recommends that both laboratory and clinical research be fostered, encouraged, and funded. For the immediate benefit of patients, the Task Force further recommends that research be aggressively pursued in organ preservation and optimal immunosuppression techniques. The Task Force also wishes to emphasize the importance of sponsoring prospective clinical trials, involving multiple institutions, to solve certain problems in patient management.

3.   The Task Force recommends that continuing attention be devoted to collecting complete information on the status and efficacy of transplantation treatments.

4.   The Task Force recommends that the National Institutes of Health and other agencies encourage the continuing free flow of information in the transplant field. We believe that better coordination of National Institutes of Health activities might be achieved by reactivating an interinstitute council on transplantation.

APPENDIX B

Report to the Secretary and the Congress on Immunosuppressive Therapies

Task Force on Organ Transplantation

EXECUTIVE SUMMARY

STATEMENT OF THE PROBLEM

Among recent developments in the field of organ transplantation has been new and more effective means of immunosuppression to prevent the body's rejection of transplanted organs. The advent of the immunosuppressant drug cyclosporin, approved by the Food and Drug Administration in 1983, brought a new set of issues to bear on the overall cost of organ transplantation. Cyclosporin costs approximately $5,000 to $7,000 per year, depending upon patient characteristics (e.g., weight) and the prescribed drug protocol, while conventional therapies (azathioprine and prednisone) average $1,000 to $2,000 per year. Earlier anecdotal reports indicated that the high costs of cyclosporin caused some patients to face severe financial problems beyond the cost of the transplant procedure itself. More important, some patients were not even considered as candidates for transplantation if they could not afford the drug regimen.

Congressional oversight hearings in 1983 and 1984 into the critical shortage of donor organs in this country ended in a debate over whether the federal government should provide some kind of assistance to transplant recipients in obtaining and paying for their immunosuppressive drugs. In passing the National Organ Transplant Act (P.L. 98-507), the

Issued by U.S. Department of Health and Human Services, Public Health Service, Health Resources and Services Administration Office of Organ Transplantation, October 1985.

Congress created the Task Force on Organ Transplantation and directed it to review the issue of immunosuppressant therapies and report its findings to Congress and the Secretary of Health and Human Services. Congress directed the Task Force to consider immunosuppressive drugs as its highest priority and report within seven months on the safety, effectiveness, and costs of immunosuppressive drugs, the extent of insurance reimbursement, problems patients encounter in obtaining the drugs, and mechanisms that might be employed to assure that individuals needing the drugs could obtain them.

The Task Force on Organ Transplantation, established by the Secretary in January 1985, established two workgroups—the Workgroup on Immunosuppressive Therapies and the Workgroup on Reimbursement—to address the various issues associated with immunosuppression and transplantation. The workgroups amassed and examined considerable data in the process of the review. Data from clinical trials were reviewed, experts were consulted, special studies were conducted, surveys conducted by others were analyzed, and a public hearing was held by the Task Force in May 1985, all of which contributed to its deliberations.

FINDINGS

Although a single agent, cyclosporin, served as a primary motivating factor for the review of immunosuppressants, the Task Force was unanimous in agreeing upon several points in developing its recommendations to assure patient access to immunosuppressive drugs:

—Any approach to resolving the problem of patient access to immunosuppressive drugs should address immunosuppressants in general, not only cyclosporin.

—The problems associated with access to immunosuppressive therapies and the cost thereof are generic to *all* transplant recipients, not just renal transplant recipients.

—Any approach to resolving the financial dilemma within which many transplant recipients have been placed must be targeted to those patients who are regarded as most needy financially.

In pursuing its review, the Task Force acknowledged that patient *access* to immunosuppressives, including the effect of patient ability to pay for immunosuppressives on access to transplantation, was its primary concern. Thus, assuring patient access to immunosuppressive drugs was the most important factor in the deliberations of the Task Force and was the driving force behind its subsequent recommendations.

Efficacy of Cyclosporin. The Task Force concluded that cyclosporin constitutes a major breakthrough in organ transplantation. While a variety of immunosuppressive therapies are in use, data from numerous clinical trials showed increased patient and graft survival rates, decreased hospital stays, and fewer episodes of infection and rejection with use of cyclosporin. Mortality and morbidity are significantly reduced with cyclosporin when compared to conventional immunosuppressive therapy.

Considerable variety exists in the protocols involving the administration of cyclosporin. Cyclosporin is used in combination with various other immunosuppressants and at different dosage levels. Opinions differ on whether and at what time after transplant cyclosporin may be discontinued and conventional immunosuppressives substituted in order to avoid accumulation of damage from toxic side effects. Although cyclosporin has some toxic side effects, principally nephrotoxicity (damage caused to the kidney), there is recent evidence that use of cyclosporin in combination with other immunosuppressive agents and reduced dosages of cyclosporin decreases this toxicity.

Cost Benefit. The Task Force found that because of the reduced rate of complications and shorter length of hospital stay, cyclosporin has a favorable impact on the cost of cadaveric renal transplantation. Even though cyclosporin is more expensive than conventional immunosuppressive therapy in the first six months posttransplant, it remains at least cost neutral over the long term, and the patient directly benefits by having fewer complications.

Patient Problems. The Task Force determined that approximately 25 percent of the transplant population has no private insurance coverage for immunosuppressive medications or coverage by a state Medicaid program or other state program. These transplant recipients experience serious difficulty in obtaining and paying for needed immunosuppressive drugs, especially cyclosporin. This has resulted in non-medically indicated changes in their drug regimens with potentially adverse consequences for the ultimate success of their transplant. The Task Force also found evidence that inability to pay for immunosuppressive medications has been a factor in the initial selection of patients for transplantation.

RECOMMENDATIONS

In view of the fact that the majority of private insurers and state Medicaid programs do provide coverage for outpatient immunosuppressive medications, and the realization that federal health care spending faces severe budgetary constraints, the Task Force concludes that *any federal funding for immunosuppressive medication should be limited to assisting only financially needy Medicare-eligible transplant patients.*

Having examined a variety of funding alternatives, *the Task Force recommends the establishment of a joint Health Care Financing Administration– Public Health Service program to provide immunosuppressive medications to transplant centers for distribution to financially needy Medicare-eligible transplant patients.* The program would be administered by the Public Health Service and supported with Medicare Trust Funds.

The Task Force takes no position at the present time on whether extrarenal transplants should be federally funded but does recommend that federal funding of immunosuppressive medications occur if the federal government funds extrarenal transplants. It further recommends that the federal government evaluate the outcomes of any program to fund outpatient immunosuppressive drugs and support demonstration projects on methods for reimbursing transplant procedures and immunosuppressive therapies.

The Task Force also recommends that private health insurance coverage of transplants include the cost of immunosuppressive therapy. Finally, the Task Force recommends that multicenter trials be conducted to evaluate the safety, efficacy, and costs of immunosuppressive medications and protocols.

APPENDIX C

Defining Death: A Report on the Medical, Legal, and Ethical Issues in the Determination of Death

President's Commission for the Study of Ethical Problems in Medicine and Biomedical and Behavioral Research, July 1981

SUMMARY OF CONCLUSIONS AND RECOMMENDED STATUTE

The enabling legislation for the President's Commission directs it to study "the ethical and legal implications of the matter of defining death, including the advisability of developing a uniform definition of death."[1] In performing its mandate, the Commission has reached conclusions on a series of questions which are the subject of this Report. In summary, the central conclusions are:

1. That recent developments in medical treatment necessitate a restatement of the standards traditionally recognized for determining that death has occurred.
2. That such a restatement ought preferably to be a matter of statutory law.
3. That such a statute ought to remain a matter for state law, with federal action at this time being limited to areas under current federal jurisdiction.
4. That the statutory law ought to be uniform among the several states.
5. That the "definition" contained in the statute ought to address general physiological standards rather than medical criteria and tests, which will change with advances in biomedical knowledge and refinements in technique.

6. That death is a unitary phenomenon which can be accurately demonstrated either on the traditional grounds of irreversible cessation of heart and lung functions or on the basis of irreversible loss of all functions of the entire brain.
7. That any statutory "definition" should be kept separate and distinct from provisions governing the donation of cadaver organs and from any legal rules on decisions to terminate life-sustaining treatment.

To embody these conclusions in statutory form the Commission worked with the three organizations which had proposed model legislation on the subject, the American Bar Association, the American Medical Association, and the National Conference of Commissioners on Uniform State Laws. These groups have now endorsed the following statute, in place of their previous proposals:

Uniform Determination of Death Act

An individual who has sustained either (1) irreversible cessation of circulatory and respiratory functions or (2) irreversible cessation of all functions of the entire brain, including the brain stem, is dead. A determination of death must be made in accordance with accepted medical standards.

The Commission recommends the adoption of this statute in all jurisdictions in the United States.

NOTE

1. 42 U.S.C. §1802 (1978).

APPENDIX D

Guidelines for the Determination of Death

Report of the Medical Consultants on the Diagnosis of Death to the President's Commission for the Study of Ethical Problems in Medicine and Biomedical and Behavioral Research.[1]

The advent of effective artificial cardiopulmonary support for severely brain-injured persons has created some confusion during the past several decades about the determination of death. Previously, loss of heart and lung functions was an easily observable and sufficient basis for diagnosing death, whether the initial failure occurred in the brain, the heart and lungs, or elsewhere in the body. Irreversible failure of either the heart and lungs or the brain precluded the continued functioning of the other. Now, however, circulation and respiration can be maintained by means of a mechanical respirator and other medical interventions, despite a loss of all brain functions. In these circumstances we recognize as dead an individual whose loss of brain functions is complete and irreversible.

To recognize reliably that death has occurred, accurate criteria must be available for physicians' use. These now fall into two groups, to be applied depending on the clinical situation. When respiration and circulation have irreversibly ceased, there is no need to assess brain functions directly. When cardiopulmonary functions are artificially maintained, neurologic criteria must be used to assess whether brain functions have irreversibly ceased.

More than half of the states now recognize, through statutes or

From *Defining Death: A Report on the Medical, Legal, and Ethical Issues in the Determination of Death.* President's Commission for the Study of Ethical Problems in Medicine and Biomedical and Behaviorial Research. U.S. Government Printing Office, 1981   356-539/9903.

judicial decisions, that death may be determined on the basis of irreversible cessation of all functions of the brain. Law in the remaining states has not yet departed from the older, common law view that death has not occurred until "all vital functions" (whether or not artificially maintained) have ceased. The language of the statutes has not been uniform from state to state, and the diversity of proposed and enacted laws has created substantial confusion. Consequently, the Amemican Bar Association, the American Medical Association, the National Conference of Commissioners on Uniform State Laws, and the President's Commission for the Study of Ethical Problems in Medicine and Biomedical and Behavorial Research have proposed the following model statute, intended for adoption in every jurisdiction:

> *Uniform Determination of Death Act*
>
> An individual who has sustained either (1) irreversible cessation of circulatory and respiratory functions or (2) irreversible cessation of all functions of the entire brain, including the brain stem, is dead. A determination of death must be made in accorance with accepted medical standards.

This wording has also been endorsed by the American Academy of Neurology and the American Electroencephalographic Society.

The statute relies upon the existence of "accepted medical standards" for determining that death has occurred. The medical profession, based upon carefully conducted research and extensive clinical experience, has found that death can be reliably determined by either cardiopulmonary or neurologic criteria. The tests used for determining cessation of brain functions have changed and will continue to do so with the advent of new research and technologies. The "Harvard criteria" (*JAMA*, 205:337, 1968) are widely accepted, but advances in recent years have led to the proposal of other criteria. As an aid to the implementation of the proposed uniform statute, we provide here one statement of currently accepted medical standards.

INTRODUCTION

The criteria that physicians use in determining that death has occurred should:

1. Eliminate errors in classifying a living individual as dead
2. Allow as few errors as possible in classifying a dead body as alive
3. Allow a determination to be made without unreasonable delay
4. Be adaptable to a variety of clinical situations, and
5. Be explicit and accessible to verification.

Because it would be undesirable for any guidelines to be mandated by legislation or regulation or to be inflexibly established in case law, the proposed Uniform Determination of Death Act appropriately specifies only "accepted medical standards." Local, state, and national institutions and professional organizations are encouraged to examine and publish their practices.

The following guidelines represent a distillation of current practice in regard to the determination of death. Only the most commonly available and verified tests have been included. The time of death recorded on a death certificate is at present a matter of local practice and is not covered in this document.

These guidelines are advisory. Their successful use requires a competent and judicious physician, experienced in clinical examination and the relevant procedures. All periods of observation listed in these guidelines require the patient to be under the care of a physician. Considering the responsibility entailed in the determination of death, consultation is recommended when appropriate.

The outline of the criteria is set forth below in capital letters. The indented text that follows each outline heading explains its meaning. In addition, the two sets of criteria (cardiopulmonary and neurologic) are followed by a presentation of the major complicating conditions: drug and metabolic intoxication, hypothermia, young age, and shock. It is of paramount importance that anyone referring to these guidelines be thoroughly familiar with the entire document, including explanatory notes and complicating conditions.

The Criteria for Determination of Death

An individual presenting the findings in *either* section A (cardiopulmonary) *or* section B (neurological) is dead. In either section, a diagnosis of death requires that *both* <u>cessation of functions</u>, as set forth in subsection 1, *and* <u>irreversibility</u>, as set forth in subsection 2, be demonstrated.

A. An individual with irreversible cessation of circulatory and respiratory functions is dead.

1. *Cessation* **is recognized by an appropriate clinical examination.**

Clinical examination will disclose at least the absence of responsiveness, heartbeat, and respiratory effort. Medical circumstances may require the use of confirmatory tests, such as an ECG.

2. *Irreversibility* **is recognized by persistent cessation of functions during an appropriate period of observation and/or trial of therapy.**

In clinical situations where death is expected, where the course has been gradual, and where irregular agonal respiration or heartbeat finally ceases, the period of observation following the cessation may be only the few minutes required to complete the examination. Similarly, if resuscitation is not undertaken and ventricular fibrillation and standstill develop in a monitored patient, the required period of observation thereafter may be as short as a few minutes. When a possible death is unobserved, unexpected, or sudden, the examination may need to be more detailed and repeated over a longer period, while appropriate resuscitative effort is maintained as a test of cardiovascular responsiveness. Diagnosis in individuals who are first observed with rigor mortis or putrefaction may require only the observation necessary to establish that fact.

B. An individual with irreversible cessation of all functions of the entire brain, including the brain stem, is dead. The "functions of the entire brain" that are relevant to the diagnosis are those that are clinically ascertainable. Where indicated, the clinical diagnosis is subject to confirmation by laboratory tests, as described in the following portions of the text. Consultation with a physician experienced in this diagnosis is advisable.

1. *Cessation* **is recognized when evaluation discloses findings of a** *and* **b:**

a. Cerebral functions are absent, and . . .

There must be deep coma, that is, cerebral unreceptivity and unresponsivity. Medical circumstances may require the use of confirmatory studies such as an EEG or blood-flow study.

b. brain stem functions are absent.

Reliable testing of brain stem reflexes requires a perceptive and experienced physician using adequate stimuli. Pupillary light, corneal, oculocephalic, oculovestibular, oropharyngeal, and respiratory (apnea) reflexes should be tested. When these reflexes cannot be adequately assessed, confirmatory tests are recommended.

Adequate testing for apnea is very important. An accepted method is ventilation with pure oxygen or an oxygen and carbon dioxide mixture for ten minutes before withdrawal of the ventilator, followed by passive flow of oxygen. (This procedure allows $Paco_2$ to rise without hazardous hypoxia). Hypercarbia adequately stimulates respiratory effort within 30 seconds when $Paco_2$ is greater than 60 mm Hg. A ten-minute period of apnea is usually sufficient to attain this level of hypercarbia. Testing of arterial blood gases can be used to confirm this level. Spontaneous breathing efforts indicate that part of the brain stem is functioning.

Peripheral nervous system activity and spinal cord reflexes may persist after death. True decerebrate or decorticate posturing or seizures are inconsistent with the diagnosis of death.

2. *Irreversibility* **is recognized when evaluation discloses findings of a** *and* **b** *and* **c:**

a. The cause of coma is established and is sufficient to account for the loss of brain functions, and . . .

Most difficulties with the determination of death on the basis of neurological criteria have resulted from inadequate attention to this basic diagnostic prerequisite. In addition to a careful clinical examination and investigation of history, relevant knowledge of causation may be acquired by computed tomographic scan, measurement of core temperature, drug screening, EEG, angiography, or other procedures.

b. the possibility of recovery of any brain functions is excluded, and . . .

The most important reversible conditions are sedation, hypothermia, neuromuscular blockade, and shock. In the unusual circumstance where a sufficient cause cannot be established, irreversibility can be reliably inferred only after extensive evaluation for drug intoxication, extended observation, and other testing. A determination that blood flow to the brain is absent can be used to demonstrate a sufficient and irreversible condition.

c. the cessation of all brain functions persists for an appropriate period of observation and/or trial of therapy.

Even when coma is known to have started at an earlier time, the absence of all brain functions must be established by an experienced physician at the initiation of the observation period. The duration of observation periods is a matter of clinical judgment, and some physicians recommend shorter or longer periods than those given here.

Except for patients with drug intoxication, hypothermia, young age, or shock, medical centers with substantial experience in diagnosing death neurologically report no cases of brain functions returning following a six-hour cessation, documented by clinical examination and confirmatory EEG. In the absence of confirmatory tests, a period of observation of at least 12 hours is recommended when an irreversible condition is well established. For anoxic brain damage where the extent of damage is more difficult to ascertain, observation for 24 hours is generally desirable. In anoxic injury, the observation period may be reduced if a test shows cessation of cerebral blood flow or if an EEG shows electrocerebral silence in an adult patient without drug intoxication, hypothermia, or shock.

Confirmation of clinical findings by EEG is desirable when objective documentation is needed to substantiate the clinical findings. Electrocerebral silence verifies irreversible loss of cortical functions, except in patients with drug intoxication or hypothermia. (Important technical details are provided in "Minimal Technical Standards for EEG Recording in Suspected Cerebral Death" [*Guidelines in EEG 1980*. Atlanta, American Electroencephalographic Society, 1980, section 4, pp. 19–24].) When joined with the clinical findings of absent brain stem functions, electrocerebral silence confirms the diagnosis.

Complete cessation of circulation to the normothermic adult brain for more than ten minutes is incompatible with survival of brain tissue. Documentation of this circulatory failure is therefore evidence of death of the entire brain. Four-vessel intracranial angiography is definitive for diagnosing cessation of circulation to the entire brain (both cerebrum and posterior fossa) but entails substantial practical difficulties and risks. Tests are available that assess circulation only in the cerebral hemispheres, namely radioisotope bolus cerebral angiography and gamma camera imaging with radioisotope cerebral angiography. Without complicating conditions, absent cerebral blood flow as measured by these tests, in conjunction with the clinical determination of cessation of all brain functions for at least six hours, is diagnostic of death.

COMPLICATING CONDITIONS

Drug and Metabolic Intoxication. Drug intoxication is the most serious problem in the determination of death, especially when multiple drugs are used. Cessation of brain functions caused by the sedative and anesthetic drugs, such as barbiturates, benzodiazepines, meprobamate, methaqualone, and trichloroethylene, may be completely reversible even though they produce clinical cessation of brain functions and electrocerebral silence. In cases where there is any likelihood of sedative presence, toxicology screening for all likely drugs is required. If exogenous intoxication is found, death may not be declared until the intoxicant is metabolized or intracranial circulation is tested and found to have ceased.

Total paralysis may cause unresponsiveness, areflexia, and apnea that closely simulates death. Exposure to drugs such as neuromuscular blocking agents or aminoglycoside antibiotics, and diseases like myasthenia gravis are usually apparent by careful review of the history. Prolonged paralysis after use of succinylcholine chloride and related drugs requires evaluation for pseudo-cholinesterase deficiency. If there is any question, low-dose atropine stimulation, electromyogram, peripheral nerve stimulation, EEG, tests of intracranial circulation, or extended observation, as indicated, will make the diagnosis clear.

In drug-induced coma, EEG activity may return or persist while the patient remains unresponsive, and therefore the EEG may be an important evaluation along with extended observation. If the EEG shows electrocerebral silence, short latency auditory or somatosensory evoked potentials may be used to test brain stem functions, since these potentials are unlikely to be affected by drugs.

Some severe illnesses (e.g., hepatic encephalopathy, hyperosmolar coma, and preterminal uremia) can cause deep coma. Before irreversible cessation of brain functions can be determined, metabolic abnormalities should be considered and, if possible, corrected. Confirmatory tests of circulation or EEG may be necessary.

Hypothermia. Criteria for reliable recognition of death are not available in the presence of hypothermia (below 32.2°C core temperature). The variables of cerebral circulation in hypothermic patients are not sufficiently well studied to know whether tests of absent or diminished circulation are confirmatory. Hypothermia can mimic brain death by ordinary clinical criteria and can protect against neurologic damage due to hypoxia. Further complications arise since hypothermia also usually precedes and follows death. If these complicating factors make it unclear whether an individual is alive, the only available measure to resolve the issue is to restore normothermia. Hypothermia is not a common cause of difficulty in the determination of death.

Children. The brains of infants and young children have increased resistance to damage and may recover substantial functions even after exhibiting unresponsiveness on neurological examination for longer periods than do adults. Physicians should be particularly cautious in applying neurologic criteria to determine death in children younger than five years.

Shock. Physicians should also be particularly cautious in applying neurologic criteria to determine death in patients in shock because the reduction in cerebral circulation can render clinical examination and laboratory tests unreliable.

Note

1. The guidelines set forth in this report represent the views of the signatories as individuals; they do not necessarily reflect the policy of any institution or professional association with which any signatory is affiliated. Although the practice of individual signatories may vary slightly, signatories agree on the acceptability of these guidelines: Jesse Barber, M.D., Don Becker, M.D., Richard Behrman, M.D., J.D., Donald R. Bennett, M.D., Richard Beresford, M.D., J.D., Reginald Bickford, M.D., William A. Black, M.D., Benjamin Boshes,

M.D., Ph.D., Philip Braunstein, M.D., John Burroughs, M.D., J.D., Russell Butler, M.D., John Caronna, M.D., Shelley Chou, M.D., Ph.D., Kemp Clark, M.D., Ronald Cranford, M.D., Michael Earnest, M.D., Albert Ehle, M.D., Jack M. Fein, M.D., Sal Fiscina, M.D., J.D., Terrance G. Furlow, M.D., J.D., Eli Goldensohn, M.D., Jack Grabow, M.D., Phillip M. Green, M.D., Ake Grenvik, M.D., Charles E. Henry, Ph.D., John Hughes, M.D., Ph.D., D.M., Howard Kaufman, M.D., Robert King, M.D., Julius Korein, M.D., Thomas W. Langfitt, M.D., Cesare Lombroso, M.D., Kevin M. McIntyre, M.D., J.D., Richard L. Masland, M.D., Don Harper Mills, M.D., J.D., Gaetano Molinari, M.D., Byron C. Pevehouse, M.D., Lawrence H. Pitts, M.D., A. Bernard Pleet, M.D., Fred Plum, M.D., Jerome Posner, M.D., David Powner, M.D., Richard Rovit, M.D., Peter Safar, M.D., Henry Schwartz, M.D., Edward Schlesinger, M.D., Roy Selby, M.D., James Snyder, M.D., Bruce F. Sorenson, M.D., Cary Suter, M.D., Barry Tharp, M.D., Fernando Torres, M.D., A. Earl Walker, M.D., Arthur Ward, M.D., Jack Whisnant, M.D., Robert Wilkus, M.D., and Harry Zimmerman, M.D.

The preparation of this report was facilitated by the President's Commission but the guidelines have not been passed on by the Commission and are not intended as matters for governmental review or adoption.

APPENDIX E

Text of State Statutes Concerning Blood Transfusions and Organ Transplantations

Alabama. Procuring, furnishing, donating, processing, distributing, or using human whole blood, plasma, blood products, blood derivatives, and other human tissues such as corneas, bones or organs for the purpose of injecting, transfusing, or transplanting any of them in the human body is declared for all purposes to be the rendition of a service by every person participating therein and whether any remuneration is paid therefor is declared not to be a sale of such whole blood, plasma, blood products, blood derivatives, or other human tissues. [Ala. Code § 7-2-314(4) (1984).]

Alaska. Implied warranties of merchantability and fitness are not applicable to a contract for the sale of human blood, blood plasma or other human tissue or organs from a blood bank or reservoir of tissue or organs. The blood, blood plasma, tissue, or organs may not, for the purposes of AS 45.02.101–45.02.725, be considered commodities subject to sale or barter, but shall be considered medical services. [Alaska Stat. § 45.02.316(e) (1980).]

Arizona. A. No physician, surgeon, hospital or person who assists a physician, surgeon or hospital in obtaining, preparing, injecting or transfusing blood or its components from one or more human beings to another human being shall be liable on the basis of implied warranty or strict tort liability for any such activity but such person or entity shall be liable for his or its negligent or willful misconduct.

B. No nonprofit blood bank, tissue bank, donor or entity who donates, obtains, processes or preserves blood or its components from one or more human beings for the purpose of transfusing or transferring blood or its components to another human being shall be liable for his or its negligent or willful misconduct. [Ariz. Rev. Stat. Ann. § 32-1481 (1976).]

• • • • •

The procurement, processing, distribution, or use of whole human blood, plasma, blood products and blood derivatives for the purpose of injecting or transfuing them into the human body shall be construed as to the transmission of serum hepatitis to be the rendition of a service by every person participating therein and shall not be construed to be a sale. [Ariz. Rev. Stat. Ann. § 36-1151 (1974).]

Arkansas. The availability of scientific knowledge, skills and materials for the transplanation [transplantation], injection, transfusion or transfer of human tissue, organs, blood and components thereof is important to the health and welfare of the people of this state. The imposition of legal liability without fault upon the persons and organizations engaged in such scientific procedures inhibits the exercise of sound medical judgment and restricts the availability of important scientific knowledge, skills and materials. It is therefore the public policy of this state to promote the health and welfare of the people by limiting the legal liability arising out of such scientific procedures to instances of negligence or willful misconduct. [Ark. Stat. Ann. § 82-1607 (1976).]

· · · · ·

No physician, surgeon, hospital, blood bank, tissue bank, or other person or entity who donates, obtains, prepares, transplants, injects, transfuses or otherwise transfers, or who assists or participates in obtaining, preparing, transplanting, injecting, transfusing or transferring any tissue, organ, blood or component thereof from one or more human beings, living or dead, to another human being, shall be liable as the result of any such activity, save and except that each such person or entity shall remain liable for negligence or willful misconduct only. [Ark. Stat. Ann. § 82-1608 (1976).]

· · · · ·

The implied warranties of merchantability and fitness shall not be applicable to a contract for the sale of human blood, blood plasma or other human tissue or organs from a blood bank or reservoir of such other tissues or organs. Such blood, blood plasma or tissue or organs shall not, for the purpose of this article, be considered commodities subject to sale or barter, but shall be considered as medical services. [Ark. Stat. Ann. § 85-2-316(3)(d)(i) (Supp. 1983).]

California. The procurement, processing, distribution, or use of whole blood, plasma, blood products, and blood derivatives for the purpose of injecting or transfusing the same, or any of them, into the human body shall be construed to be, and is declared to be, for all purposes whatsoever, the rendition of a service by each and every person, firm, or corporation participating therein, and shall not be construed to be, and is declared not to be, a sale of such whole blood, plasma, blood products, or blood derivatives, for any purpose or purposes whatsoever. [Cal. Health & Safety Code § 1606 (West 1979).]

Colorado. (1) The availability of scientific knowledge, skills, and materials for the transplantation, injection, transfusion, or transfer of human tissue, organs, blood, or components thereof is important to the health and welfare of the people of this state. Equally important is the duty of those performing such service or providing such materials to exercise due care under the attending circumstances to the end that those receiving health care will benefit and adverse results therefrom will be minimized by the use of available and proven scientific safeguards. The imposition of legal liability without fault upon the persons and organizations engaged in such scientific procedures may inhibit the exercise of sound medical judgment and restrict the availability of important scientific knowledge, skills, and materials. It is, therefore, the public policy of this state to promote the health and welfare of the people by emphasizing the importance of exercising due care, and by limiting the legal liability arising out of such scientific procedures to instances of negligence or willful misconduct.

(2) The donation, whether for or without valuable consideration, the acquisition, preparation, transplantation, injection, or transfusion of any human tissue, organ, blood, or component thereof for or to a human being is the performance of a medical service and does not, in any way, constitute a sale. No physician, surgeon, hospital, blood bank, tissue bank, or other person or entity who donates, obtains, prepares, transplants, injects, transfuses, or otherwise transfers, or who assists or participates in donating, obtaining, preparing, transplanting, injecting, transfusing, or transferring any tissue, organ, blood, or component thereof from one or more human beings, living or dead, to another living human being for the purpose of therapy or transplantation needed by him for his heatlh or welfare shall be liable for any damages of any kind or description directly or indirectly caused by or resulting from any such activity; except that each such person or entity remains liable for his or its own negligence or willful misconduct. [Colo. Rev. Stat. § 13-22-104 (1973).]

Connecticut. The implied warranties of merchantability and fitness shall not be applicable to a contract for the sale of human blood, blood plasma, or other human tissue or organs from a blood bank or reservoir of such other tissues or organs. Such blood, blood plasma, and the components, derivatives or fractions thereof, or tissue or organs shall not be considered commodities subject to sale or barter, but shall be considered as medical services. [Conn. Gen. Stat. Ann. § 19a-280 (West Supp. 1985).]

Delaware. The implied warranties of merchantability and fitness shall not be applicable to a contract for the sale of human blood, blood plasma or other human tissue or organs from a blood bank or reservoir of such other tissues or organs. Such blood, blood plasma or tissue or organs shall not for the purposes of this Article be considered commodities or goods subject to sale or barter, but shall be considered as medical services. [Del. Code Ann. tit. 6, § 2-316(5) (1975).]

District of Columbia. No statute directly addresses liability for blood transfusions or organ transplants. Case law holds blood transfer to be a service for which implied warranties are not recognized rather than a sale. [*Fisher* v. *Sibley Memorial Hospital,* 403 A.2d 1130, 1133 (D.C. Cir. 1979).]

Florida. The procurement, processing, storage, distribution or use of whole blood, plasma, blood products, and blood derivatives for the purpose of injecting or transfusing the same, or any of them, into the human body for any purpose whatsoever is declared to be the rendering of a service by any person participating therein and does not constitute a sale, whether or not any consideration is given therefor and the implied warranties of merchantability and fitness for a particular purpose shall not be applicable as to a defect that cannot be detected or removed by a reasonable use of scientific procedures or techniques. [Fla. Stat. Ann. § 672.316(5) (West Supp. 1983).]

The procurement, processing, testing, storing, or providing of human tissue and organs for human transplant, by an institution qualified for such purposes, the rendering of a service; and such service does not constitute the sale of goods or products to which implied warranties of merchantability or fitness for a particular purpose are applicable. No implied warranties exist as to defects which cannot be detected, removed, or prevented by reasonable use of available scientific procedures or techniques. [Fla. Stat. Ann. § 672.316(6) (West Supp. 1985).]

Georgia. The implied warranty of merchantability under Code Section 11-2-314 and the implied warranty of fitness for a particular purpose under Code Section 11-2-315 shall not be applicable to the procurement, processing, storage, distribution, or use of whole human blood, blood plasma, blood products, blood derivatives, or other human tissue or organs for the purpose of injecting, transfusing, incorporating, or transplanting any of them into the human body. The injection, transfusion, or other transfer of blood, blood plasma, blood products, or blood derivatives and the transplanting or other transfer of any tissue, bones, or organs into or onto the human body shall not be considered, for the purpose of this article, commodities subject to sale or barter, but shall be considered as medical services. [Ga. Code Ann. § 11-2-316(5) (1982).]

• • • • •

The injection, transfusion, or other transfer of human whole blood, blood plasma, blood products, or blood derivatives and the transplanting or other transfer of any tissue, bones, or organs into or onto the human body shall not be considered a sale of any commodity, goods, property, or product subject to sale or barter but, instead, shall be considered as the rendition of medical services. No implied warranties of any kind or description shall be applicable thereto and no person, firm, or corporation participating in such services shall be liable for damages unless negligence is proven. [Ga. Code Ann. § 51-1-28(a) (1982).]

Hawaii. In the procuring, furnishing, donating, processing, distributing or using of human whole blood, plasma, blood products or blood derivatives for the purpose of injecting or transfusing in the human body, there shall be no implied warranty that the blood, plasma, products or derivatives are free from the virus of serum hepatitis as long as there is no known scientific test to detect the virus of serum hepatitis. [Hawaii Rev. Stat. § 325-91 (1976).]

• • • • •

No physician, surgeon, hospital, blood bank, tissue bank, or other person or entity who donates, obtains, prepares, transplants, injects, transfuses, or otherwise transfers, or who assists or participates in obtaining, preparing, transplanting, injecting, transfusing, or otherwise transferring any tissue, organ, blood or component thereof, from one or more persons, living or dead, to another person, shall be liable as a result of any such activity, save and except that each such person or entity shall remain liable for his or its own negligence or willful misconduct. [Hawaii Rev. Stat. § 327-51 (1976).]

Idaho. "Product" means any object possessing intrinsic value, capable of delivery either as an assembled whole or as a component part or parts, and produced for introduction into trade or commerce. Human tissue and organs, including human blood and its components, are excluded from this term. The "relevant product" under this chapter is that product, or its component part or parts, which gave rise to the product liability claim. [Idaho Code § 6-1302(3) (Supp. 1984).]

• • • • •

The procurement, processing, storage, distribution, or use of whole blood, plasma, blood products and blood derivatives for the purpose of injecting or transfusing the same, or any of them, into the human body for any purpose whatsoever is declared to be the rendering of a service by any person or entity (except a paid blood donor or a blood bank operated for profit) participating therein and does not constitute a sale, whether or not any consideration is given therefor, and the implied warranties of merchantability and fitness for a particular purpose shall not be applicable as to a defect that cannot be detected or removed by reasonable use of standard established scientific procedures or techniques, except such person or entity shall remain liable for his or its own negligence or willful misconduct only. [Idaho Code Ann. § 39-3702 (1977).]

Illinois. *Declaration of public policy.* The availability of scientific knowledge, skills and materials for the purpose of injecting, transfusing or transplanting human whole blood, plasma, blood products, blood derivatives and products, corneas, bones, or organs or other human tissue is important to the health and welfare of the people of this state. The imposition of legal liability without fault upon the persons and organizations engaged in such scientific procedures inhibits the exercise of sound medical judgment and restricts the availability of important scientific knowledge, skills and materials. It is therefore the public policy of this State to promote the health and welfare of the people by limiting the legal liability arising out of such scientific procedures to instances of negligence or willful misconduct. [Ill. Ann. Stat. ch. 111½, § 5101 (Smith-Hurd Supp. 1985).]

Limitation of liability. The procuring, furnishing, donating, processing, distributing or using human whole blood, plasma, blood products, blood derivatives and products, corneas, bones, or organs or other human tissue for the purpose of injecting, transfusing or transplanting any of them in the human body is declared for purposes of liability in tort or contract to be the rendition of a service by every person, firm or corporation participating therein, whether or not any remuneration is paid therefor, and is declared not to be a sale of any such items and no warranties of any kind or description nor strict tort liability shall be applicable thereto, except as provided in Section 3. [Ill. Ann. Stat. ch. 111½, § 5102 (Smith-Hurd Supp. 1985).]

Imposition of liability. Every person, firm or corporation involved in the rendition of any of the services described in Section 2 warrants to the person, firm or corporation receiving the service and to the ultimate recipient that he has exercised due care and followed professional standards of care in providing the service according to the current state of the medical arts, and in the case of a service involving blood or blood derivatives that he has rendered such service in accordance with "The Blood Labeling Act," effective October 1, 1972. [Ill. Ann. Stat. ch. 111½, § 5103 (Smith-Hurd Supp. 1985).]

Indiana. The procurement, processing, distribution or use of whole blood, plasma, blood products, blood derivatives, or other human tissue, such as corneas, bones or organs by a bank, storage facility or hospital and the injection, transfusion, or transplantation of any of them into the human body by a hospital, physician or surgeon, whether or not any remuneration is paid is declared to be for all purposes the rendition of a service and not the sale of a product. No such services shall give rise to an implied warranty of merchantability or fitness for a particular purpose, nor give rise to strict liability in tort. [Ind. Code Ann. § 16-8-7-2 (West 1984).]

Iowa. The procurement, processing, distribution or use of whole blood, plasma, blood products, blood derivatives and other human tissues such as corneas, bones or organs for the purpose of injecting, transfusing or transplanting any of them into the human body is declared to be, for all purposes, the rendition of a service by every person participating therein and, whether or not any remuneration is paid therefor, is declared not to be a sale of such whole blood, plasma, blood products, blood derivatives or other tissues, for any purpose, subsequent to July 1, 1969. However, any person or entity that renders such service warrants only under this section that due care has been exercised and that acceptable professional standards of care in providing such service according to the current state of the medical arts have been followed. Strict liability, in tort, shall not be applicable to the rendition of such service. [Iowa Code Ann. § 142A.8 (West Supp. 1984).]

Kansas. The procuring, furnishing, donating, processing, distributing or using human whole blood, plasma, blood products, blood derivatives and products for the purpose of injecting or transfusing any of them in the human body is declared for all purposes to be the rendition of a service by every person, firm or corporation participating therein, whether or not any remuneration is paid therefor, and is declared not to be a sale of any such items and no warranties of any kind or description shall be applicable thereto. No such person, firm or corporation participating in rendering such services shall be liable for damages unless negligence is proven. [Kan. Stat. Ann. § 65-3701 (1980).]

Kentucky. The procurement, processing, distribution or use of whole blood, plasma, blood products, blood derivatives and other human tissues such as corneas, bones or organs for the purpose of injecting, transfusing or transplanting any of them into the human body is declared to be, for all purposes, the rendition of a service by every person participating therein and, whether or not any remuneration is paid therefor, is declared not to be a sale of such whole blood, plasma, blood products, blood derivatives or other tissues, for any purpose, subsequent to enactment of this section. [Ky. Rev. Stat. Ann. § 139.125 (Bobbs-Merrill 1982).]

Louisiana. Strict liability, or liability of any kind without negligence shall not be applicable to physicians, hospitals, hospital blood banks, or nonprofit community blood banks in the screening, processing, transfusion, or medical use of human blood and blood components of any kind and the transplantation or medical use of any human organ, human tissue, or approved animal tissue which results in transmission of viral diseases undetectable by appropriate medical and scientific laboratory tests. [La. Rev. Stat. Ann. § 9:2797 (West Supp. 1985).]

• • • • •

     Notwithstanding the provisions of Paragraph (A)(2) of this Article, the implied warranties of merchantability and fitness shall not be applicable to a contract for the sale of human blood, blood plasma or other human tissue or organs from a blood bank or reservoir of such other tissues or organs. Such blood, blood plasma or tissue or organs shall not for the purposes of this Article be considered commodities subject to sale or barter but shall be considered as medical services. [La. Civ. Code Ann. art. 1764 B. (West Supp. 1985).]

Maine. The procurement, processing, distribution or use of whole blood, plasma, blood products, blood derivatives, and other human tissues such as corneas, bones or organs for the purpose of injecting, transfusing or transplanting any of them into the human body is declared to be, for all purposes, the rendition of a service by every person participating therein and, whether or not any remuneration is paid therefor, is declared not to be a sale of such whole blood, plasma, blood products, blood derivations or other tissues, for any purpose, subsequent to October 1, 1969. [Me. Rev. Stat. Ann. tit. 11, § 2-108 (Supp. 1984).]

Maryland. A person who obtains, processes, stores, distributes, or uses whole blood or any substance derived from blood for injection or transfusion into an individual for any purpose may not be held liable for the virus of serum hepatitis under:

     1. Strict liability in tort;
     2. The implied warranty of merchantability; or
     3. The implied warranty of fitness.

[Md. Health-Gen. Code Ann. § 18-402 (1982).]

Massachusetts. The implied warranties of merchantability and fitness shall not be applicable to a contract for the sale of human blood, blood plasma or other human tissue or organs from a blood bank or reservoir of such other tissues or organs. Such blood, blood plasma or tissue or organs shall not for the purpose of this Article be considered commodities subject to sale or barter, but shall be considered as medical services. [Mass. Ann. Laws ch. 106, § 2-316(5) (Michie/Law. Co-op. 1976).]

Michigan. (1) The department shall establish standards pursuant to section 9133 to regulate the procurement, processing, distribution, and use of blood, blood plasma, blood products, blood derivatives, and human and artificial tissues.

(2) The procurement, processing, distribution, and use of whole blood, blood plasma, blood products, blood derivatives, and human and artificial tissues such as corneas, bones, or organs for the purpose of injecting, transfusing, or transplanting into a human body, is declared to be, for all purposes, the rendition of a service by a person participating therein and, whether or not remuneration is paid therefor, is declared not to be a sale thereof for any purpose.

(3) An express, implied, or other warranty does not attach to these services. A person involved in the rendition of the service is not liable as a result thereof, except for the person's own negligence or willful misconduct. [Mich. Stat. Ann. § 14.15(9121) (Callaghan 1980).]

Minnesota. The use of any part of a body for the purpose of transplantation in the human body shall be construed, for all purposes whatsoever, as a rendition of a service by each and every person participating therein and shall not be construed as a sale of such part for any purpose whatsoever. [Minn. Stat. Ann. § 525.928 (West. 1975).]

Mississippi. The procurement, processing, storage, distribution and/or use of whole blood, plasma, blood products and blood derivatives for the purpose of injecting or transfusing the same or any of them into the human body for all purposes whatsoever, constitutes the rendering of a service by every person participating therein, whether or not any remuneration is paid therefor, and does not constitute a sale. The maximum usable life span or shelf life for human blood preserved in citrate phosphate dextrose shall be governed by federal regulations promulgated and adopted by the Food and Drug Administration. [Miss. Code Ann. § 41-41-1 (1972).]

Missouri. The procurement, processing, distribution or use of whole blood, plasma, blood products, and blood derivatives and other human tissues, including but not limited to corneas, bones, hearts or other organs for the purpose of injecting, transfusing or transplanting any of them into the human body is declared to be, for all purposes, the rendition of a service by every person, firm, or corporation participating therein and, whether or not any remuneration is paid therefor, is declared not to be a sale of such whole blood, plasma, blood products, blood derivatives or other tissues, bones or organs for any purpose subsequent to enactment of this section. It is further declared that any implied warranties of merchantability and fitness for a particular purpose shall not be applicable as to a defect that cannot be detected or removed by reasonable use of scientific procedures or techniques. Nothing herein shall relieve any person, firm or corporation from negligence. [Mo. Ann. Stat. § 431.069 (Vernon Supp. 1985).]

Montana. The furnishing of and the injecting or transfusing into the human body of whole blood, plasma, blood products, and blood derivatives by a hospital, long-term care facility, or doctor of any such substances obtained from any source which said hospital, long-term care facility, or doctor is not directly or indirectly financially interested in or has any control over is hereby declared not to be a sale of such whole blood, plasma, blood products, or blood derivatives for any purpose. [Mont. Code Ann. § 50-33-102 (1983).]

No physician, long-term care facility, or hospital may be held liable, in the absence of fault or negligence on the part of such a hospital, long-term care facility, or doctor, for injuries resulting from the furnishing or performing of such services. [Mont. Code Ann. § 50-33-103 (1983).]

No blood bank may be held liable in the absence of fault or negligence for injuries resulting from the injecting or transfusing of whole blood, plasma, blood products, or blood derivatives supplied by any such blood bank to any hospital or physician if such blood products have been tested by the latest testing procedures in accordance with recommendations of the American Association of Blood Banks and by such test are not found to be dangerous to the health of the recipient of such blood products. [Mont. Code Ann. § 50-33-104 (1983).]

Nebraska. Procuring, furnishing, donating, processing, distributing, or using human whole blood, plasma, blood products, blood derivatives, and other human tissues such as corneas, bones, or organs for the purpose of injecting, transfusing, or transplanting any of them into the human body is declared for all purposes to be the rendition of a service by every person participating therein and whether or not any remuneration is paid therefor is declared not to be a sale of such whole blood, plasma, blood products, blood derivatives, or other human tissues. [Neb. Rev. Stat. § 71-4001 (1981).]

Nevada. The procurement, processing, distribution or use of whole human blood, plasma, blood products and blood derivatives for the purpose of injection or transfusion into the human body constitutes, as to the transmission of serum hepatitis, the rendition of a service and not a sale by every person participating therein, and no implied warranty of merchantability or fitness, nor any doctrine of liability other than negligence or willful misconduct, shall apply to such service. [Nev. Rev. Stat. § 460.010 (1983).]

New Hampshire. It is expressly declared that no strict liability in tort, nor any implied warranty, attaches to the procurement, furnishing, donation, processing, distributing, or use of whole blood, plasma, blood products or blood derivatives for the purpose of administering, injecting or transfusing any of them into the human body, whether or not remuneration is paid therefor, and no person, firm, or corporation participating therein shall be liable for damages, except for negligence. [N.H. Rev. Stat. Ann. § 507:8-b (1983).]

New Jersey. No statute directly addresses liability for blood transfusions or organ transplants. Case law has held the providing of blood transfusions to be services, rather than sales. Therefore negligence principles, and not strict liability claims, are applicable in this area. [*See, e.g., Brody* v. *Overlook Hospital,* 127 N.J. Super. 331, 317 A.2d 392, *aff'd,* 66 N.J. 448, 332 A.2d 596 (1974); *Baptista* v. *Saint Barnabas Medical Center,* 109 N.J. Super. 217, 262 A.2d 902 (1970).]

New Mexico. The procuring, furnishing, donating, processing, distributing or using of human whole blood, plasma or blood products shall not give rise to any implied warranties of any type and the doctrine of strict tort liability shall not be applicable to the transmission of hepatitis in the blood, plasma or blood products. Nothing in this section shall be construed as affecting the liability of any person, firm, corporation or other organization for negligence or willful misconduct. [N.M. Stat. Ann. § 24-10-5 (1981).]

New York. The collection, processing, storage, distribution or use of blood or a blood derivative for the purpose of diagnosis, prevention or treatment of disease or the assessment of medical condition is hereby declared to be a public health service and shall not be construed to be, and is declared not to be, a sale of such blood or blood derivative, for any purpose or purposes whatsoever. [N.Y. Pub. Health Law § 580.4 (McKinney Supp. 1984).]

North Carolina. The procurement, processing, distribution or use of whole blood, plasma, blood products, blood derivatives and other human tissues such as corneas, bones or organs for the purpose of injecting, transfusing or transplanting any of them into the human body is declared to be, for all purposes, the rendition of a service by every person or institution participating therein and, whether or not any remuneration is paid therefor, is declared not to be a sale of such whole blood, plasma, blood products, blood derivatives or other human tissues, for any purpose. No person or institution shall be liable in warranty, express or implied, for the procurement, processing, distribution or use of said items but nothing herein shall alter or restrict the liability of such person or institution in negligence or tort in consequence of said service. [N.C. Gen. Stat. § 90-220.10 (1981).]

North Dakota. The implied warranties of merchantability and fitness shall not be applicable to a contract for the sale of human blood, blood plasma, or other human tissue or organs from a blood bank or reservoir of such other tissues or organs. Such blood, blood plasma, or tissue or organs shall not for the purposes of this chapter be considered commodities subject to sale or barter, but shall be considered as medical services. [N.D. Cent. Code § 41-02-33(3)(d) (1983).]

• • • • •

No physician, surgeon, hospital, blood bank, tissue bank, or other person or entity who donates, obtains, prepares, transplants, injects, transfuses, or otherwise transfers, or who assists or participates in obtaining, preparing, transplanting, injecting, transfusing, or transferring any tissue, organ, blood, or component thereof from one or more human beings, living or dead, to another human being, shall be liable as the result of any such activity, save and except that each such person or entity shall remain liable for his or its own negligence or willful misconduct only.

The availability of scientific knowledge, skills, and materials for the transplantation, injection, transfusion, or transfer of human tissue, organs, blood, and components thereof is important to the health and welfare of the people of this state. The imposition of legal liability without fault upon the persons and organizations engaged in such scientific procedures inhibits the exercise of sound medical judgment and restricts the availability of important scientific knowledge, skills and materials. It is therefore the public policy of this state to promote the health and welfare of the people by limiting the legal liability arising out of such scientific procedures to instances of negligence or willful misconduct. [N.D. Cent. Code § 43-17-40 (1978).]

Ohio. The procuring, furnishing, donating, processing, distributing, or using human whole blood, plasma, blood products, blood derivatives, and products, corneas, bones, organs, or other human tissue except hair, for the purpose of injecting, transfusing, or transplanting any of them in the human body, is declared for all purposes to be the rendition of a service by every person, firm, or corporation participating therein, whether or not any remuneration is paid therefor, is declared not to be a sale of any such items, and no warranties of any kind or description are applicable thereto. [Ohio Rev. Code Ann. § .2108.11 (Page 1976).]

Oklahoma. The procurement, processing, distribution or use of whole blood, plasma, blood products, blood derivatives and other human tissues such as corneas, bones or organs for the purpose of injecting, transfusing or transplanting any of them into the human body, for compensation or otherwise, shall be deemed a transaction for the purpose of this act. No such transaction shall give rise to any implied warranty of the fitness, quality, suitability of purpose, safety, acceptability to the body of the patient or of any other characteristic or circumstance incident to the transaction involved bearing upon the propriety of the transaction, as applied to the recipient, on the part of the person or persons rendering such service, in the absence of negligence. Provided, that the provisions of this act shall in no way be deemed to affect the operations of the Oklahoma State Penitentiary. [Okla. Stat. Ann. tit. 63, § 2151 (West 1984).]

Oregon. 1. The procuring, processing, furnishing, distributing, administering or using of any part of a human body for the purpose of injecting, transfusing or transplanting that part into a human body is not a sales transaction covered by an implied warranty under the Uniform Commercial Code or otherwise.

2. As used in this section, "part" means organs, tissues, eyes, bones, arteries, blood, other fluids and any other portions of a human body. [Or. Rev. Stat. § 97.300 (1983).]

Pennsylvania. Notwithstanding any other law, no hospital, blood bank, or other entity or person shall be held liable for death or injury resulting from the lawful transfusion of blood, blood components or plasma derivatives, or from the lawful transplantation or insertion of tissue, bone or organs, except upon a showing of negligence on the part of such hospital, blood bank, entity or person. For the purposes of this act negligence shall include but not be limited to any failure to observe accepted standards in the collection, testing, processing, handling, storage, transportation, classification, labeling, transfusion, injection, transplantation or other preparation or use of any such blood, blood components, plasma derivatives, tissue, bone or organs. Specifically excluded hereunder is any liability by reason of implied warranty or any other warranty not expressly undertaken by the party to be charged. [Pa. Stat. Ann. tit. 35, § 10021 (Purdon 1977).]

Rhode Island. No statute directly addresses liability for blood transfusions or organ transplants.

South Carolina. The implied warranties of merchantability and fitness shall not be applicable to a contract for the sale, procurement, processing, distribution or use of human tissues such as corneas, bones or organs, whole blood, plasma, blood products or blood derivatives. Such human tissues, whole blood, plasma, blood products or blood derivatives shall not be considered commodities subject to sale or barter and the transplanting, injection, transfusion or other transfer of such substances into the human body shall be considered a medical service. [S.C. Code Ann. § 44-43-10 (Law. Co-op. 1985).]

South Dakota. The implied warranties of merchantability and fitness shall not be applicable, so far as the transmission of serum hepatitis is concerned, to a contract for the sale of human blood, blood plasma, or other human tissue or organs from a blood bank or reservoir of such other tissue or organs. Such blood, blood plasma or tissue or organs shall not for purposes of this chapter be considered commodities subject to sale or barter, but shall be considered as medical services. [S.D. Codified Laws Ann. § 57A-2-315.1 (1980).]

Tennessee. The implied warranties of merchantability and fitness shall not be applicable to a contract for the sale, procurement, processing, distribution or use of human tissues (such as corneas, bones, or organs), whole blood, plasma, blood products, or blood derivatives. Such human tissues, whole blood, plasma, blood products, or blood derivatives shall not be considered commodities subject to sale or barter, and the transplanting, injection, transfusion or other transfer of such substances into the human body shall be considered a medical service. [Tenn. Code Ann. § 47-2-316(5) (1979).]

Texas. The implied warranties of merchantability and fitness shall not be applicable to the furnishing of human blood, blood plasma, or other human tissue or organs from a blood bank or reservoir of such other tissues or organs. Such blood, blood plasma or tissue or organs shall not for the purpose of this Title be considered commodities subject to sale or barter, but shall be considered as medical services. [Tex. Bus. & Com. Code Ann. § 2-316(e) (Vernon 1968).]

• • • • •

The availability of scientific knowledge, skills and materials for the transplantation, injection, transfusion or transfer of human tissue, organs, blood and components thereof is important to the health and welfare of the people of this State. The imposition of legal liablity without fault upon the persons and organizations engaged in such scientific procedures inhibits the exercise of sound medical judgment and restricts the availability of important scientific knowledge, skills and materials. It is therefore the public policy of this State to promote the health and welfare of the people by limiting the legal liability arising out of such scientific procedures to instances of negligence. [Section 1, Tex. Rev. Civ. Stat. Ann. art. 4590-3 (Vernon 1976).]

No physician, surgeon, hospital, blood bank, tissue bank, or other person or entity who donates, obtains, prepares, transplants, injects, transfuses or otherwise transfers, or who assists or participates in obtaining, preparing, transplanting, injecting, transfusing or transferring any tissue, organ, blood or component thereof from one or more human beings, living or dead, to another human being, shall be liable as the result of any such activity, save and except that each such person or entity shall remain liable for his or its own negligence. [Section 2, Tex. Rev. Civ. Stat. Ann. art. 4590-3 (Vernon 1976).]

Utah. The procurement, processing, distribution, or use of whole human blood, plasma, blood products, and blood derivatives for the purpose of injecting or transfusing them into the human body together with the process of injecting or transfusing the same shall be construed to be the rendition of a service by every person participating therein and shall not be construed to be a sale. [Utah Code Ann. § 26-31-1 (Supp. 1983).]

Vermont. No statute directly addresses liability for blood transfusions or organ transplants.

Virginia. No action for implied warranty shall lie for the procurement, processing, distribution or use of whole blood, plasma, blood products, blood derivatives and other human tissue such as corneas, bones, or organs for the purpose of injecting, transfusing or transplanting any of them into the human body except where any defects or impurities in the said whole blood, plasma, blood products, blood derivatives and other human tissue such as corneas, bones, or organs are detectable by the use of established medical and technological procedures employed pursuant to the standards of local medical practice. [Va. Code § 32.1-297 (1979).]

Washington. The procurement, processing, storage, distribution, administration, or use of whole blood, plasma, blood products and blood derivatives for the purpose of injecting or transfusing the same, or any of them, into the human body is declared to be, for all purposes whatsoever, the rendition of a service by each and every person, firm, or corporation participating therein, and is declared not to be covered by any implied warranty under the Uniform Commercial Code, Title 62A RCW, or otherwise, and no civil liability shall be incurred as a result of any of such acts, except in the case of wilful or negligent conduct: *Provided, however,* That this section shall apply only to liability alleged in the contraction of hepatitis and malaria and shall not apply to any transaction in which the blood donor receives compensation: *Provided further,* That this section shall only apply where the person, firm or corporation rendering the above service shall have maintained records of donor suitability and donor identification similar to those specified in Sections 73.301 and 73.302(e) as now written or hereafter amended in Title 42, Public Health Service Regulations adopted pursuant to the Public Health Service Act, 42 U.S.C. 262; *Provided further,* That nothing in this section shall be considered by the courts in determining or applying the law to any blood transfusion occurring before the effective date hereof and the court shall decide such case as though this section had not been passed. [Wash. Rev. Code Ann. § 70.54.120 (1975).]

West Virginia. The procuring, furnishing, donating, processing, distributing or the using of human whole blood, blood plasma, blood products, blood derivatives, corneas, bones or organs or other human tissue for the purpose of injecting, transfusing or transplanting any of them in the human body, is declared for all purposes to be the rendition of a service by every person, firm or corporation participating therein, whether or not any remuneration is paid therefor, and is declared not to be a sale of any such items and no warranties of any kind or description shall be applicable thereto. [W. Va. Code § 16-23-1 (1979).]

Wisconsin. The procurement, processing, distribution or use of whole blood, plasma, blood products, blood derivatives and other human tissues such as corneas, bones or organs for the purpose of injecting, transfusing or transplanting any of them into the human body is declared to be, for all purposes, the rendition of a service by every person participating therein and, whether or not any remuneration is paid therefor, is declared not to be a sale of such whole blood, plasma, blood products, blood derivatives or other tissues, for any purpose. No person involved in the procurement, processing, distribution or use of whole blood, plasma, blood products or blood derivatives for the purpose of injecting or transfusing any of them into the human body shall be liable for damages resulting from these activities except for his own negligence or willful misconduct. [Wis. Stat. Ann. § 146.31(2) (West Supp. 1984).]

No hospital, nonprofit tissue bank, physician, nurse or other medical personnel acting under the supervision and direction of a physician involved in the procurement, processing, distribution or use of human tissues such as corneas, bones or organs for the purpose of transplanting any of them into the human body shall be liable for damages resulting from those activities except for negligence or willful misconduct by that hospital, nonprofit tissue bank, physician, nurse or other medical personnel. [Wis. Stat. Ann. § 146.31(3) (West Supp. 1984).]

Wyoming. The implied warranties of merchantability and fitness shall not be applicable to a contract for the sale of human blood, blood plasma or other human tissue or organs from an individual or a blood bank or reservoir of such other tissues or organs. Such blood, blood plasma or tissue or organs shall not for the purpose of this article be considered commodities subject to sale or barter, but shall be considered as medical services. [Wyo. Stat. § 34-21-233(c)(iv) (1977).]

• • • • •

A physician, surgeon, hospital, blood bank, tissue bank, or other person or entity who donates, obtains, prepares, transplants, injects, transfuses, or otherwise transfers, or who assists or participates in obtaining, preparing, transplanting, injecting, transfusing or transferring any tissue, organ, blood, or component thereof from one (1) or more human beings, living or dead, to another human being, is not liable as the result of any such activity except for his or its own negligence or misconduct. [(Wyo. Stat. § 35-5-110 (1977).]

APPENDIX F

Required Consent Laws
of California, New York, and Oregon

CALIFORNIA

REGULAR SESSION

Chapter 779, Law 1985

Assembly Bill No. 631

An act to add Section 7184 to the Health and Safety Code, relating to anatomical donors.

The people of the State of California do enact as follows:

SECTION 1. Section 7184 is added to the Health and Safety Code, to read:
    7184. Each general acute care hospital shall develop a protocol for identifying potential organ and tissue donors. The protocol shall require that any deceased individual's next of kin or other individual, as set forth in Section 7151.5, at *or near* the time of notification of death be asked whether the deceased was an organ donor or if the family is a donor family. If not, the family shall be informed of the option to donate organs and tissues pursuant to Chapter 3.5 (commencing with Section 7150) of Part 1 of

California Regular Session, 1985; New Laws, pages 3205–3206.

EXPLANATION—Matter in *italics* is new; matter in brackets [ ] is old law to be omitted.

Division 7. With the approval of the designated next of kin or other individual, as set forth in Section 7151.5, the hospital shall then notify an organ and tissue procurement organization and cooperate in the procurement of the anatomical gift or gifts. *The protocol shall encourage reasonable discretion and sensitivity to the family circumstances in all discussions regarding donations of tissue or organs.* The protocol may take into account the deceased individual's religious beliefs or obvious nonsuitability for organ and tissue donation. *In the event an organ and tissue procurement organization does not exist in a region, the hospital shall contact an organ or a tissue procurement organization, as appropriate.* Laws pertaining to notification of the coroner shall be complied with in all cases of reportable deaths.

SECTION 2. No reimbursement is required by this act pursuant to Section 6 of Article XIII B of the California Constitution because the local agency or school district has the authority to levy service charges, fees, or assessments, pursuant to Sections 1177 and 1473 of the Health and Safety Code, sufficient to pay for the program or level of service mandated by this act.

Approved, September 19, 1985

NEW YORK

REGULAR SESSION

Chapter 801, Laws 1985

Senate Int. No. 4925-C

AN ACT to amend the public health law, in relation to anatomical gifts; consents

The People of the State of New York, represented in Senate and Assembly, do enact as follows:

New York Regular Session, 1985; New Laws, pages 857–858.

Section 1. The public health law is amended by adding a new article forty-three-A to read as follows:

ARTICLE 43-A
REQUEST FOR CONSENT TO AN ANATOMICAL GIFT

Section 4351. Duties of hospital administrator.

§*4351. Duties of hospital administrator. 1. Where, based on accepted medical standards, a patient is a suitable candidate for organ or tissue donation, the person in charge of such hospital, or his designated representative, other than a person connected with the determination of death, shall at the time of death request any of the following persons, in the order of priority stated, when persons in prior classes are not available and in the absence of (1) actual notice of contrary intentions by the decedent, or (2) actual notice of opposition by a member of any of the classes specified in paragraph (a), (b), (c), (d), or (e) hereof or (3) other reason to believe that an anatomical gift is contrary to the decedent's religious beliefs, to consent to the gift of all or any part of the decedent's body for any purpose specified in article forty-three of this chapter:*

   (a) the spouse;
   (b) a son or daughter twenty-one years of age or older;
   (c) either parent;
   (d) a brother or sister twenty-one years of age or older;
   (e) a guardian of the person of the decedent at the time of his death.

Where said hospital administrator or his designee shall have received actual notice of opposition from any of the persons named in this subdivision or where there is otherwise reason to believe that an anatomical gift is contrary to the decedent's religious beliefs, such gift of all or any part of the decedent's body shall not be requested. Where a donation is requested, consent or refusal need only be obtained from the person or persons in the highest priority class available.

   2. Where a donation is requested, said person in charge of such hospital or his designated representative shall complete a certificate of request for an anatomical gift, on a form supplied by the commissioner. Said certificate shall include a statement to the effect that a request for consent to an anatomical gift has been made, and shall further indicate thereupon whether or not consent was granted, the name of the person granting or refusing the consent, and his or her relationship to the decedent. Upon completion of the certificate, said person shall attach the certificate of request for an anatomical gift to the death certificate required by this chapter or, in the city of New York, to the death certificate required by the administrative code of the city of New York.

   3. A gift made pursuant to the request required by this section shall be executed pursuant to applicable provisions of article forty-three of this chapter.

   4. The commissioner shall establish regulations concerning the training of hospital employees who may be designated to perform the request, and the procedures to be employed in making it.

5. The commissioner shall establish such additional regulations as are necessary for the implementation of this section.

§2. The commissioner of health shall conduct a study of existing transplant services in New York state and prepare projections regarding future need and the availability of such services. On or before July first, nineteen hundred eighty-seven, the commissioner of health shall submit a report to the governor and the legislature regarding the implementation of this act, including the result of the study required herein and such recommendations as the commissioner may deem appropriate.

§3. This act shall take effect on the first day of January next succeeding the date on which it shall have become a law.

Approved, August 1, 1985

OREGON

REGULAR SESSION

Chapter 379, Laws 1985

House Bill No. 2909

AN ACT

Relating to organ transplants.

Be It Enacted by the People of the State of Oregon:

SECTION 1. (1) When death occurs in a hospital to a person who has not made an anatomical gift, the hospital administrator or designated representative shall request the person described in ORS 97.265(2), in order of priority stated when persons in prior classes are not available at the time of death, and in the absence of actual notice of contrary indication by the decedent or one in a prior class, to consent to the gift of all or any part of the decedent's body as an anatomical gift.

(2) Where such request is made, pursuant to this section, the request and its disposition shall be noted in the patient's medical record and on the death certificate and shall be documented as provided in ORS 97.275(5).

(3) Where, based on medical criteria, such request would not yield a donation which would be suitable for use, the Assistant Director for Health may, by rule, authorize an exception to the request required by this section.

(4) The Assistant Director for Health shall establish rules concerning the training of hospital employees who may be designated to perform the request, and the procedures to be employed in making it. In addition, the assistant director shall establish such rules as are necessary to implement appropriate procedures to facilitate the delivery of donations from receiving hospitals to potential recipients.

(5) The Assistant Director for Health shall establish such additional rules as are necessary for the implementation of this section.

Approved, July 3, 1985

APPENDIX G

Transplants: Quality We Can Afford

Senator Albert Gore, Jr.

At a congressional hearing on the National Organ Transplant Act, in 1984, a panel of transplant surgeons was asked why they wanted to let the government stick its nose into transplantation. "It already does," replied Dr. Oscar Salvatierra.

Dr. Salvatierra and his colleagues, Dr. Norm Shumway and Dr. Tom Starzl, went on to describe just how much transplant technology owes to "government interference." Public research laid the foundation for transplantation. When Congress decided in 1972 to extend Medicare benefits to patients with end-stage kidney failure, it set the stage for a new technology. Today, kidney transplants dramatically improve more than 7000 lives every year, largely because the government was willing to help. Liver, heart, heart-lung, and pancreas transplants as well are all products of government support.

Unfortunately, the current administration has chosen to ignore these facts. During congressional hearings, federal officials insisted that government had no right to address the shortage of organ donors and other obstacles that patients in need of this remarkable new medical technology must confront.

Experts testified that the entire current system of organ procurement in the United States was 100 percent federally funded. Medicare was spending about $70 million dollars each year to support a system that was not working. Four of the most important groups in transplantation—the American Society of Transplant Surgeons, the North American Transplant Coordinators Organization, the Southeastern Organ Procurement Foundation, and the Association of Independent Organ Procurement Agencies—helped write the National Organ Transplant Act, and enlisted government aid. Yet the administration steadfastly maintained that public funds and responsible government leadership should not be part of the solution of this public health problem.

Three years ago, a patient who needed a heart, liver, or heart-lung transplant to stay alive had to turn to the media for help. A national plea on prime-time TV was the only way to find the funds or the organ to save a life. It was an unpleasant and uncomfortable sight.

A young black mother from North Carolina called my office in tears asking what she had done wrong. Her child died still awaiting a donor. They had tried to get the media interested. Now, as she watched her TV each night and saw other children receiving national attention, followed by dramatic tales in which donors were found, she had a sick feeling inside; she had not been able to do this for her child and that had killed him.

Her story, and others like it, led Congress to move quickly. Democrats and Republicans, congressmen and senators joined in an effort that produced legislation in a remarkably short time. Congress passed the National Organ Transplant Act to force government to take responsibility for a difficult problem that government had helped create.

Organ transplantation, like most new medical technologies, was developed at taxpayer expense. Through government-supported research and the extraordinary commitment embodied in the End-Stage Renal Disease (ESRD) program, kidney transplants have grown from one scientist's dream into a medically accepted therapy, with a better than 80 percent one-year survival rate. But when transplant surgeons began using this life-saving technology on a regular basis, the government started having second thoughts about whether or not to pay for it.

The cost of health care is a very real problem, but it is certainly not unique to organ transplantation. Modern science offers us the prospect of health care far beyond what is easily affordable. Transplants caused those new to the debate to begin talking about rationing. Those who were more familiar with the problem spoke about allocating resources among competing health needs.

Most government officials would prefer not to ration health care resources by selecting among individuals who could benefit from a particular treatment. And the ESRD program demonstrates that society supports government efforts to avoid rationing.

The allocation of health care resources is an important form of planning. It makes sense to decide how much we want to spend on health care, then choose to spend so much on research, so much on primary care, so much on preventive care, and so much on tertiary care. Allocation should make our health care system much more efficient and decrease the need to ration. But under this administration, the transplant debate has strayed from these central questions. Officials have approached medical technologies on an ad hoc, case-by-case basis, treating transplantation as somehow unique from all other available forms of health care.

Medicare officials claim that liver transplants and heart transplants are "experimental" and are therefore not covered under Medicare. This use of the word "experimental" is a sham—an excuse to dodge paying for a reasonable and necessary service. This attitude undermines public confidence in our entire health care technology assessment system, which has become too sensitive to political pressures and lacks a scientific basis.

Under the current system, Medicare will pay $100,000 to aggressively treat pancreatic cancer in a terminal patient, but will deny another patient the same $100,000 for a heart transplant that could save his or her life. The explanation given is that the heart transplant is "experimental."

During the deliberations on liver transplants, the NIH Consensus Development Conference concluded that "liver transplantation is a therapeutic modality for end-stage liver disease that deserves broader application." It went on to recommend "expansion of this technology to a limited number of centers where performance of liver transplantation can be carried out under optimal conditions." Congress endorsed these conclusions in legislation to provide liver transplants for CHAMPUS beneficiaries just as the NIH had suggested.

After waiting another six months, however, the administration reached a different conclusion. Officials announced at a February 9, 1984, congressional hearing that they supported recognition of liver transplantation as a nonexperimental procedure for children under age eighteen with congenital abnormalities as the cause of liver failure. These officials claimed that only in this group were liver transplants no longer "experimental"—even though there was no scientific basis whatsoever for their decision.

For purely political reasons, the Administration deliberately chose to include a group of patients not covered under Medicare. The decision was a great disappointment to all of us who have worked on this issue. It was so far out of touch with the scientific facts that counsel for CHAMPUS rejected the approach and continued to cover both adults and children in line with the NIH recommendations.

One of the most disturbing aspects of the manner in which the administration evaluated liver transplantation is that the same thing could happen again with heart transplantation. Medicare's decision to cover heart transplants will not create an end-stage heart disease program similar to the kidney program, but will merely add heart transplants as an accepted benefit for those who are already eligible for Medicare. As part of Battelle's National Heart Transplantation Study, commissioned by the Department of Health and Human Services, Medicare paid for fifteen heart transplants, but only for Medicare beneficiaries. It took more than a year to find fifteen patients who were both eligible for Medicare and who met the rigorous medical criteria for transplantations.

There are two ways to become eligible for Medicare before age sixty-five—one is to have end-stage renal disease, which is a contraindication for a heart transplant, and the other is to collect Social Security disability for two years. Unfortunately, not many people who need a heart transplant live long enough to qualify through the disability provision. In fact, the National Heart Transplantation Study predicts, using the most liberal assumptions, that Medicare will not have to pay for more than 100 heart transplants per year. That works out to less than $10 million per year. Medicare spends over $70 billion each year—$2 billion on the ESRD program alone. Clearly, Medicare can afford the $10 million.

We can hope to learn from this experience. As a nation, more and more of us have recognized the need for society to answer some basic questions. Congress recently endorsed my proposal to establish a National Commission on Bioethics as a forum for such discussions. We must consider how the debate over allocation of resources will affect decisions such as whether a medical center will undertake a heart transplant program.

I expect Medicare coverage of heart transplants to be limited not only to certain patients, but also to certain "designated centers." Recently CHAMPUS published their final proposal for covering liver transplants. Under this proposal, a center must demonstrate two years experience with liver transplants in which a center performs at least ten per year, and must demonstrate a one-year survival rate of better than 50 percent. This approach follows the lead of private insurers such as Blue Shield of California.

I predict that Medicare coverage of heart transplants will follow a similar path. Centers with heart transplant programs or those eager to start one will have to demonstrate three years experience with heart transplants with a two-year survival rate of about 70 percent. Of the 70 centers now doing heart transplants, maybe only a dozen would meet this tough standard.

This is a tough policy, but it is one I support. The alternative is to continue Medicare's current all-or-nothing coverage policy which, in this instance, would mean deciding not to cover heart transplants. The "designated centers" policy will not prevent other centers from doing heart transplants, but I think some programs will be forced to close down.

If we are to avoid rationing medical care we need to allocate our resources carefully. Improving efficiency is a critical piece of that process. While I oppose singling out individual technologies on an ad hoc basis, as has happened with transplants, I do believe we must develop a methodology that allows us to say no to certain technologies, or to decide to shift more resources to preventive care. Only after we develop this methodology will we have the tool to assess individual technologies intelligently, and intelligent choices can then be made. But it would be wrong to continue to assess technologies without agreeing first on the methodology by which they will be judged.

The National Heart Transplantation Study concluded that the United States needs about twenty heart transplant programs. But there are already more than seventy programs in existence, and many other hospitals are starting new ones. Meanwhile, the supply of donor organs remains limited. Even under the most optimistic circumstances, no more than 1500 hearts would be available for transplants in a given year. With such a relatively small donor organ pool upon which to draw, it hardly makes sense to let a hundred different hospitals across the country set up heart transplant programs. There simply are not enough hearts to go around. With so many hospitals competing for the organs, most programs will never get enough opportunities to develop the necessary expertise. Such duplication drives up costs, wastes valuable hearts, and reduces success rates.

Whether we like it or not, the assessment of new medical technologies—and other efforts to control health care costs—will require a federal role. The federal government is already involved through Medicare and federally funded medical research and development. The government and the Congress have a responsibility to make sure taxpayers get the most from their money.

The choice is ours. Through designated centers, careful technology assessment, and better organ procurement we can design a system that offers high-quality care at a reasonable price. Or we can let chaos continue to reign, and risk turning the world's finest health care system into one that is merely the world's most expensive. The sooner we start planning for the future, the better life will be for all of us.

Selected Bibliography

Books

R. Calne, A Gift of Life: Observations on Organ Transplants (Basic Books, New York, N.Y.) (1970).

F. Kissmeyer-Nielsen, E. Thorsby, Human Transplantation Antigens (Williams & Wilkins Company, Baltimore, Md.) (1970).

G. Miller, Moral and Ethical Implications of Human Organ Transplants (Charles C. Thomas, Springfield, Ill.) (1971).

W. Nolen, Spare Parts for the Human Body (Random House, New York, N.Y.) (1971).

C. Pallia, ABC of Brain Stem Death (The Devonshire Press, Torquay, U.K.) (1983).

F. Rapaport, A Second Look at Life: Transplantation and Dialysis Patients: Their Own Stories (Grune & Stratton, New York, N.Y.) (1973).

R. Scott, The Body as Property (Viking Press, New York, N.Y.) (1981).

R. Simmons, S. Klein, R. Simmons, Gift of Life: The Social and Psychological Impact of Organ Transplantation (John Wiley & Sons, New York, N.Y.) (1977).

Artificial Organs and Cardiopulmonary Support Systems (F. Rapaport, J. Merrill, eds.) (Grune & Stratton, New York, N.Y.) (1972).

Human Transplantation (F. Rapaport, J. Dausset, eds.) (Grune & Stratton, New York, N.Y.) (1968).

Machine at the Bedside: Strategies for Using Technology in Patient Care (S. Reiser, M. Anbar, eds.) (Cambridge University Press, Cambridge, U.K.) (1984).

Articles

Annas, G., *Allocation of Artificial Hearts in the Year 2002:* Minerva v. National Health Agency, American Journal of Law and Medicine 3(1):59–76 (Spring 1977).

Annas, G., *Life, Liberty, and the Pursuit of Organ Sales,* Hastings Center Report 14(1):22–23 (February 1984).

Annas, G., *The Prostitute, the Playboy, and the Poet: Rationing Schemes for Organ*

Transplantation, AMERICAN JOURNAL OF PUBLIC HEALTH 75(2):187–89 (February 1985).

Annas, G., *Regulating Heart and Liver Transplants in Massachusetts: An Overview of the Report of the Task Force on Organ Transplantation*, LAW, MEDICINE AND HEALTH CARE 13(1):4–7 (February 1985).

Annas, G., *Regulating the Introduction of Heart and Liver Transplantation*, AMERICAN JOURNAL OF PUBLIC HEALTH 75(1):93–95 (January 1985).

Annas, G., *Selling Organs*, CENTERSCOPE 15(2):20–22 (July 1984).

Arnet, W., *The Criteria for Determining Death in Vital Organ Transplants—A Medico-Legal Dilemma*, MISSOURI LAW REVIEW 13(1):152–74 (Summer 1979).

Austen, W., Cosimi, A., *Heart Transplantation After 16 Years*, NEW ENGLAND JOURNAL OF MEDICINE 311(22):1436–38 (November 28, 1984).

Baron, C., et al., *Live Organs and Tissue Transplants from Minor Donors in Massachusetts*, BOSTON UNIVERSITY LAW REVIEW 55(1):159–93 (January 1975).

Behney, C., Sisk, J., *Organ Transplantation, Medical Technology Assessment and Resource Allocation*, CONNECTICUT MEDICINE 48(12):797–800 (December 1984).

Black, P., *Brain Death: Part I*, NEW ENGLAND JOURNAL OF MEDICINE 299(7):338–44 (August 17, 1978).

Black, P., *Brain Death: Part II*, NEW ENGLAND JOURNAL OF MEDICINE 299(8):393–401 (August 24, 1978).

Black, P., *Clinical Problems in the Use of Brain-Death Standards*, ARCHIVES OF INTERNAL MEDICINE 143:121–23 (January 1983).

Black, P., Zervas, N., *Declaration of Brain Death in Neurosurgical and Neurological Practice*, NEUROSURGERY 15(2):170–74 (1983).

Bloomers, J., et al., *Transplant and Dialysis: The Cost/Benefit Question*, IOWA MEDICINE 74(1):15–17 (January 1984).

Bosso, J., *Considerations of the Institutional Review Board in Artificial Organ Development*, JOURNAL OF CONTEMPORARY LAW 11(1):61–65 (1984).

Boyce, R., *Organ Transplantation Crisis: Should the Deficit Be Eliminated Through Inter Vivos Sales?* AKRON LAW REVIEW 17(2):283–302 (Fall 1983).

Bowker, W., *Experimentation on Humans and Gifts of Tissue: Articles 20–23 of the Civil Code*, McGILL LAW JOURNAL 19(2):161–94 (1973).

Burt, R., *Coercion and Communal Morality*, JOURNAL OF HEALTH POLITICS, POLICY AND LAW 9(2):323–24 (Summer 1984).

Caplan, A., *If There's A Will, Is There A Way?* LAW, MEDICINE AND HEALTH CARE 13(1):32–34 (February 1985).

Caplan, A., et al., *Mrs. X and the Bone Marrow Transplant*, HASTINGS CENTER REPORT 13(3):17–19 (June 1983).

Caplan, A., *Organ Procurement: It's Not in the Cards*, HASTINGS CENTER REPORT 14(5):9–12 (October 1983).

Caplan, A., *Organ Transplants: The Costs of Success*, HASTINGS CENTER REPORT 13(6):23 (December 1983).

Caplan, A., *Sounding Board: Ethical and Policy Issues in the Procurement of Cadaver Organs for Transplantation*, NEW ENGLAND JOURNAL OF MEDICINE 311(15):981–83 (October 11, 1984).

Capron, A., *Transplants: Begging for Life*, The Washington Post, A-15, column 2 (Tuesday, August 9, 1983).

Capron, A., *When Well-Meaning Science Goes Too Far,* HASTINGS CENTER REPORT 15(1):8–9 (February 1985).

Casscells, W., *A Clinician's View of the Massachusetts Task Force on Organ Transplantation,* LAW, MEDICINE AND HEALTH CARE 13(1):27–28 (February 1985).

Chapman, D., *Retailing Human Organs Under the Uniform Commercial Code,* JOHN MARSHALL LAW REVIEW 16(2):393–418 (Spring 1983).

Cowan, D., Bertsch, E., *Innovative Therapy: The Responsibility of Hospitals,* THE JOURNAL OF LEGAL MEDICINE 5(2):219–51 (June 1984).

DeVries, W., *et al., Clinical Use of the Total Artificial Heart,* NEW ENGLAND JOURNAL OF MEDICINE 310(5):273–78 (February 2, 1984).

Englehardt, H., *Shattuck Lecture—Allocating Scarce Medical Resources and the Availability of Organ Transplantation: Some Moral Suppositions,* NEW ENGLAND JOURNAL OF MEDICINE 311(1):66–71 (July 5, 1984).

Evans, R., *Transplantation: A Public Policy Dilemma,* BUSINESS AND HEALTH 3(5):5–8 (April 1986).

Francis, L., *Artificial and Transplanted Organs: Movable Parts and the Unmoving Law,* JOURNAL OF CONTEMPORARY LAW 11(1):29–59 (1984).

Friedman, F., *et al., Life and Death in a Policy Vacuum,* HOSPITALS 58(10):79–80 (May 16, 1984).

Galletti, P., *Replacement of the Heart with a Mechanical Device: The Case of Dr. Barney Clark,* NEW ENGLAND JOURNAL OF MEDICINE 310(5):312–14 (February 2, 1984).

Gerber, P., *Some Medico-Legal Implications of the Human Tissue Transplant Act,* MEDICAL JOURNAL OF AUSTRALIA 2(10):533 (November 17, 1979).

Gore, A., *The Need for a New Partnership,* HASTINGS CENTER REPORT 5(1):13 (February 1985).

Gore, A., *Transplants Can Improve Quality of Care,* BUSINESS AND HEALTH 3(5):9–10 (April 1986).

Gorovitz, S., *Against Selling Body Parts,* REPORT FROM THE CENTER FOR PHILOSOPHY AND PUBLIC POLICY 4(2):9–12 (Spring 1984).

Gorovitz, S., *The Artificial Heart: Questions to Ask, and Not to Ask,* HASTINGS CENTER REPORT 4(5):15–17 (October 1979).

Green, H., *An NIH Panel's Early Warnings,* HASTINGS CENTER REPORT 4(5):13–15 (October 1984).

Greifer, I., *Transplantation Surgery,* MOUNT SINAI JOURNAL OF MEDICINE 51(1):52–53 (January-February 1984).

Griese, O., *Organ Transplants—Is Presumed Consent the Answer? Part I: How Serious is the Shortage?* ETHICS AND MEDICS 9(6):2–3 (June 1984).

Griese, O., *Organ Transplants—Is Presumed Consent the Answer? Part II: Is the Cost Beyond the Reach of the Needy?* ETHICS AND MEDICS 9(7):2–4 (July 1984).

Griese, O., *Organ Transplants—Is Presumed Consent the Answer? Part III: Is Equitable Distribution Possible?* ETHICS AND MEDICS 9(8):2–4 (August 1984).

Gunby, P., *Organ Transplant Improvements, Demands Draw Increasing Attention,* JOURNAL OF THE AMERICAN MEDICAL ASSOCIATION 251(12):1521–23, 1527 (March 23–30, 1984).

Guttman, F., *Organ Transplants in Children,* PEDIATRIC ANNALS 11(11):910–12, 914–15 (November 1982).

Hartman, T., *The Buying and Selling of Human Organs From the Living: Why Not?* AKRON LAW REVIEW 13(1):152–74 (Summer 1979).

Iglehart, J., *The Politics of Transplantation,* NEW ENGLAND JOURNAL OF MEDICINE 310(13):864–68 (March 29, 1984).

Iglehart, J., *Transplantation: The Problems of Limited Resources,* NEW ENGLAND JOURNAL OF MEDICINE 309(2):123–28 (July 14, 1983).

Jonsen, A., *Organ Transplants and the Principle of Fairness,* LAW, MEDICINE AND HEALTH CARE 13(1):37–39, 44 (February 1985).

Kissick, W., *Organ Transplantation and the Art of the Possible,* LAW, MEDICINE AND HEALTH CARE 13(1):34–35 (February 1985).

Kolata, G., *Organ Shortage Clouds New Transplant Era,* SCIENCE 221(4605):32–33 (July 1, 1983).

Koop, C., *Increasing the Supply of Solid Organs for Transplantation,* PUBLIC HEALTH REPORTER 98(6):566–72 (November-December 1983).

Koop, C., *Promoting Organs for Transplantation,* JOURNAL OF THE AMERICAN MEDICAL ASSOCIATION 251(12):1591–92 (March 23–30, 1984).

Lamb, J., *Organ Transplantation: Recognizing the Donor,* AMERICAN JOURNAL OF NURSING 80(9):1600–01 (September 1980).

Lansing, P., *The Conflict of Patient Privacy and the Freedom of Information Act,* JOURNAL OF HEALTH POLITICS, POLICY AND LAW 9(2):315–22 (Summer 1984).

Levafour, G., *et al., Renal Transplant Associated Malaria,* JOURNAL OF THE AMERICAN MEDICAL ASSOCIATION 244(16):1820–21 (October 17, 1980).

Levine, R., *Total Artificial Heart Implantation—Eligibility Criteria,* JOURNAL OF THE AMERICAN MEDICAL ASSOCIATION 252(11):1458–59 (September 21, 1984).

Lombardo, P., *Consent and "Donations" from the Dead,* HASTINGS CENTER REPORT 11(6):9–11 (December 1981).

Marshall, V., *Organ and Tissue Transplantation: Past, Present and Future,* MEDICAL JOURNAL OF AUSTRALIA 2(9):411–14 (October 30, 1984).

Matis, A., *et al. A Proposal for Cadavers Organ Procurement: Routine Removal with Right of Informed Refusal,* JOURNAL OF HEALTH POLITICS, POLICY AND LAW 10(2):231–44 (Summer 1985).

Maugh, T., *Transplants (II): Altering the Donor Organ,* SCIENCE 210(4466):177–79 (October 1980).

Marx, J., *Improving the Success of Kidney Transplants,* SCIENCE 209(4457):673–74 (August 8, 1980).

May, W., *Religious Justifications for Donating Body Parts,* HASTINGS CENTER REPORT 15(1):38–42 (February 1985).

Merrikin, K., Overcast T., *Patient Selection for Heart Transplantation: When is Discriminating Choice Discrimination?* JOURNAL OF HEALTH POLITICS, POLICY AND LAW 10(1):7–32 (Spring 1985).

Miller, F., *Reflections on Organ Transplantation in the United Kingdom,* LAW, MEDICINE AND HEALTH CARE 13(1):31–32 (February 1985).

Murray, K., Olsen, D., *The Utah Artificial Heart: Success in the Laboratory and its Application to Man,* JOURNAL OF CONTEMPORARY LAW 11(1):3–65 (1984).

Muyskens, J., *An Alternative Policy for Obtaining Cadaver Organs for Transplantation,* PHILOSOPHY AND PUBLIC AFFAIRS 8:88–99 (Fall 1978).

Najarian, J., Ascher, N., *Liver Transplantation,* NEW ENGLAND JOURNAL OF MEDI-
CINE 311(18):1179–81 (November 1, 1984).

Nathanson, M., *Health Care Community Recoils from "Free Market" for Transplant
Organs,* MODERN HEALTHCARE 14(1):89–92 (January 1984).

Norton, M., *et al., Organ Transplantation: Medico-Legal Considerations,* MEDICINE
AND LAW 2(4):291–315 (1983).

Opelz, G., Terasaki, P., *Absence of Immunization Effect in Human-Kidney Retransplan-
tation,* NEW ENGLAND JOURNAL OF MEDICINE 299(8):367–74 (August 24, 1978).

Overcast, T., *et al., Problems in the Identification of Potential Organ Donors—Misconceptions and Fallacies Associated With Donor Cards,* JOURNAL OF THE AMERICAN
MEDICAL ASSOCIATION 251(12):1559–62 (March 23–30, 1984).

Overcast, T., Merrikin, K., Evans, R., *Malpractice Issues in Heart Transplantation,*
AMERICAN JOURNAL OF LAW AND MEDICINE 10(4):363–95 (Winter 1985).

Pauly, M., *Equity and Costs,* LAW, MEDICINE AND HEALTH CARE 13(1):28–31 (February 1985).

Perry, C., *The Right of Public Access to Cadaver Organs,* SOCIAL SCIENCE AND MED-
ICINE [F] 15F(4):163 (December 1981).

Porter, S., *Organ Transplants. Part One: Ohio Physicians Getting Involved,* OHIO STATE
MEDICAL JOURNAL 80(1):29 (January 1984).

Porter, S., *Organ Transplants. Part Two: Questions and Controversy,* OHIO STATE MED-
ICAL JOURNAL 80(1):33 (January 1984).

Preston, T., *Who Benefits from the Artificial Heart?* HASTINGS CENTER REPORT 15(1):5–
7 (February 1985).

Prottas, J., *Obtaining Replacements: The Organizational Framework of Organ Procurement,* JOURNAL OF HEALTH POLITICS, POLICY AND LAW 8(2):235–50 (Summer
1983).

Rachels, J., *Barney Clark's Key,* HASTINGS CENTER REPORT 13(2):17–19 (April
1983).

Robertson J., *Organ Donations by Incompetents and the Substituted Judgment Doctrine,*
COLUMBIA LAW REVIEW 76(1):48–78 (January 1976).

Rose, E., *Medicolegal Problems Associated with Organ and Tissue Transplantation,* MED-
ICAL TRIAL TECHNIQUE QUARTERLY 31(1):99–118 (Summer 1984).

Russell, P., Cosimi, A., *Transplantation: Medical Progress,* NEW ENGLAND JOURNAL
OF MEDICINE 301(9):470–79 (August 30, 1979).

Sadler, A., Sadler, B., *A Community of Givers, Not Takers,* HASTINGS CENTER REPORT
14(5):6–9 (October 1984).

Sanbar, S., *Medicolegal Aspects of Human Organ Transplantation: Ethics and Economics,*
LEGAL ASPECTS OF MEDICAL PRACTICE 12(4):1–5 (April 1984).

Schaal, P., *Nurses' Response to Transplants: A Systems View,* AORN JOURNAL 39(1):42
(January 1984).

Schwartz, H., *Bioethical and Legal Considerations in Increasing the Supply of Transplantable Organs: From UAGA to 'Baby Fae',* AMERICAN JOURNAL OF LAW AND
MEDICINE 10(4):397–437 (Winter 1985).

Skelley, L., *Practical Issues in Obtaining Organs for Transplantation,* LAW, MEDICINE
AND HEALTH CARE 13(1):35–27 (February 1985).

Sophie, L., *et al., Intensive Care Nurses' Perceptions of Cadaver Organ Procurement,* HEART AND LUNG 12(3):261 (May 1983).

Steinbrook, R., *Kidneys for Transplantation,* JOURNAL OF HEALTH POLITICS, POLICY AND LAW 6(3):504–19 (Fall 1981).

Starzl, T., *Implied Consent for Cadaveric Organ Donation,* JOURNAL OF THE AMERICAN MEDICAL ASSOCIATION 251(12):1592 (March 23–30, 1984).

Strauss, M., *Special Report: The Political History of the Artificial Heart,* NEW ENGLAND JOURNAL OF MEDICINE 310(5):332–36 (February 2, 1984).

Tendlor, M., *Rabbinic Comment: Transplantation Surgery,* MOUNT SINAI JOURNAL OF MEDICINE 51(1):54–57 (January-February 1984).

Trent, B., *Is Media Hype Necessary for Organ Transplants?* CANADIAN MEDICAL ASSOCIATION JOURNAL 120(6):774 (1984).

Toole, W., Toole, F., *Heart Transplants and the Legal and Ethical Problems Surrounding Organ Retrieval,* NORTH CAROLINA MEDICAL JOURNAL 44(12):783–85 (December 1983).

Veith, F., *et al., Brain Death: I. A Status Report of Medical and Ethical Considerations,* JOURNAL OF THE AMERICAN MEDICAL ASSOCIATION 238(10):1651–55 (October 10, 1977).

VanThiel, D., *et al., Post Mortem Organ Procurement for Transplantation,* ANNALS OF INTERNAL MEDICINE 99(3):498 (September 1983).

West, J., *et al., Ethical Dilemmas in Transplantation,* JOURNAL OF THE IOWA MEDICAL SOCIETY 71(9):379 (September 1984).

White, J., *A Review of Organ Transplantation Policy,* HEALTH AFFAIRS 109–14 (Winter 1985).

Wilkinson, L., *Legal Resolution of Denial of Access to Medical Technology,* GOLDEN GATE UNIVERSITY LAW REVIEW 14(2):203–56 (Summer 1984).

Winslow, G., *A Test of Ethical Principles,* BUSINESS AND HEALTH 3(5):11–17 (April 1986).

Woolley, F., *Ethical Issues in the Implantation of the Total Artificial Heart,* NEW ENGLAND JOURNAL OF MEDICINE 310(5):292–96 (February 2, 1984).

American Medical Association 1980 Interim Meeting Report: Organ Donation and Transplantation, JOURNAL OF THE TENNESSEE MEDICAL ASSOCIATION 74(7):507–09, 515 (July 1981).

Blythe v. Seagraves: *North Carolina Treats the Issue of Whether a Minor and Her Parents May Legally Consent to the Minor's Participation as Donor, in a Kidney Transplant,* NORTH CAROLINA CENTRAL LAW JOURNAL 9(2):216–26 (Spring 1978).

Current Opinions of the Judicial Council of the American Medical Association: Organ Transplantation, Section 2.13 (American Medical Association, Chicago, Ill.) (June 1984).

First Congress of the European Society for Organ Transplantation, TRANSPLANTATION PROCEEDINGS 16(5):1149 (October 1984).

On Harmonization of Legislations of Member States Relating to Removal, Grafting and Transplantation of Human Substances, MEDICINE, SCIENCE AND THE LAW (19)2:141 (April 1984).

The Implications of Cost-Effectiveness Analysis of Medical Technology: Case Study #6: The Cost Effectiveness of Bone Marrow Transplant Therapy and its Policy Implications (Office of Technology Assessment, Washington, D.C.) (May 1981).

The Implications of Cost-Effectiveness Analysis of Medical Technology: Case Study #9: The Artificial Heart: Cost, Risks, and Benefits (Office of Technology Assessment, Washington, D.C.) (May 1982).

Liver Transplantation (National Institutes of Health Consensus Development Conference Summary, Washington, D.C.) (U.S. Government Printing Office: 381-132:3164) (1983).

The Morality of Buying Organ Transplants, PROGRESS IN CLINICAL AND BIOLOGICAL RESEARCH 38:127 (1980).

Patient Selection for Artificial and Transplanted Organs, HARVARD LAW REVIEW 82(6):1322–42 (April 1968).

Standards for Tissue Banking (American Association of Tissue Banks, Arlington, Va.) (1984).

The Use of Immunosuppressive Drugs in Kidney Transplantation (Staff Memorandum) (Office of Technology Assessment, Washington, D.C.) (March 1984).

Index

Veterans Administration
—transplant reimbursement, 240

warranty, see liability

TABLE OF CASES

About the Editors

DALE H. COWAN is a practicing physician and attorney. In addition, to a private medical practice in hematology and medical oncology and directorship of the Division of Hematology/Oncology at Marymount Hospital in Cleveland, he is involved in health care delivery and financing activities. Dr. Cowan played a major role in establishing a physician-sponsored Preferred Provider Organization at Marymount Hospital, helped create the Emerald Health Network, and authored a book on Preferred Provider Organizations. He is a clinical professor of environmental health sciences at Case Western Reserve University School of Medicine, a fellow of the American College of Physicians and the American College of Legal Medicine, and a member of the Ohio State and American Bar Associations. He recently completed a four-year term as a member of the National Advisory Council of the National Heart, Lung, and Blood Institute. Dr. Cowan received his M.D. from Harvard Medical School and his J.D. from Case Western Reserve University School of Law.

JO ANN KANTOROWITZ is former acting executive director of the American Society of Law & Medicine. She served as attorney for the Society as well as offering private legal counsel on health care law and tax law to a Public Broadcasting System affiliate and a local Massachusetts tenant's union. In addition to authoring several articles in *Law, Medicine & Health Care,* she has several forthcoming books and articles in the health care law field. Ms. Kantorowitz received her J.D. from Northeastern University School of Law and is a member of the Massachusetts Bar and the District of Columbia Bar.

JAY MOSKOWITZ is associate director for Program Planning and Evaluation, Office of the Director, National Institutes of Health. He has also been associate director of Scientific Program Operation and associate director for Program Planning and Evaluation of the National Heart, Lung, and Blood Institute, program coordinator and acting chief of the Division of Lung Diseases, the National Heart and Lung Institute; and a grants associate of the National Institutes of Health's Division of Research Grants. Dr. Moskowitz received his Ph.D. from Brown University and is a member of the Society for Experimental Biology and Medicine, the American Association for the Advancement of Science, and the Society of Sigma Xi.

PETER H. RHEINSTEIN is director of the Office of Drug Standards in the Center for Drugs and Biologics at the Food and Drug Administration. He is immediate past president of the Drug Information Association and treasurer and member of the Board of Governors of the American College of Legal Medicine. He is a past chairman of the Food and Drug Committee of the Federal Bar Association, a fellow of the American Academy of Family Physicians, and a member of the American Bar Association and the American Medical Association. Before joining the FDA, Dr. Rheinstein served on the faculty of internal medicine at the University of Maryland. He was medical director for a chain of investor-owned health care facilities, a founder of a company providing physicians for hospital emergency departments, and is board certified in family practice. Dr. Rheinstein earned his M.D. at Johns Hopkins University School of Medicine and his J.D. from the University of Maryland.